Continuing Care
Retirement Communities
An Empirical, Financial,
and Legal Analysis

Other publications of the
PENSION RESEARCH COUNCIL

Fundamentals of Private Pensions—*Dan M. McGill*
Concepts of Actuarial Soundness in Pension Plans—*Dorrance C. Bronson*
Social Aspects of Retirement—*Otto Pollak*
Positive Experiences in Retirement—*Otto Pollak*
Ensuring Medical Care for the Aged—*Mortimer Spiegelman*
Legal Protection of Private Pension Expectations—*Edwin W. Patterson*
Legal Status of Employee Benefit Rights under Private Pension
     Plans—*Benjamin Aaron*
Decision and Influence Processes in Private Pension Plans—*James E.
     McNulty, Jr.*
Fulfilling Pension Expectations—*Dan M. McGill*
Collectively Bargained Multi-Employer Pension Plans—*Joseph J. Melone*
Actuarial Aspects of Pension Security—*William F. Marples*
Status of Funding under Private Pension Plans—*Frank L. Griffin, Jr.* and
     Charles L. Trowbridge (out of print)
Guaranty Fund for Private Pension Obligations—*Dan M. McGill*
Preservation of Pension Benefit Rights—*Dan M. McGill*
Retirement Systems for Public Employees—*Thomas P. Bleakney*
Employer Guarantee of Pension Benefits—*Dan M. McGill*
Reciprocity among Private Multiemployer Pension Plans—*Maurice E.
     McDonald*
A New Look at Accounting for Pension Costs—*William D. Hall* and *David
     L. Landsittel*
Social Security and Private Pension Plans: Competitive or
     Complementary?—*Dan M. McGill* (ed.)
Pension Mathematics—*Howard E. Winklevoss*
Indexation of Pension and Other Benefits—*Robert J. Myers*
Joint Trust Pension Plans—*Daniel F. McGinn*
Financing the Civil Service Retirement System—*Dan M. McGill* (ed.)
Social Investing—*Dan M. McGill,* (ed.)

Continuing Care Retirement Communities
An Empirical, Financial, and Legal Analysis

Howard E. Winklevoss
Senior Vice President
Johnson & Higgins
Adjunct Associate Professor
of Insurance and Actuarial Science
Wharton School

Alwyn V. Powell
Assistant Professor of
Actuarial Science and Insurance
Georgia State University

in collaboration with

David L. Cohen, Esq.
Associate
Ballard, Spahr, Andrews & Ingersoll

Ann Trueblood-Raper
Consultant in Gerontology

1984
Published for the
Pension Research Council
Wharton School
University of Pennsylvania
by
RICHARD D. IRWIN, INC.   Homewood, Illinois   60430

To our children:
Amanda, Cameron, & Tyler
and
Thandi & Sibongile

ISBN 0-256-03125-8
Library of Congress Catalog Card No. 83–81175

Printed in the United States of America

1 2 3 4 5 6 7 8 9 0 M P 1 0 9 8 7 6 5 4

PENSION RESEARCH COUNCIL

PURPOSE OF THE COUNCIL

The Pension Research Council was formed in 1952 in response to an urgent need for a better understanding of the private pension mechanism. It is composed of nationally recognized pension experts representing leadership in every phase of private pensions. It sponsors academic research into the problems and issues surrounding the private pension institution and publishes the findings in a series of books and monographs. The studies are conducted by mature scholars drawn from both the academic and business spheres.

Foreword

Those familiar with the interests and past activities of the Pension Research Council may be surprised that it is publishing a book on continuing care retirement communities. Over the years, the Council has been concerned principally with the actuarial and financial soundness of pension plans and the protection of the rights of individuals who look to them as a source of old-age financial support. In other words, the Council has traditionally sponsored research with the underlying purpose of strengthening those mechanisms designed to provide the financial resources needed for a secure old age. In contrast, this book is concerned with a relatively recent institutional arrangement that seeks to provide old-age security and health care *in kind*.

Almost from the moment The Commonwealth Fund and the Robert Wood Johnson Foundation approved a grant to the Wharton School to study continuing care retirement communities, the Council expressed an interest in reviewing the findings of the study, with a view toward its publication. The sponsors of the project had the same concerns about this new institution that the Pension Research Council has about the pension institution—its ability to deliver the benefits and services promised. The nature of the arrangement raises questions about its actuarial soundness, financial stability, and protection of members' rights.

The author of this Foreword participated in the study in an oversight capacity and was in a position to judge the quality of the research involved. The project director, Dr. Howard E. Winklevoss, a member of the Wharton School faculty and the Council, kept the Council fully apprised of developments and of progress being made on the project. The final draft of the report was reviewed by members of the Council—and by the project's advisory committee—who recommended publication by the Council, if permissable. The project sponsors (The Commonwealth Fund and the Robert Wood Johnson Foundation) suggested several guidelines for selecting an entity to publish the study results but left the choice to the dean of the Wharton School. On the basis of his knowledge of and confidence in the Pension Research Council, Dean Donald C. Carroll designated the Council to publish the study.

The Council is proud to publish the results of this pioneering study. The study and its recommendations should be a constructive influence on the future growth of this new social organism, embodying an innovative approach to old-age financial security.

The Council extends its congratulations to The Commonwealth Fund and the Robert Wood Johnson Foundation for conceiving this project, and it expresses its profound gratitude to them for making the necessary financial resources available.

Funds for the publication of this volume were drawn from the Ralph H. Blanchard Memorial Endowment of the Pension Research Council. Mr. Blanchard was one of the founders of the organization now known as the National Health and Welfare Mutual Life Insurance Association, which provides pension and insurance facilities for the staffs of social welfare agencies. Mr. Blanchard served as president of the organization for 14 years, and at the time of his death in 1972 he was honorary president. The Memorial Endowment was established and funded by the NHW Mutual Life Insurance Association to perpetuate the memory of Mr. Blanchard and to further the social goals to which he was so deeply committed. The subject matter of this study epitomizes the concern for the elderly that occupied the thoughts and energy of Mr. Blanchard throughout his life.

It should be understood, of course, that the statements made and the views expressed in this volume are solely the responsibility of the authors and should not be attributed to the funding agencies.

Dan M. McGill

Preface

Today there are about 275 continuing care retirement communities (CCRCs) in the United States where some 90,000 elderly people (average age about 80) live independently in their own apartments but have the opportunity for eating together, group recreation, and other activities that comes from being part of an organized community. Most important, in addition to having immediately available a variety of health and social services which they can call on according to their desires and needs, the residents have a virtual guarantee that they will be adequately taken care of no matter what happens to their health. The fear of someday being a burden on relatives or friends or of finding oneself helpless among uncaring strangers is effectively removed.

It is this health care guarantee that principally distinguishes CCRCs from other retirement communities. CCRCs provide insurance against the cost of long-term care, and supplement coverage of acute health care costs paid for largely by Medicare and private insurance. Their unique feature is that they provide this otherwise unobtainable full insurance in combination with independent living arrangements that the resident can enjoy as long as health permits.

CCRCs are intended to be fully self-supporting, and therein lies the origin of this book. The study is the first detailed analysis of the actuarial, financial, and legal issues involved in keeping existing CCRCs financially sound and providing for the formation of new communities in ways that protect the rights of residents while assuring the perpetuation of the community.

CCRCs provide essentially a new form of insurance, but until now this type of insurance has not been subjected to rigorous examination. It is fortunate that such an examination has begun, and it is to be hoped that this book will be followed quickly by other work in the field. The members of the Advisory Committee who worked closely with the research team believe that the CCRC field may be on the threshold of a major expansion, principally because for the first time large numbers of older Americans will be able to meet the cost.

The financing method combines a sizable entrance fee (average $35,000 single and $39,000 couple at the time of the study) with a monthly payment which is adjusted from time to time for inflation and occasionally other factors (average $600 single and $850 couple). About 70 percent of older people now own their homes, and in many cases they have enough equity in those homes to meet the required entrance fees. And inflation-proof Social Security plus some additional income from private pensions and investments can form a basis for meeting the monthly fee for many older people, although undoubtedly considerably less than a majority.

It is true that many who can afford CCRCs will nevertheless prefer other retirement arrangements, but for a considerable number the full health insurance, including long-term care, combined with independent living in a community setting will make CCRCs attractive.

On behalf of the other 12 members of the Advisory Committee, I wish to commend the research team—Howard E. Winklevoss, Ph.D., project director; Alwyn V. Powell, MAAA; David L. Cohen, Esq.; Ann Trueblood-Raper; and Amy R. Karash—for their efforts to address the comments and suggestions of the Advisory Committee throughout the past 18 months and for diligently pursuing the research which has produced this book. We also wish to thank Dr. Dan M. McGill, who served the study as consultant to the research team and as chairman of the Wharton School Insurance Department and the Pension Research Council.

It is our hope that the book will be useful to public policymakers, to corporations and foundations with an interest in older people and their health, to the financial community, and to potential sponsors of CCRCs.

The Robert Wood Johnson Foundation of Princeton and The Commonwealth Fund of New York City provided financial support for the work of the research team and the Advisory Committee. We are grateful for their backing and hope that the philanthropic community will continue to support important research on CCRCs and related topics.

Robert M. Ball

Chairman of the Advisory Committee
Continuing Care Retirement Community Study

Authors' Preface

Nearly four years have passed since we completed our first comprehensive actuarial study of a continuing care retirement community (CCRC). At that time, the application of actuarial science to set fees in this growing field was nonexistent. Most of the assumptions and methodologies used to set fees and establish financing were not based on scientific analysis but instead were rules of thumb or anecdotal approaches. Moreover, the literature about the industry dealt with social and health-related issues, and rarely with the financial issues associated with operating a facility.

To some degree, the limited financial sophistication was due to the newness of the concept and a misconception regarding its true nature. Many of the early marketing efforts concentrated on the real estate component of the services provided. The central theme of providing a way to finance long-term health care needs privately was a secondary and rarely emphasized issue. Actuaries and other financial analysts were basically unaware of this industry prior to publicity about the financial distress of some communities that made national headlines in the late 1970s. Even then, there was considerable controversy over the correct pricing methodologies and the appropriate types of contractual guarantees. It was even suggested that the continuing care financing arrangement to ensure lifetime health care for small groups of elderly was not viable, or was possible only with fees that were prohibitively expensive.

Recognizing that the service goals of the continuing care concept may be one answer to the growing needs of the independent elderly for housing and health care, the Robert Wood Johnson Foundation and The Commonwealth Fund solicited proposals to conduct research to address the question of financial viability for the concept. In April 1981, they agreed to fund jointly a research grant to the Wharton School of the University of Pennsylvania, with Howard E. Winklevoss, Ph.D., and Alwyn V. Powell, MAAA, as the primary investigators. So that the research would be timely, the authors decided to concentrate on the following three areas: (1) a definition and survey of the general characteristics of the CCRC industry, (2) a detailed development and explanation of the actuarial principles underlying the pricing and long-term financial characteristics of CCRCs, and (3) a discussion of the legal issues arising from the continuing care contract with suggestions for their legislative treatment.

This book is the culmination of 18 months of research. Its primary objectives are to set forth normative guidelines for pricing and evaluating continuing care retirement communities and to provide a reference that will assist legislators in assessing the advantages and disadvantages of various components of continuing care regulation. This book is not designed as a "how-to" book on the financial operation of CCRCs; rather, it is intended to provide the management and board members of CCRCs with a broad understanding of the financial intricacies of their communities. Furthermore, this book provides guidelines to analysts who wish to conduct similar research by explaining in detail the methodologies developed during the course of the study.

Chapter 1 presents an overview of the industry's growth and explains why the industry is worthy of research; the rest of the book is divided into three parts, corresponding to the study's three research topics. Part One consists of Chapters 2 and 3, which summarize the empirical findings of the survey of 207 CCRCs (75 percent of the defined universe). Part Two consists of Chapters 4 through 11, which will interest those readers whose concerns embrace financial issues. These chapters develop the actuarial methodology proposed for evaluating the long-term financial condition of a CCRC. The results of applying this methodology to six existing CCRCs are discussed in each of the chapters. Part Three consists of Chapters 12 and 13. Chapter 12 discusses relevant legal issues and how they are treated by existing legislation. Chapter 13 presents the authors' recommendations for state-level legislation on each of these issues. Finally, Chapter 14 summarizes the significant research findings and recommendations and suggests a number of areas that merit further research. The appendixes contain technical explanations of the methodologies developed by the authors.

We would like to offer thanks to the members of the study's Advisory Committee, who reviewed all preliminary drafts of the book and attended 11 days of seminars to guide the research staff in the conduct of the study. Other valuable advice was contributed by members of the review panel, which consisted of providers of continuing care and legal experts practicing in the field; the members of both groups are listed on the following pages. Several members of the Pension Research Council also offered their comments prior to publication, and Dr. Dan M. McGill, chairman of the Pension Research Council, is owed special thanks for his review of the book and for his helpful guidance throughout the study.

Our collaborators made important contributions to this volume. They include Ann Trueblood-Raper, consultant in gerontology, who wrote Chapters 2 and 3; David L. Cohen, Esq., associate at Ballard, Spahr, Andrews & Ingersoll, who researched and wrote Chapters 12 and 13; Dr. Robert A. Zelten, associate professor of insurance and health care systems, who contributed to Chapter 10; and Mitchell Leon, public relations consultant, who contributed to Chapter 1.

We are grateful to the American Association of Homes for the Aging for its assistance in developing our 24-page survey instrument, for encouraging its members to complete the instrument, and for its helpful comments and support.

The authors are particularly indebted to the following staff members, whose collective contributions were essential for the timely completion of this project: Robert Goodrich; Roger W. Hallowell; Joseph Marant; Jayaram Muthuswamy; and Catherine C. Singer. We extend our special thanks to Amy R. Karash, our administrator, who planned the logistics associated with the survey questionnaire, word-processed and edited innumerable versions of the book, and provided day-to-day support from the inception of the study.

Finally, and most important, we are grateful to our wives, Carol and Keitumetse, whose encouragement and acceptance of additional responsibilities during the course of the study enabled us to devote our time to the research and writing of this book.

Naturally, the authors remain solely responsible for any conceptual or technical errors that may remain.

Howard E. Winklevoss

Alwyn V. Powell

UNIVERSITY OF PENNSYLVANIA
CONTINUING CARE RETIREMENT COMMUNITY STUDY
REVIEW PANEL

Rev. R. Arthur Wagner, *President,* Methodist Manor, Inc., West Allis,
Wisconsin
Paul White, *President,* Philadelphia Presbyterian Homes, Inc., Wayne,
Pennsylvania
Ellis G. Willard, *President,* The Presbyterian Homes of New Jersey,
Princeton, New Jersey

Contents

Part Three
Legal Analysis, 223

List of Tables

List of Figures

Chapter One

Introduction

■ Of all the challenges facing American society, none is more dramatic than the one created by the unprecedented "age bulge" in the population. The number of Americans aged 60 and over has increased nearly sevenfold so far this century. Moreover, the number of Americans aged 65 and over is expected to approach 50 million by the year 2025, nearly double the current figure of 26 million.

The elderly now account for 11.6 percent of the population. However, projections by the Census Bureau are that the elderly will account for 13.1 percent of the population in the year 2000 and 21.7 percent in 2050.

The aging of the American population has understandably been the focus of attention and concern, and has accounted for a major portion of the government's health care and income security dollars in recent years. At the same time, health service delivery planners, providers of care, advocates for the elderly, and the philanthropic community active in health affairs have been instrumental in drawing attention to the need for well-conceived living and health care arrangements for the growing number of older Americans.

That concern and need are being expressed against the backdrop of a remarkable economic and social accomplishment which has taken place over the past four decades—the provision of nearly universal Social Security benefits for Americans over 65. At this time, nearly 95 percent of people over 65 are eligible to receive monthly Social Security benefits indexed to climb at the rate of inflation. In 1982, an estimated $156 billion in Social Security benefits was paid out to 36 million

Americans. An estimated 25 percent of those over 65 are eligible for private pensions which supplement their Social Security benefits.

As the economic well-being of most members of the older American community has continued to improve, much more attention has been paid to the need for a broad range of shelter and care options.

In many cases, the ideal option is a combination of community-based medical and nonmedical assistance which permits the elderly person to remain in his or her own home. In other cases, the alternative of living in the homes of other family members or moving to a nursing home may be preferable or necessary. However, for a growing number of retired Americans, a practical and attractive solution to the problem of where to live with maximum independence and readily available social and medical services has been the continuing care retirement community.

Continuing care retirement communities provide lifetime residence to people after retirement. These communities offer long-term contracts which typically guarantee shelter, health care, and various other social services for the rest of the resident's life, through the same risk-sharing principles on which commercial insurance policies are based. Retirement homes founded on the continuing care concept have been in existence, in varying forms, for over half a century, but they have been a growing phenomenon since the 1960s.[1]

During the past two decades, the demand for continuing care accommodations has increased markedly. Retirees are attracted to the notion of having both independence and security together in a campus-like setting. The homes encourage residents to lead full, active lives as long as possible, yet offer access to various kinds of assistance, including full-time nursing care, when needed.

This study was undertaken in recognition of the fact that in order to provide the quality services they wish to offer, it is incumbent upon retirement facilities to have the soundest financial management. Although sound financial management is the primary subject of this book, it is first useful to place in perspective the issues associated with retirement living and the reasons why it is a subject of growing importance.

ECONOMIC ISSUES

As Joseph Pechman, director of economic studies at the Brookings Institution, has described the situation:

> Twenty or thirty years ago the elderly were a disadvantaged group in the population. As a result of public policies, primarily Social Security, they

---

[1] Aldersly, Inc., also known as the Danish Home, in San Raphael, California, has been in continuous operation as a continuing care retirement community since 1921.

have improved their relative status compared with the nonelderly to the point where, right now, on the average, the elderly are as well off as the nonelderly. That's a great national achievement.[2]

According to data from the Social Security Administration, 26 percent of the elderly derive at least 90 percent of their income from Social Security and two thirds of the elderly derive at least half of their income from Social Security.[3]

The changes now being considered in the scope and direction of government activities threaten the very tangible accomplishments of the last several decades in providing a base of economic, health, and social supports for America's elderly.

Many states have increased taxes and/or reduced spending in an attempt to trim their multimillion-dollar shortfalls. Expansion of public services and programs under these conditions has become ever more difficult, even as demands have risen.

The federal government is currently spending over $210 billion in major programs for the elderly, with Social Security accounting for three quarters of that amount and Medicare, the health program for the elderly, accounting for another $50 billion.

Estimates of the federal deficit for 1983 range upwards of $200 billion. Unemployment rates of 10 percent and high interest rates, as well as inflation of 14 percent in the nation's health care bill, have brought calls for reductions in the rate of growth in the economic security and health programs. Our national commitment to the continued economic and social well-being of our elderly is being sorely tested.

In addition to the need for continuing public support, there is a need to identify private sources of financing for retirement living, sources that allow the elderly themselves, as a group, to use the resources available to them to help finance their later years affordably. The continuing care retirement community, with its exclusive reliance on private financing, is one of the attractive options being developed to meet this need.

THE CHALLENGE OF AN AGING SOCIETY

Retirement living is an issue of extreme importance to an increasing number of Americans, especially as more workers retire before age 65 and as life expectancy continues to grow. Labor force participation over the past three decades has been tending toward earlier retirement; rates of labor force participation for men over age 65 are now less than half the rates in 1950.

---

[2] *New York Times,* December 19, 1982, p. 4.

[3] Ibid.

Between 1980 and 2030, the total population is expected to grow by 40 percent. In contrast, the number of people over 65 will double. The over-75 group is growing at an even faster rate. Currently, 38 percent of the elderly are 74 years of age or older. By 2030, this figure will increase to 45 percent. Those aged 85 and older now number about 2 million. By 2030, this figure will triple to 6 million.[4] This demographic upheaval will create an unprecedented demand for services, especially long-term care services.

There will continue to be large numbers of older people who cannot afford their retirement years, though in general the next elderly generation will be wealthier than any before it. The number of elderly persons living in poverty, according to Census Bureau estimates, dropped from 35.2 percent in 1959 to 25.3 percent in 1969 to 14.6 percent in 1974. Since then, the figure has remained within the 14–16 percent range.

America's current system of housing and long-term care is being deeply affected by the speed with which these societal changes are occurring. The elderly are demanding high-quality services. They are better educated, longer living, more active, and better off financially than any elderly group before them. They are giving providers of housing and health care new challenges to guarantee not only shelter and services but also creative avenues for their interests and a new definition of quality of life.

CHOICES IN SHELTER AND SERVICES

Most older people want to live independently for as long as possible, but until fairly recently, few options were available to those older persons who could not, or did not wish to, maintain their own homes. Increasingly, the available options have not been limited to private residence at one extreme and institutional care at the other. More than a matter of preference, however, the choice of where to live is often complicated by the presence or absence of a spouse, the proximity of adult children, and questions of health needs, income limitations, and housing supply. The available options may include renting an apartment or space in a private home, sharing living quarters, or living with or near relatives. More independent but impaired elderly may take advantage of home health or other in-home support services, where available. In some areas, adult day care and respite care help families keep elderly relatives at home. Federal housing projects combined with rental assistance offer affordable shelter to some low-income persons, but support for these programs has been reduced. Congregate

---

[4] Health Care Financing Administration, *Long-Term Care Background and Future Directions* (Washington, D.C., 1981).

living arrangements offer independent living accommodations and such non-medical amenities as meals and housekeeping. Other alternatives exist as well, though most are not yet available on a wide scale.

A number of relatively new alternatives to existing federal and state programs have developed. Among these are communities that offer rental housing, communities that offer housing and guaranteed access to health care at a daily rate, and the aforementioned continuing care retirement communities, which treat housing and services as an integral set of concerns.

As the elderly population grows, and pressures for housing and services mount accordingly, more imaginative, cost-effective approaches to traditional forms of care will be needed, combining private, community, and voluntary commitments with available government resources to meet the growing demand.

FINANCING OF LONG-TERM CARE

Public demand on the future direction of long-term care and the means to finance that demand often focus on alternatives to institutional settings for the provision of care. Yet the existing health care system provides far greater support for institutional and medically oriented care than for any of these alternatives.

The complexity and fragmentation of federal and state programs, moreover, make it difficult for elderly persons to get the services they need in order to remain at home. In addition, certain elderly persons will always require the ongoing medical care, nursing services, continual supervision, and assistance with daily living that institutions, chiefly nursing homes, provide.

Although only 5 percent of the elderly, about 1.3 million persons, live in nursing homes today, that number is expected to increase by more than 50 percent in the next 20 years. The great majority of nursing home residents are over 75, female, and single, widowed, or divorced. It is estimated that about 20 percent of people over 65 may be in a nursing home at some point during the remainder of their lives.

Medicaid, the federal health program for the poor, is the principal public funding mechanism for care in nursing homes. Government funds paid for nearly 70 percent of nursing home costs in 1979, with private payments accounting for the rest.[5] At the current rate of increase, the total cost of nursing care will triple by 1990, from the current $25 billion to more than $75 billion. The actual annual national nursing home bill should be much lower than this projection, however. States are taking steps to reduce the growth of nursing home beds and

---

[5] Health Care Financing Administration, unpublished data.

to increase the availability of skilled nursing care in the home and other community settings.

The high costs, as much as $18,000 to $20,000 a year, quickly deplete the savings of many persons who enter nursing homes on a private-paying basis. Only a small percentage of nursing home residents can afford to be private payors for an extended period of time. The rest often turn to Medicaid, which accounts for 87 percent of government expenditures for nursing home care. However, Medicaid is a means-tested welfare program, and federal and state governments are taking steps to restrict its growth. Medicare, which accounts for less than 4 percent of government expenditures for nursing home care, pays very little because of a 100-day limit on benefits and, currently, a prior hospitalization requirement.

At present, only about 1 percent of nursing home payments are made by third parties. However, insurance companies are beginning to recognize a potentially expanded role for themselves in the provision of long-term care. Insurers are testing the market for long-term health care insurance policies and analyzing the financial risks associated with such coverage. Another insurance option is the formation of residential communities into risk-sharing groups, spreading the potential health care liability over a number of individuals. An existing example of this self-insurance approach is the continuing care retirement community (CCRC), the subject of this book.

CCRCs, which combine the insurance principle of risk pooling, private capital, and a management system, are likely to become an increasingly important option for financially self-sufficient retirees as greater emphasis is placed on developing private financing alternatives to address pressing needs.

HISTORY AND GROWTH OF CCRCs

The continuing care retirement community represents a further step in the evolution of public and private involvement in caring for the aged, including the provision of pension or assistance programs under governmental and private sector auspices.

The concept of continuing care is the result of the cross-pollination of related ideas and disciplines, many of which have their roots in the social programs of England, Germany, and the Scandinavian countries.

Among the precursors of the CCRC were the medieval guilds, which were the beginnings of premodern times of attempts by self-reliant people, through prior contributions, to insure themselves against losses arising from death, injury, and old age. Mutual aid societies and the English friendly societies were organized for such purposes.

As immigration to the United States increased during the 18th and 19th centuries, the English, Welsh, Irish, Scottish, Germans, French, Swiss, Jews, Belgians, Italians, Dutch, and Scandinavians organized mutual aid societies.

The increase in immigration also gave rise to a religious revival movement, especially in the cities where many immigrants congregated. As a social historian has written of this period:

> In a healthy parish the families could help one another over many everyday emergencies, and parish acquaintance was the foundation of many mutual-benefit societies like those federated into the German Central Verein (1855) and the Irish Catholic Benefit Union (1869). But the resources of parish families and their priest were limited, and the benefit associations were mostly interested in helping their contributing members. Very soon the bishop had to think about a second, institutional line of defense against need. So were founded a variety of charities, all of them conceived to supplement the home. Hospitals were for the sick poor who could not be treated at home; some were for "incurables," but in any case the treatment was likely to fail, leaving the family without a breadwinner or his wife. Hence the orphanage and a home for the aged.[6]

During this same period, the county poorhouse or township poor farm, which reflected the growth of public responsibility for the indigent aged, became part of the American landscape.

Subsequently, but before the development of compulsory old-age insurance systems, some consideration was given to the establishment of industrial pension systems for aging workers and state-administered old-age assistance laws.

> The early years of the depression focused public attention upon the plight of the needy aged, many of whom would never have been in the relief category if it had not been for the loss of savings through bank failures, deterioration of investments, and unemployment. Old-age assistance promised a more humane care of aged dependent persons than commitment to the poorhouse. By 1935, old-age assistance legislation had been provided by the laws of twenty-eight states and two territories.[7]

At the same time that states were struggling to provide for elderly residents who met certain residence and financial qualifications, church groups and other private organizations were developing community-based homes for their aging members.

A 1929 Bureau of Labor Statistics survey of homes for the aged found that religious or private organizations operated 80 percent of the

---

[6] James Leiby, *A History of Social Welfare and Social Work in the United States* (New York: Columbia University Press, 1978), pp. 80–81.

[7] Earl L. Muntz, *Growth and Trends in Social Security* (New York: National Industrial Conference Board, 1949), p. 66.

homes for which data were obtained. Many of these homes would not be recognized as continuing care retirement communities by today's standards, but they embodied many of the same principles used by religious and community groups to develop housing and medical care arrangements for the elderly.

Often, churches did not have pensions for their ministers and missionaries and felt that it was their responsibility to provide for the housing and care of these people on their retirement. Two communities quite similar to continuing care retirement communities were established for these purposes: Pilgrim Place in Claremont, California, begun in 1915; and Penney Retirement Community in Penney Farms, Florida, begun in 1925 by James Cash Penney. In the 1929 Bureau of Labor Statistics survey, 16 of 26 national church groups reported having a pension or relief fund for aged ministers.[8]

Most of the communities included in this study that offered continuing care contracts to residents prior to 1934 were originally homes for the aging (and sometimes children) sponsored by the United Methodists in Oregon, the Presbyterians, the United Church of Christ, and private foundations.

Pacific Homes Corporation also belongs in this category. According to information distributed by United Methodist Communications in 1979, Pacific Homes has its roots in the German Methodist Conference that established a home for retired ministers at a campground, now the site of Kingsley Manor, in Hollywood in 1912. In 1928, the German Conference merged with the Southern California Conference of the Methodist Episcopal Church, and in 1929 the Pacific Old Peoples Home was incorporated as a California nonprofit corporation. Kingsley Manor was the only property operated by the corporation until 1949. Presumably the success and ambiance of these communities for ministers and missionaries had appeal and application to the wider church population and the growing number of people who retired to southern California.

From 1949 to 1964,

> six additional properties were acquired by the corporation which came to be known as Pacific Homes Corporation. Pacific Homes historically operated its business on the basis of prepaid life-care contracts which essentially promised residents lifetime care, including comprehensive health care services. Residents paid an "accommodations fee" to cover the cost of the residence and a "life care fee" designed to cover the cost of health care. In later years, Pacific Homes also entered into continuing

---

[8] Florence E. Parker, Estelle M. Stewart, and Mary Conymgton, compilers, *Care of Aged Persons in the United States* (New York: Arno Press, 1976), p. 110. Originally published by the U.S. Department of Labor in 1929.

care agreements which included an accommodations fee and a monthly care fee.[9]

The funding of CCRCs through a one-time life care fee has proven to be an unstable situation, and all CCRCs now utilize a combination of an entry fee and a monthly maintenance fee.

Several other communities have offered continuing care contracts for over 30 years, including Brethren Hillcrest Homes in La Verne, California (1947): Dorothy Love Retirement Community in Sidney, Ohio (1922); and Park Vista Presbyterian Home in Youngstown, Ohio (1947). The Heritage in San Francisco, California, founded by the San Francisco Ladies' Protection and Relief Society in 1853, has offered continuing care contracts since 1955.

Homes for the aging which provided care and services to their residents under a policy of receiving all present and future assets in return for a lifetime of total care ("asset turnover" or "total care") gradually changed to a more marketable payment schedule based on actual costs.

In the first decades of the 20th century the principles of insuring oneself against accident, sickness, and for one's retirement began to take hold in the United States. These developments were instrumental in paving the way for the growth of CCRCs as an affordable option for retired persons.

This period also saw progress in the establishment of pensions for various categories of retired workers, primarily civil servants, veterans, and railroad workers and industrial workers to a lesser extent. It was the Depression which impelled American political and social leaders to consider the idea of old-age insurance more seriously. Great pressure developed on government in the early 1930s to enact a program of economic security for citizens in their old age. Efforts to add compulsory national health insurance to the program which eventually became known as Social Security were dropped because of intense opposition from physicians.

Throughout the period of debate over the extent of public responsibility for older citizens, including the level of financial support provided, the concept of CCRCs, frequently sponsored by religious organizations and supported by contributions from residents to the extent of their financial resources, continued to grow.

The existence of pensions for a larger number of retired workers made it possible for many of them to enter continuing care retirement communities over the years. A religious revival occurred in the United States between 1940 and 1960, as church membership rose from 49

---

[9] Edwin H. Maynard, *A Summary of Events* (United Methodist Communications, 1979).

percent to 69 percent of the population, and this period coincided with an expansion in the number of CCRCs.

In the 1950s, such church groups as the Northern California Presbyterians, the United Church of Christ, and the American Baptists, sought an alternative to the traditional "home," which was neither attractive nor suitable for the growing numbers of fairly independent, financially secure people living along the Pacific Coast and in the Bay area of California.

During this period, churches in Oregon organized and established several CCRCs, including Willamette View Manor in Portland, sponsored by the United Methodists in Oregon in 1955, and Rogue Valley Manor in Medford, sponsored jointly by the Episcopal, Presbyterian, and Methodist churches.

In 1954, the National Retired Teachers Association built Grey Gables in Ojai, California, and operated it as a CCRC. Villa Gardens in Pasadena, California, was established for teachers by the California Teachers Association in 1927. Although neither of these communities currently offers continuing care contracts, both remain operating retirement communities.

The federal government also influenced the growth and development of continuing care in the late 1950s and early 1960s. In 1959, the National Housing Act created the Section 231 program, providing federal mortgage insurance to aid in the development of new or substantially rehabilitated rental housing for elderly individuals. A number of CCRCs built in the early 1960s, among them the two communities known as The Sequoias, were constructed with Section 231 federally insured mortgages. In 1964, however, the program rules were revised to exclude the use of Section 231 in conjunction with "founder's fees" or any type of admission payment.

Nearly all CCRCs are owned and operated by nonprofit organizations, many sponsored or affiliated with a religious body. Nearly 300 CCRCs were identified in the United States by the empirical study reported in this volume.

Although continuing care retirement communities have existed for many decades, their median age is only 14 years, where age means the number of years since the community first offered a continuing care contract to a resident.

A distinct regional pattern emerges in comparing opening dates of communities by regional location, as illustrated in Figure 1–1. Cross-tabulation of these two factors shows that the oldest communities were built primarily in the North Central region and in the West. Steady growth in CCRCs has occurred throughout the past two decades in the North Central area, while the Western region experienced explosive growth between 1960 and 1969 with less growth in recent years. The largest number of communities opened between 1970 and 1979 were in

FIGURE 1–1
Opening Dates by Regional Location

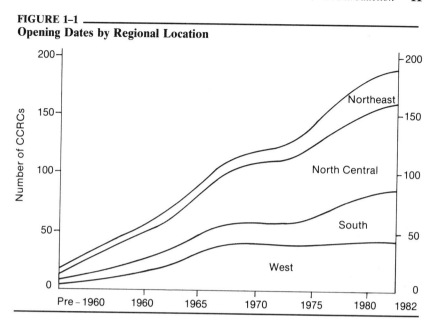

the Northeastern region. The South is the site of most recent growth; most of the new communities (73 percent of those opened in 1980 and 1982) are located in the Sun Belt.

CHARACTERISTICS OF CCRCs

CCRCs are organizations established to provide housing and services, including health care, to people of retirement age. These communities typically offer independent living in a campus-like setting, which may also contain health care facilities such as congregate living, personal care, and intermediate nursing care or skilled nursing care. The communities offer residents the guarantee of shelter and various health care services, usually for life.

CCRCs have an average of 165 independent living units and two or three other levels of on-site care, in either a campus or high-rise design. The physical facilities of CCRCs vary in style and structure and may feature studios, one- and two-bedroom apartments, high- or low-rise buildings, or duplexes. Some communities offer only skilled nursing care, to which residents transfer when they are no longer able to maintain their apartments independently. Others also have intermediate care facilities, consisting of congregate living and/or personal care units. Some offer home nursing programs or other optional health care services such as physical, occupational, or speech therapy. Many communities have built their levels of care in phases, some by original plan and others by converting or extending an existing facility.

Communities tend to build independent living units (ILU) first and skilled nursing units later. The study data showed that many communities have added personal care facilities (PCF) recently or have started with PCFs and added ILUs.

Most communities have a menu of social activities available to residents. Communities vary in size from under 50 to over 2,000 residents, but they typically house between 200 and 500—a population large enough to provide healthy social interaction without being overwhelming. The average resident population is 245. The average age of residents in independent living units is 80.2 years and that of residents in intermediate nursing care units is 85.4 years. Most CCRCs have active resident associations.

To enter a CCRC, residents usually meet a minimum age requirement (often 62 years) and are able to pay a relatively large one-time entry fee and an additional monthly fee, both of which can vary greatly, depending on region and the economic climate. Entry fees are usually dependent upon the size of the living unit occupied, and some portion of the fee is usually refunded if the resident vacates within a given period. The monthly fee may increase if inflation causes living costs to rise, but the fee will not increase by the full amount of any health care costs the resident might incur. In many cases, there is no additional charge for health care.

The range of entry fees and monthly fees in CCRCs is quite broad, reflecting a wide variation in services, guarantees, and the effects of inflation. This study found that average entry and monthly fees are comparatively moderate and that the potential universe of CCRC residents is much larger than had been previously thought. For one person, the average entry fee is $34,689 and the average monthly fee is $562. For a couple, the average fees rise to $38,682 and $815, respectively.

These figures support the proposition that CCRCs are within the financial reach of many middle-income individuals, especially elderly homeowners with substantial equity in their private residences and persons with inflation-indexed retirement pensions.

Approximately 70 percent of couples over 65 and 35 percent of single persons over 65 own their homes, and 80 percent of the homes are owned outright. However, housing expenses for older persons have doubled in the past decade as the costs of energy, real estate taxes, insurance, and maintenance have increased, and these costs now represent about 42 percent of the income of older homeowners.[10] Selling one's home can, for many Americans of retirement age, create

---

[10] American Association of Retired Persons, *Report on 1981 White House Conference on Aging* (Washington, D.C., 1981).

all or the major part of the lump-sum payment necessary to enter a CCRC.

The growth of retirement systems, including pensions for retired private and public employees and inflation-indexed Social Security benefits, which alone can provide a couple $1,000 per month, is likely to make the CCRC a more viable option for increasing numbers of retirees. And it appears that the CCRC's self-pay approach will become more attractive as the financial burdens of home ownership begin to outweigh the advantages.

In short, then, CCRCs can offer a significant number of elderly people of varying economic means a contract for lifetime health insurance, virtually assuring them of financial security for the remainder of their lifetimes. CCRCs represent an important alternative to nursing homes and other long-term care facilities in that they reverse the trend of alienation experienced by many isolated older people by providing an opportunity for social interaction with peers, a variety of activities, physical security, and a continuum of nursing care as it is required—features which reverse the trend of alienation suffered by people confined to freestanding nursing homes.

Illness and death rates are lower for CCRC residents than for the general population, and there are undoubtedly several reasons for this. For example, healthy individuals may be more willing to pay a larger entry fee; middle- and upper-income individuals may have had better health care earlier in life; and the entry requirements of many communities preclude the acceptance of nonhealthy individuals. A number of studies have confirmed that good housing and adequate health care are conducive to long life, and it may be that the communal spirit and variety of activities offered by a CCRC may foster a lower incidence of illness and an increased life expectancy among residents.

The CCRC is able to offer the attractive package of independent living and health care because it is based on an insurance concept to fund its health care liability. A portion of the entry fees and monthly fees paid by residents is utilized by the community to pay health care expenses; since only a relatively small proportion of the community's residents require health care at any one time, these fees represent an insurance premium paid by the entire community for health care which will be used currently only by a small group. In addition, some portion of fees is often set aside to provide subsidies for residents who cannot continue to pay their monthly fee. It is almost unheard of for a resident to be evicted from a community because of an inability to pay fees due to uncontrollable circumstances.

Since every CCRC resident is guaranteed health care whenever he or she needs it, management must generate a continuing influx of new entrants to fund the community's health care liability. This strong commitment to the lifelong security of CCRC residents typifies the intensity of management's responsibility to maintain the financial well-being of the community itself through health care reserves, and represents the critical distinction between continuing care retirement communities and other arrangements, which operate strictly on a month-to-month, or rental, basis.

One of the unique aspects of initiating a CCRC is the substantial inflow of funds from the lump-sum entry fees paid by the initial group of residents. For example, a community with 300 residents would collect $9 million if the average entry fee were $30,000. The usual arrangement is to use these funds to finance a portion of the facility and to secure an additional amount in the form of a mortgage or bond issue to finance the remainder. Monthly fees are often set to cover operating expenses, with mortgage payments being supported by the resale of apartments when individuals either die or are permanently transferred to the health care center.

Potential Problems

This financing arrangement and pricing methodology appear relatively simple, but a number of precautions must be taken to assure a community's financial stability. Double-digit inflation in recent years has spelled financial trouble for some CCRCs and required them to take corrective action to cover their unfunded liabilities. A crucial element in the financing structure is the turnover or resale of apartments, since the funds obtained in this way are often needed to meet the community's debt service. However, because of the small number of residents, random deviations can cause the number of deaths and/or the number of residents who transfer permanently to the health care center to vary significantly from year to year. If only a few apartments are released in a given period of time, significant cash flow problems can develop—due to an "unlucky" deviation in mortality and morbidity rates. Yet another factor that can cause CCRCs to experience lower than expected turnover is the low mortality and morbidity associated with CCRC residents. Thus, apartment turnover rates may be considerably lower than anticipated from published mortality tables.

If a community avoids these first problems, there is another, more subtle one. From a health care utilization standpoint, a new community requires 10 to 15 years to mature before its health care center becomes fully occupied (that is, mature). Unless the CCRC management establishes a health care reserve in anticipation of this eventuality, monthly fees will have to be increased by a rate greater than inflation, a rate that residents may find unpalatable or unaffordable.

Because the CCRC depends so heavily on the group insurance concept to fund its health care liability, it seems natural that the industry should develop actuarially based guidelines to assure that its reserving methodologies are appropriate. Until now, however, the accounting and actuarial professions have not developed the appropriate methodology for determining health care reserve requirements for CCRCs. The newness of the industry and the lack of a perceived need on the part of many CCRC managers are the primary reasons for the lack of development in this area. Moreover, boards of directors of nonprofit organizations are generally reluctant to allow revenues to exceed expenses in a manner that would allow the accumulation of a health care reserve (even if they knew its correct value) because such a pricing structure gives the appearance of a "profit" at the residents' expense.

Another barrier to actuarially based pricing structures is that the first community in an area to introduce actuarially based prices may become uncompetitive with respect to other communities in its area. Thus, the tendency to set prices according to the fees set by other communities is a problem that must be solved in future years.

In addition to the health care reserve, a CCRC, like many other business organizations, should hold reserves for the continual modernization and refurbishment of the facility and for its eventual replacement. This is a particularly difficult problem in an inflationary environment, because such future expenditures require that substantial sums be accumulated.

A third area in which reserves are required is the financial aid liability associated with residents who currently, or in the future, cannot meet their monthly fees. Although continuing care contracts generally reserve the right to expel individuals who cannot meet monthly fees, as a practical matter this is seldom, if ever, done. Many communities attempt to solicit contributions from the surrounding area to support such individuals; but this may not be a sufficient solution in uncertain economic times when high levels of inflation may cause more and more residents to fall short of funds.

A final note should be made on the contribution of high, and, especially, varying inflation to the unsatisfactory financial status of some communities. The prepayment of any future cost that cannot be predicted with confidence naturally increases the probability of financial difficulty. During the last decade, inflation has been particularly damaging with respect to the prepayment aspects of continuing care, and it is necessary for CCRCs to develop methods to deal with this problem in the future.

Legislation has been enacted at the state level to attempt to control the financial management of CCRCs, but so far only 10 states have statutes regulating any aspect of continuing care communities. In those states that have developed some continuing care regulation, the methodology and underlying assumptions associated with the laws appear inadequate. Mortality assumptions included in such legislation are not appropriate for CCRCs, since they assume higher death rates than actually occur. In addition, the "small group" problem is not addressed and the inflation problem faced by communities accepting prepayment is not dealt with in regulations.

OVERVIEW OF CHAPTERS

This book is divided into three parts: (1) an empirical survey of CCRCs that describes in detail the various characteristics of existing communities; (2) a financial analysis of CCRCs that examines current financial management practices and discusses extensively the ways in which actuarial science can be applied to developing appropriate fees and ensuring the long-term financial health of CCRCs; and (3) a legal analysis that first describes the current status of CCRC regulation and then examines those areas where the authors believe regulation is appropriate or inappropriate.

The empirical analysis is presented in Chapters 2 and 3. These chapters analyze the results obtained from a 24-page survey instrument that was completed by more than 200 CCRCs. Several characteristics are discussed, including institutional definition; geographic location; organization, affiliation, and tax status; contract provisions; fees; refunds; resident population; health care utilization; services and special features; management and financial policies; capital financing; and reserves.

The financial analysis follows in the next eight chapters. Chapter 4 discusses the appropriateness of applying actuarial science to the evaluation of the long-term financial status of CCRCs. Several pricing methodologies are described, and the cash flow implications of each approach are illustrated for a hypothetical nonprofit community offering an extensive health care guarantee (i.e., the resident continues to pay the same monthly fee after permanent transfer to the health care center). Only one approach to fee-setting, the closed-group method, is used in the remaining analysis, but the alternative methods are compared with the closed-group approach for five characteristics.

Chapter 5 sets forth the assumptions required for financial analyses of CCRCs and presents a methodology for developing these assumptions. This methodology is applied to several actual communities, and the results of the studies are summarized.

The actuarial model used to translate the actuarial assumptions into projections of future population flows is described in Chapter 6. Population flows are used to determine several statistics useful in financial analyses, such as apartment turnover and apartment density ratio (number of residents in apartments to total number of apartments). Also, these flows generate information regarding nonfinancial planning issues, such as the ultimate health care capacity requirements. Since the underlying assumptions regarding new entrants will vary, the model is used to illustrate the consequences of changes in entry age distributions and health care transfer policies for future population flows. Chapter 6 also contains the results of applying the population projection methodology to actual communities.

Chapter 7 introduces the discussion on actuarial pricing, describing the closed-group methodology for determining the actuarial costs of offering continuing care contracts to new entrants. These costs are the basis for developing fees that are actuarially adequate and equitable (i.e., that reflect differentials according to age, sex, apartment type, number of occupants, and so forth). Moreover, the actuarial costs are also the basis by which management can set fees that are *actuarially adequate in aggregate* for a group of entrants, even though individual fees may not themselves meet this goal.

The actuarial adequacy of fees for a group of entrants must be monitored over time. If experience differs from the underlying assumptions, then fees must be adjusted to maintain actuarial balance. The actuarial valuation methodology, presented in Chapter 8, is the basic tool used for such monitoring. In addition to determining whether the community is in overall actuarial balance, the actuarial valuation generates information regarding fee adjustments that should be made to keep the community in actuarial balance and information on the reserves (in terms of liquid and fixed assets) that should be held in order to provide for the future liabilities associated with current residents. Illustrative cases are presented at the end of this chapter.

Chapter 9 presents an illustration of the cash flows for a community maintaining actuarially adequate fees and discusses how the new entrant pricing and valuation methodologies, combined with cash flow projections, can be used to assess the financial health of a community at a given point in time. These methodologies are applied to six actual communities to determine their long-term financial position.

Chapter 10 contains an introduction to external financial statements for CCRCs. This chapter describes the objectives of various types of financial statements and the generally accepted accounting principles by which they are prepared. The limitations of using these statements for making management financial decisions are also pointed out. If the reader is familiar with such statements, this chapter may be omitted.

The last chapter in this part, Chapter 11, contains the authors' recommendations for modifying statements of generally accepted accounting principles (GAAP) to bring them closer to the community's actuarial position. These recommendations cover the amortization of entry fees, expensing fixed assets, and establishing fund accounting for health care reserves. Several illustrations are presented to compare current practices with such modifications.

The legal analysis is covered in Chapters 12 and 13. Chapter 12 presents a comprehensive overview of the regulatory status of CCRCs as of June 1982. This chapter describes the components of regulation in eight states with detailed statutes as well as two model acts prepared by interested groups. The elements of regulation in those states with less comprehensive legislation and the impact of attempts at federal regulation are also examined.

The authors' recommendations in Chapter 13 are based on the assumption that they will be applied in a state statute. In several areas, our best judgment was used, combined with consultation from our Advisory Committee and other interested parties. This chapter is intended to be used as a framework from which legislators might draft reasonable and useful statutes that would avoid the errors of prior efforts. It is not intended to be an absolute guideline for all states to follow.

Chapter 14 contains a summary of the findings of this research and suggests other areas for future research. ■

Part One

Empirical Analysis

Chapter Two

An Empirical Survey of CCRCs I

■ The results of a massive data collection effort undertaken to define the characteristics of continuing care retirement communities are presented in this and the following chapter. It provides a nationwide "snapshot" of the industry, a picture unavailable prior to this study. This general overview should be useful to state legislators, current and potential sponsors, developers of CCRCs, researchers and academicians in related fields of study, prospective residents of CCRCs, and other individuals interested in continuing care retirement communities.

In an effort to contact every continuing care retirement community in operation or under construction, a mailing list was compiled utilizing a number of sources, including the *Directory of Members, 1981* of the American Association of Homes for the Aging, the *Directory of Life Care Communities* compiled by Nora Adelmann and published by Kendal-Crosslands (1980 edition), and the *1980 Directory of California Association of Homes for the Aging*. In addition, specialists in the industry and executive directors of state associations of nonprofit homes for the aging were consulted. Six hundred communities of one type or another were initially identified for questioning as to whether they met the description of a CCRC as defined in this study (see next section, "Institutional Definition").

A self-administered survey questionnaire, designed to gather information from each community on such characteristics as organizational structure, fee schedules, management and financial policies, resident census, services, and contract provisions, was mailed to the 600 communities, following a pretest by a 24-member review panel and appropriate questionnaire revisions.

Extensive follow-up measures were taken to collect completed surveys from all communities. A second mailing was sent to nonrespondents. Nonrespondent community administrators were called and urged to return the survey. In some cases, nonrespondent communities were surveyed by telephone to ascertain whether or not they did, in fact, offer continuing care as defined by the study. This effort reduced the nonresponse list by eliminating the communities that did not meet the criteria.

A total of 274 continuing care retirement communities currently operating or under construction were identified positively; of these, survey questionnaires were obtained from 207 communities, a response rate of over 76 percent. A list of all 274 communities identified as of December 31, 1981, is included in Appendix A. It was determined that, in addition to these communities, over 120 of the original universe list of 600 were offering services similar to continuing care but not meeting the study's strict definition of continuing care.

The characteristics of these communities are discussed in this chapter. Several independent variables are used in the analysis:

1. *Community age:* The year in which continuing care contracts were first offered by the community.
2. *Resident population size:* The number of residents holding continuing care contracts.
3. *Nursing care ratio:* The percentage of all continuing care residents receiving nursing care.
4. *Health care ratio:* The percentage of all continuing care residents receiving health care (which includes nursing and personal care).
5. *Region:* Geographic location.
6. *Health care guarantee:* The extent to which fees charged to contractholders for nursing care are less than the daily rate charged those without continuing care contracts.
7. *Fees:* Total expected combined entry and monthly fees over a typical resident's expected lifetime in the community.

Definitions of each of these variables can be found at the beginning of the appropriate section.

INSTITUTIONAL DEFINITION

A precise definition of continuing care was difficult to formulate, since the industry is virtually embryonic. Many communities offer comparable packages of services but call themselves by different names, often depending on regional custom. Conversely, many communities that claim to provide continuing care in fact offer a distinctly separate menu of services. As a result, some communities that describe themselves as CCRCs, as well as communities that "look like" CCRCs but do not meet the study's definition, are not included in the analysis.

For purposes of this study, a continuing care retirement community is defined by its *contract,* the legal agreement between the individual (resident) and the organization (community) established to provide housing, services, and health care; by the *type of accommodations* available; and by the way *fees* are paid by the resident. By definition, a continuing care contract (1) remains in effect for more than one year, (2) guarantees the resident access to nursing care whenever needed, and (3) covers fees paid by the resident for some or all nursing care, which is on a less than fee-for-service basis. All 207 communities (the number that returned completed questionnaires) included in the data base as well as the 67 communities not in the data base meet the following definition.

CCRC Definition

A continuing care retirement community is an organization established to provide housing and services, including health care, to people of retirement age. At a minimum, the community meets each of the following criteria:

Campus consists, at least, of independent living units; it may also contain health care facilities such as congregate living, personal care, and intermediate or skilled nursing care.

Community offers a contract that lasts for more than one year and guarantees shelter and various health care services.

Fees for health care services are less than the full cost of such services and have been partly prepaid by the resident.

While all the CCRCs in the data base (n = 207) meet this functional definition, they use different terms in describing themselves. About half (50 percent)[1] describe themselves as "retirement communities," "retirement residences," "retirement villages," or "retirement centers"; another quarter refer to themselves as "life care communities"; and 13 percent use the expression "continuing care retirement community." A few are self-described as "total care retirement," "life care retirement residence," "independent living," "long-term health care," or "home for the aging." The question asked and the tabulated responses are given below:

Phrase most often used to describe facility

Retirement community	45.4%
Life care community	24.2
Continuing care retirement community	13.0
Other	10.1
Home for the aging	3.5
Life/continuing care community	1.4
Continuing care community	1.9
Nursing home	0.5
	100.0%

[1] This includes the 45.4 percent that checked "Retirement Community" plus half of the 10 percent responses checking "Other."

Types of Housing

Most CCRCs have a combination of independent living and health care units. For almost half of the communities (46.9 percent), this combination includes independent living and nursing care levels only, while another 40.1 percent have personal care. A small group of CCRCs (3.4 percent) do not have nursing care units but do have personal care units and independent living. Very few communities have only independent living units. Those communities that do not have an on-site health care center are defined as CCRCs if they have formal arrangements with an outside health care facility to provide services for their continuing care contractholders.

Facilities

Independent living and nursing care only	46.9%
Independent living, personal care, and nursing care	40.1
Independent living and personal care only	3.4
Independent living only	2.9
No response	6.7
	100.0%

The median number of independent living units per community is 165, with a fairly even distribution between 50 and 300 units. The median number of ILUs has been increasing over time, from 110 for communities constructed before 1960 to 217 for communities built after 1970. Only four communities were found to have more than 400 units. Figure 2–1 shows the distribution of independent living units for all communities.

Two models or styles of physical plant design are predominant among CCRCs. The first, designated the *garden* or *campus* style, is represented by 44.4 percent of CCRCs. These have six or more buildings laid out in a campus setting, presumably in suburban locations or on generous portions of city land. Typically, the buildings are one-story or low-rise structures.

The second model, referred to as *high rise,* is typical of at least 27 percent of CCRCs with less than five buildings and six or more stories per building. Such high-rise communities are found in urban locations or among newer communities built on expensive land. Figure 2–2 shows the distribution of CCRCs by the number of buildings and the maximum number of stories.

Contract

One of the distinctive features of a CCRC is that both the resident and the community organization make a long-term commitment. In fact, when asked how long their contract actually remains in effect, 94.2 percent of CCRCs responded, "For the resident's lifetime." No com-

FIGURE 2–1
Distribution of Number of Independent Living Units

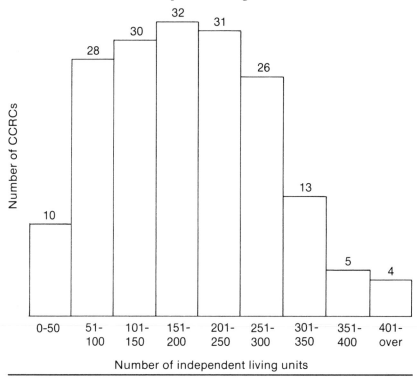

Number of independent living units

munity reported ever asking a resident to leave because of his or her inability to pay fees (unless this occurred through willful and intentional dissipation of funds).

In a limited-choice question, CCRCs checked the phrase that best described the contract they currently offer to new residents. A fairly even split between "life care" and "continuing care" is evident, while a few communities use such expressions as "life lease," "fee for service," and "rental":

Describe current contract

Life care	39.6%
Continuing care	34.8
Other	14.0
Life lease	7.8
Fee-for-service	2.4
Rental	1.4
	100.0%

The various names for these functionally similar contracts reflect regional and historical differences within the field. "Life care" is more

FIGURE 2–2
Frequency Block Chart

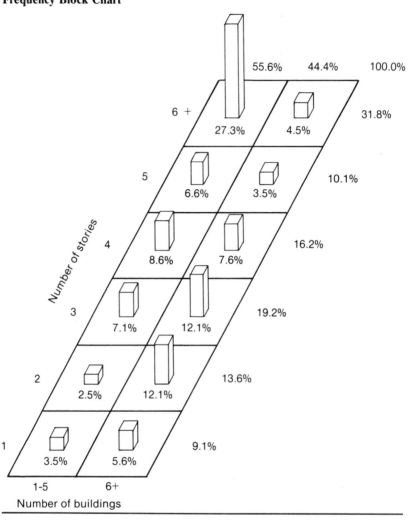

prevalent in the Northeastern section of the country, particularly in Pennsylvania. Communities in the West, represented mainly by those in California, are more likely to use "continuing care" because this term is included in the definition contained in the California regulation (California Health and Safety Code) as a result of the negative connotation of "life care" or "total care" associated with an older type of home for the aging which required an entrant to turn over all assets to the home for "care for life." Current continuing care contracts are mutually terminable (can be terminated by the resident or the community) and thus quite different from traditional life care in this sense.

Beyond this historical variance within the field over terminology, the distinction between "life care" and "continuing care" is not meaningful. All 274 communities identified by the study meet the definition of a continuing care retirement community and are increasingly recognized by this term.

Health Care Guarantee

The third definitional criterion of a CCRC concerns the fee schedule (entry and monthly fees) and cost allocation for health care provided under the terms of the continuing care contract. On this point, there is virtual unanimity among the CCRCs studied with respect to the *guarantee of access* to nursing care:

> **Do currently offered contracts guarantee an independent living unit and access to nursing care whenever needed?**
>
> | | |
> |---|---|
> | Yes | 97.6% |
> | No | 0.5 |
> | No response | 1.9 |

However, some communities offer contracts covering almost all health care costs incurred in the health care center, while others have contracts that cover only a limited portion.[2] To distinguish between these two types, a variable called the *health care guarantee* was created, based on a community's response to several questions.

Health Care Guarantee Definition

The health care guarantee is the degree to which costs for nursing care are covered by the continuing care contract and are shared among all residents ("pooled risk") so that fees paid by an individual resident are less than those paid on a fee-for-service basis.

Communities were categorized into two groups based on their health care guarantee. Communities in which all residents pay the same monthly fee for temporary or permanent nursing care as they were charged when they were in an independent living unit *or* communities in which all residents pay the same basic rate, typically less than 80 percent of per diem rates (even if this is different from the rate they were charged while in an independent living unit), are classified as offering an *extensive* health care guarantee. Fifty-four percent of

---

[2] Almost all hospital, as opposed to health care center, costs are covered under Medicare Part A, and a considerable amount of physicians' costs is covered under Medicare Part B. If the community requires insurance supplementary to Medicare, that combination covers all hospital costs and most physicians' costs, leaving the costs of nursing care to the community.

CCRCs are in this group. The second group, classified as offering a *limited* health care guarantee, includes all communities in which residents receiving nursing care are charged the rate that is paid on a per diem basis by individuals not holding contracts (i.e., paying on a fee-for-service basis) after a specified length of stay that typically ranges from 10 to 180 days. The various plans and fee schedules used by communities in this category are discussed in more detail at a later point in this chapter. Forty-four percent of CCRCs are in this group.[3]

GEOGRAPHIC LOCATION

Continuing care retirement communities are found throughout the country, although some states have relatively large numbers, while other states have none. Figure 2–3 shows the distribution of the 274 CCRCs identified by the study.

The states with more than 1 million elderly people also have the most CCRCs, with one notable exception. New York, which has the

FIGURE 2–3
Regional Distribution

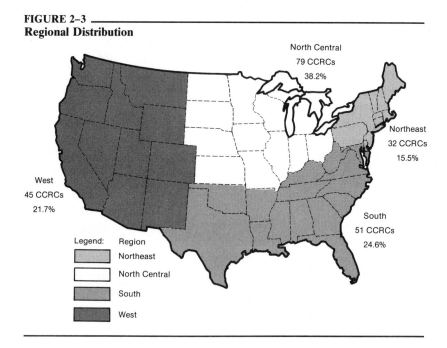

North Central
79 CCRCs
38.2%

Northeast
32 CCRCs
15.5%

West
45 CCRCs
21.7%

South
51 CCRCs
24.6%

Legend: Region
Northeast
North Central
South
West

---

[3] In some cases, judgment had to be used in classifying the community; the basic distinction between limited and extensive guarantees was preserved to the extent made possible by a community's responses. Two percent of the communities remained unclassified.

second largest elderly population among the states, does not permit the operation of CCRCs.[4] In rank order, the other states are California with 36 CCRCs, Florida with 33, Pennsylvania with 31, Ohio with 22, and Illinois with 16.

In order to facilitate data analysis, the 50 states and the District of Columbia were grouped into four regions, as follows:

Northeast
Connecticut	New Hampshire	New York	Rhode Island
Maine	New Jersey	Pennsylvania	Vermont
Massachusetts			

North Central
Illinois	Kansas	Missouri	Ohio
Indiana	Michigan	Nebraska	South Dakota
Iowa	Minnesota	North Dakota	Wisconsin

South
Alabama	Georgia	Mississippi	Tennessee
Arkansas	Kentucky	North Carolina	Texas
Delaware	Louisiana	Oklahoma	Virginia
District of Columbia	Maryland	South Carolina	West Virginia
Florida			

West
Alaska	Hawaii	Nevada	Utah
Arizona	Idaho	New Mexico	Washington
California	Montana	Oregon	Wyoming
Colorado			

The distribution of CCRCs among these four regions is shown in Figure 2–3.

Several of the factors and characteristics presented in the following sections are analyzed according to these regional groupings to determine whether they vary by geographic location. In reviewing such figures, however, one should keep in mind that (1) Pennsylvania, (2) Florida and Virginia, and (3) California dominate the Northeastern, Southern, and Western groups, respectively. CCRCs in the North Central region are more evenly distributed: Ohio, Illinois, Iowa, Kansas, and Missouri each have more than 10 CCRCs.

ORGANIZATION, AFFILIATION, AND TAX STATUS

All but a few continuing care retirement communities (97.1 percent) have nonprofit federal income tax status. Only two proprietary communities have been identified by the study. More than 93 percent (93.2

---

[4] New York's nursing home regulations prohibit any residential health care facility operator from accepting prepayment for basic services for more than a three-month period.

percent) own their buildings, 2.9 percent lease them, and 1 percent both own and lease buildings.

The concept of "sponsorship" and the legal relationship between a community and its "sponsoring" body have been scrutinized and defined in recent court cases, and the sponsoring organization's financial responsibility—implied or real—has been under particular review. As a result, changes in sponsoring philosophy and practice are being made by many organizations providing continuing care. With this in mind, several questions about CCRCs' affiliations were included in the survey questionnaire.

About two thirds of all CCRCs are affiliated with another institution, typically a nonprofit, religious organization. Only a few are affiliated with proprietary organizations. One third of the communities are inde-

FIGURE 2–4

Tax Status and Sponsorship of Continuing Care Retirement Communities

All communities (100%)			
Nonprofit status (97%)			*
Affiliated with another organization (63%)		Independent (36%)	†
Nonprofit sponsor or affiliation (59%)	‡		
Sponsor appoints controlling share of board members (35%)	Sponsor does not appoint controlling share of board (28%)		
Owned by sponsor (25%)	Not owned by sponsor (38%)		
Managed by sponsor (24%)	Not managed by sponsor (39%)		
Sponsor financially responsible (24%)	Sponsor not financially responsible (39%)		

* 1% = proprietary; 2% = no response.
† 1% = no response.
‡ 4% = affiliated with proprietary organization.

pendent. Figure 2–4 displays the tax and affiliation characteristics of all the CCRCs studied.

Considering for the moment only those CCRCs that are affiliated with another organization (n = 131), one sees that almost all of the "parent" organizations are nonprofit, religious bodies:

**Federal income tax status
of affiliated organization
(n = 131)**

Nonprofit	92.3%
Profit	6.9
No response	0.8

**If nonprofit, type of
affiliated organization
(n = 122)**

Religious	89.3%
Foundation	0.8
Other	9.9

In more than half (56.2 percent) of communities with an affiliation (n = 131), the affiliated "parent" organization appoints a controlling share of the board of directors or trustees; it also may reserve the right to approve major program changes and/or indebtedness by the community organization. Another group of respondents have a more distant relationship, characterized as historical or philosophical, with their affiliated organizations. Almost 40 percent of communities with an affiliation are owned by, managed by, and/or financially responsible to their parent organization. The concept and fact of sponsorship and affiliation are not the same for all communities; indeed, the entire spectrum of affiliation from distant, historical ties to a close, symbiotic relationship is evidenced among CCRCs nationwide.

**Relationship between community and affiliated organization
(n = 131)**

Owned by	39.2%*
Managed by	37.7
Financially responsible for	38.5
Appoints controlling share of board membership	56.2

* Percentages sum to more than 100 percent since responses are not mutually exclusive.

In some states, nonprofit CCRCs are seeking exemption from real estate taxes; in other states they are already exempt. Survey data provide a profile of these exempt communities:

**Community exempt from
state real estate taxes**

Yes	65.2%
No	27.1
N/A	1.0
No response	6.7

Smaller communities and communities that offer limited health care guarantees are more likely to have tax-exempt status.

Since real estate taxes are under the jurisdiction of state governments, it is not surprising that exemption from state real estate tax varies by region.

**Regional location by percentage
exempt from state real estate taxes**

Region	Percent CCRCs exempt
Northeast*	50.0%
North Central	72.7
South	63.6
West†	88.1

* Represented primarily by Pennsylvania, which does not exempt CCRCs from its real estate tax.
† Represented primarily by California, which exempts CCRCs from its real estate tax.

CONTRACT PROVISIONS

All communities included in the data base, by definition, offer contracts that remain in effect for more than one year. In fact, almost all of the CCRCs (94.2 percent) stated that their continuing care contracts remain in effect for the resident's lifetime (1.4 percent have contracts that last for one year only, and 4.4 percent have contracts specifying some other duration).

Over half of the communities studied offer one contract, but a sizable minority (40.1 percent) offer more than one contract type, complicating the pricing, accounting, and financial management of these communities. Most of these communities (n = 83) have two or three types of contracts.

**If multiple contracts are offered, how many
contract types are held? (n = 83)**

Two contract types	42.2%
Three contract types	28.9
Four contract types	6.0
Five contract types	6.0
More than five contract types	9.6
No response	7.3

In a large majority of CCRCs (80.9 percent), nearly all residents (over 90 percent) hold continuing care contracts. Facilities are either totally identified as continuing care retirement communities, or they offer a continuum of services on another basis entirely; few facilities combine residents holding contracts with residents of independent living units paying on some other basis. (In 13.3 percent of CCRCs, 90 percent or less of the resident population holds contracts; 5.8 percent did not respond.)

Probationary Period

More than half (54.6 percent) of the communities have contracts that provide for an adjustment or probationary period during which the community can terminate a contract by giving written notice to a resident. Communities in the Western and Northeastern regions are more likely to have such a probationary period than are those in the other two regions. There is a slight trend away from providing a probationary period in the contracts offered by newer communities.

Contract Termination Policies

Many contracts held by residents of CCRCs are archaic and not well defined, though the contracts offered by newer communities tend to be clearer and more specific. In particular, the conditions surrounding termination of a contract between community and resident are spelled out more carefully in the new contracts.

Contracts can be terminated by most CCRCs (72.9 percent) *if a resident cannot be cared for* in the community's facilities (e.g., if care for mental illness or skilled nursing care is needed where the community does not provide such); 23.2 percent cannot terminate contracts under this condition (3.9 percent no response).

As shown in Table 2–1, communities are much less likely to terminate a contract because of a *resident's inability to pay the fees*. This is

TABLE 2–1
Contract Termination by Community Age Due to Inability to Pay Fees

	Percent CCRCs	
Community age	Able to terminate contract	Unable to terminate contract
Pre-1960	29.4%	70.6%
1960–69	33.3	66.7
1970–79	43.8	56.2
1980–post	66.7	33.3
All years	40.2	59.8

due in part to IRS regulations relating to their nonprofit tax status and in part to the moral commitment of continuing care providers. The majority of CCRCs (96.1 percent) have contracts that do not allow them to ask residents to leave if they run out of money under any conditions or only on the condition that the resident has willfully dissipated his or her financial resources. Moreover, only 1 percent of all communities indicated that a resident had ever been asked to leave because of lack of funds. There is a trend toward including a "willful dissipation" provision in the contracts being offered by communities built since 1980, as the data below illustrate. The section on "Financial Aid" shows how communities and their resident populations deal with this potentially difficult situation.

FEES

Two different types of fees are paid by residents of continuing care retirement communities: an *entry fee* (a lump-sum payment, also called a "founder's fee" or an "accommodation fee") and a *monthly fee*. In addition, communities have developed a variety of fee schedules to accommodate residents who want continuing care contracts for personal care or nursing care, married couples who need different levels of service, and to meet other situations arising out of the aging process which demand a flexible, human approach in providing a continuum of care. These schedules are addressed under the heading "Health Care Fees."

An indication of the complexity of fee schedules among CCRCs is the response to the question "Do you allow residents to choose from a variety of entry fee and/or monthly fee combinations for residence in a particular apartment type?" Forty percent said yes; 60 percent said no.

Entry Fees

In most communities (91.8 percent), entry fees are established and paid according to the size and type of living unit. Entry fees depend on the entrant's age in only 7.7 percent of CCRCs. The practice of basing fees on the unit size (real estate basis) rather than an entrant's age or physical condition (actuarial basis) persists despite industry-wide agreement that the product is the intangible, insurance-like concept of continuing care and not the living unit itself.

Although the range of entry fees charged by communities is broad, reflecting a wide variation in services and guarantees and the effects of inflation, the *average* fee is moderate, refuting critics' claims that continuing care is only for the rich. The median differential between the entry fees charged a single individual and the entry fees charged for two persons in one unit is only 16 percent (see Table 2–2). In fact, few communities vary the entry fee for more than one person in a particular apartment.

TABLE 2–2
Range of Entry Fees

	One-person fees (n = 1,028)	Two-person fees (n = 845)
Minimum	$ 1,000	$ 1,000
10th percentile	13,700	15,680
25th percentile	20,500	24,400
Median	32,500	38,000
75th percentile	49,500	55,000
90th percentile	66,675	72,250
Maximum	178,000	178,000
Average	$ 34,689	$ 38,582

Entry fees tend to vary by region. North Central communities typically have lower entry fees; Southern communities have entry fees slightly higher than the average. Entry fees are related, of course, to construction and financing costs, which are higher for new communities, most of which are located in the Southern region. As these costs have escalated in recent years, the entry fee charged per square foot has also increased (see Table 2–3).

TABLE 2–3
Entry Fees—Charges per
Square Foot

Range of charges	
10th percentile	$29
25th percentile	42
50th percentile	56
75th percentile	69
90th percentile	81
Average charge	$60
Construction before 1975	55
Construction after 1975	70

Entry fees are higher in CCRCs with larger resident populations and in CCRCs offering an extensive health care guarantee, as shown in Table 2–4.

TABLE 2–4
Summary Table:
CCRC Entry Fees for One-Bedroom Unit
(n = 285)

	Percent of all units	Less than $20,000	$20,001– $30,000	$30,001– $40,000	$40,001– $50,000	$50,001 and over
Region						
Northeast	15.4%	0.0%	9.3%	18.0%	26.2%	18.0%
North Central	35.4	59.6	53.4	34.4	20.0	18.0
South	30.6	24.6	14.0	32.8	38.4	40.0
West	18.6	15.8	23.3	14.8	15.4	24.0
	100.0%	100.0%	100.0%	100.0%	100.0%	100.0%
Resident population						
200 and less	40.7%	49.1%	41.9%	52.5%	27.7%	30.0%
201 to 300	22.5	31.6	30.2	21.3	9.2	28.0
301 and more	36.8	19.3	27.9	26.2	63.1	42.0
	100.0%	100.0%	100.0%	100.0%	100.0%	100.0%
Health care guarantee						
Extensive	58.9%	24.6%	37.2%	57.4%	84.6%	84.0%
Limited	41.1	75.4	62.8	42.6	15.4	16.0
	100.0%	100.0%	100.0%	100.0%	100.0%	100.0%

Entry Fee Increases

Since entry fees are present payments for future services, they must be calculated carefully and, in times of high inflation, adjusted frequently. They are constrained, however, by the market and, in some cases, by the policy or tradition of a sponsoring organization. According to the data, entry fees are increased once a year by a little over half of CCRCs (54.1 percent). Few communities (4.3 percent) increase fees more often than annually or on a regular, biannual basis (8.7 percent). A relatively large number of communities (24.2 percent) increase fees on some other basis, such as "as needed," depending on the market demand, costs, or new construction. Some communities adjust fees for each new resident, and a few increase fees monthly, quarterly, or "to meet state requirements." Eight communities indicated that entry fees had never been changed or had changed only once in the past 5–18 years.

For the period June 30, 1980, to July 2, 1981, the average increase in entry fees was 12 percent. As the following data show, the range of percentage increases varied from 0 percent to over 30 percent. The median is slightly below the average at 10 percent:

Approximate percentage increase in entry fees from June 30, 1980, to July 2, 1981:

No response and 0%	37.2%
1–10%	40.1
11–20%	20.3
21–30%	1.9
Over 30%	0.5

Amortization of Entry Fees

About one third (35.6 percent) of communities amortize entry fees into their financial statements based on the *individual life expectancy of each resident;* another third (32 percent) amortize entry fees within a specified number of years;[5] and 11.9 percent amortize entry fees based on the average expected lifetime of a *group of residents*. A variety of schedules are followed by 9.8 percent of CCRCs, yet another example of the complexity and dissimilarity of continuing care communities. (No response was received from 10.7 percent.)

Illustrative examples of methods used by communities to amortize entry fees are:

"According to the Colorado State Law regulating reserve requirements."

"Treated as nonoperating income for capital use as needed."

---

[5] Typically tied to a community's entry fee refund schedule. Within 5 years (11.9 percent), within 10 years (13.9 percent), and more than 10 years (6.2 percent).

"Received upon death of resident."

"At time of payment."

"Not amortized—considered as a gift."

"Earn 1 percent a month or over nine years."

Monthly Fees

Monthly fees vary depending upon the size and type of dwelling unit, the number of occupants, and the number of meals included. A wide range of monthly fees are charged among CCRCs, as demonstrated in Table 2–5. These figures support the proposition that fees charged by CCRCs can be afforded by middle-income individuals.

TABLE 2–5
Range of Monthly Fees

	One person (n = 1,052)	Two persons (n = 853)
Minimum	$ 70	$ 70
10th percentile	320	349
25th percentile	453	610
Median	580	835
75th percentile	742	1,075
90th percentile	900	1,312
Maximum	2,762	3,026
Average	$ 562	$ 815

Monthly fees in half of the communities (50.3 percent) include three meals per day, while in 44.4 percent such fees include just one meal per day. Only 5.3 percent of CCRCs base their monthly fees on two meals per day.

The cross-tabulations presented in Table 2–6 were performed to determine whether monthly fees vary by geographic region, size of resident population, or health care guarantee. They show that monthly fees (for a one-bedroom unit) are associated with region and health care guarantee and are somewhat related to size of resident population. Monthly fees are lower in the North Central region, where entry fees are also lower than average. Communities in the Northeast have higher monthly fees, but they also tend to provide more services, as discussed later. Understandably, communities offering extensive health care guarantees have higher monthly fees than those with limited guarantees.

Monthly Fee Increases

Asked if current continuing care contracts limited the amount of increase allowed in monthly fees, 72.5 percent of CCRC respondents

TABLE 2-6
Summary Table:
CCRCs Monthly Fees for One-Bedroom Unit
(n = 285)

	Percent of all units	$500 and under	$501–$700	$701 and over
Region				
Northeast	15.4%	10.5%	3.0%	33.3%
North Central	35.4	54.8	30.3	22.6
South	30.6	26.3	36.4	28.6
West	18.6	8.4	30.3	15.5
	100.0%	100.0%	100.0%	100.0%
Resident population				
200 and less	40.7%	40.0%	46.5%	33.3%
201 to 300	22.5	30.5	26.3	10.8
301 and more	36.8	29.5	27.2	55.9
	100.0%	100.0%	100.0%	100.0%
Health care guarantee				
Extensive	58.9%	48.4%	60.6%	67.9%
Limited	41.1	51.6	39.4	32.1
	100.0%	100.0%	100.0%	100.0%

answered no, 25.1 percent answered yes, and 2.4 percent did not respond. Of those who replied affirmatively, most made statements like the following:

"The limit depends upon Social Security increases."

"Is determined by an independent auditor."

"Is set by a specified table included in the contract."

"Is dependent upon operating costs less endowment earnings."

"Is limited to a total of five increases."

"Limit determined by legislation."

Communities offering contracts limiting the amount of increase in monthly fees do not vary by size, health care ratio, or type of financing, but they do vary somewhat by region. North Central communities are least likely and Western communities are most likely to specify limits. Older communities are slightly more likely to specify limits on monthly fees.

A majority of communities (64.7 percent) give 1–30 days' notice prior to an increase in monthly fees; 18.4 percent give 46–60 days' notice; and the remaining respondents give more than 60 days' notice (12.1 percent did not respond). Whether limited or not, monthly fees are increased once a year by 83.1 percent of CCRCs, twice a year by

4.8 percent, and as needed or on some other schedule by the remaining CCRCs.

The distribution by percentage increase in monthly fees during the period June 30, 1980, to July 2, 1981, is given below. It indicates that a fairly large number (42.5 percent) experienced increases of between 11 and 20 percent. The average increase, however, was 10.4 percent (n = 176), in line with inflation for the same period.

Approximate percentage increase in monthly fees from June 30, 1980, to July 2, 1981

No response and 0%	15.1%
1–10%	39.6
11–20%	42.5
21–30%	1.4
Over 30%	1.4

Health Care Fees

Fee schedules for health care in continuing care retirement communities are complex and nonstandard. There are almost as many schedules as there are communities, especially when one considers that many communities have more than one fee schedule. Some CCRCs also offer continuing care contracts to individuals entering directly into their personal care (29 percent) or nursing care (34 percent) facilities.

Communities in the data base were categorized as offering either limited or extensive health care guarantees to residents, depending upon the communities' responses to several questions on temporary and permanent nursing care utilization fees. A CCRC was categorized as offering an *extensive* guarantee if its plan was similar to any one of the following:

1. A resident's monthly fee for temporary and/or permanent nursing care is the same as the monthly rate for his or her apartment.
2. A resident's monthly fee for nursing care is equal to that paid for the smallest independent living unit.
3. All residents pay the same rate for nursing care (e.g., middle of fee range) regardless of the type of independent living unit occupied previously.

All other communities were categorized as offering a limited health care guarantee. Examples of limited guarantee fees for temporary utilization are:

"Same monthly fee plus an additional charge for skilled nursing care but less than daily rate."

"Monthly fee for apartment is reduced and pay daily SNF (skilled nursing facility) rate."

"Discount on SNF fees for first 10 years of residency."

"Monthly fee plus 40 percent of difference between regular monthly fee and current SNF daily rate for first 180 days; thereafter, 80 percent of difference between monthly fee and current SNF daily rate."

Some of the fee schedules or formulas for permanent health care are as unique as those for temporary health care. These include:

"Basic rate minus rebate of $\frac{1}{66}$ of membership fee per month."

"Special continuing care contract with outside nursing home; resident pays monthly fee plus costs above $800 to nursing home."

"Pay SNF rate minus $\frac{1}{60}$ of entry fee per month forever."

"Credits remaining on the apartment [prorated schedule for earning fee][6] are used up at the prevailing rate before the resident has to pay.

Rates charged by CCRCs to individuals receiving nursing care who *do not* have continuing care contracts (called "outside admissions" in this report) range from a median of $36 for personal care to a median of $50 for skilled nursing care. The numbers of units by levels of care used by outside admissions to CCRCs are presented in Table 2–7. During the period June 30, 1980, to July 2, 1981, the rates for these units were raised 1–10 percent by 21.3 percent of CCRCs, 11–20 percent by 23.7 percent of CCRCs, and over 20 percent by 4.9 percent of CCRCs. The remaining 50.1 percent either did not raise their rates during this period or did not respond.

TABLE 2–7
Level of Care, Number of Beds, and Fees for Outside Admissions

Level of care	Number of beds (total CCRCs)		Median semiprivate rates	
Personal care	3,146	(n = 75)	$36	(n = 18)
Intermediate care	4,048	(n = 77)	42	(n = 43)
Skilled nursing care	8,269	(n = 132)	50	(n = 100)
Other	519	(n = 11)	—	—

Double-Occupancy Fees

One of the attractions of a continuing care retirement community for married couples is the security of knowing that a continuum of care is

---

[6] Explanation added.

provided, so that if one spouse needs health care sooner than the other, they can still be physically near each other. Thus, fee schedules must account for this fairly frequent occurrence. But not all communities approach this situation in the same way.

In most communities (72.5%), the surviving member of a double-occupancy unit can continue to reside in the unit *alone* by paying the monthly fee rate for a single person. Some communities require the survivor to pay 1½ times the single-person fee (4.8 percent) or the two-person fee (4.8 percent) or to move to a smaller unit (2.4 percent). An additional 12.6 percent have some other plan, and 2.9 percent did not respond.

If one member of a double-occupancy couple must move permanently to the health care center, in 59.4 percent of CCRCs the other member can remain in the independent unit alone by paying the single-person fee. In 14 percent of CCRCs, the remaining member is required to pay the two-person fee. This response may indicate that the question was misinterpreted to mean the total fees paid by the couple, in which case the response is the same as that described first (i.e., single-person fee). Almost one fifth (16.4 percent) of CCRCs have some other payment schedule which covers this situation.

When one spouse is in ILU and the other is in HCC, does HCC resident pay the same fee as he or she did prior to:

Temporary transfer	
Yes	48.8%
No	43.5
Yes and no	0.5
N/A	1.9
No response	5.3
Permanent transfer	
Yes	35.7%
No	58.5
Yes and no	0.5
N/A	1.4
No response	3.9

Financial Aid

Financial aid is available to residents in about three quarters (73.4 percent) of all communities, a considerable number.[7] In many of these communities, residents raise or contribute part or all of the funds available to residents who "outlive their financial resources."

Although one might expect to find financial aid more widely available in communities with older resident populations and higher per-

---

[7] Financial aid is not available in 20.3 percent of CCRCs; 6.3 percent did not respond.

42

centages of residents receiving health care, this is not the case. These factors were determined to be not significantly related to the financial aid available in any particular community.

More important, one might expect financial aid to be more widely available to residents of communities with limited health care guarantees, since these residents have less assurance of medical cost coverage than do residents in communities with extensive guarantees. Table 2–8, however, shows no significant difference between these two types of communities with respect to financial aid.

TABLE 2–8
Financial Aid by Health
Care Guarantee

Aid available	Extensive	Limited
Yes	80.4%	76.1%
No	19.6	23.9

The availability of financial aid is related significantly to the level of monthly fees charged by a community, but not to the entry fees charged. Communities with monthly fees in the $401–$600 range and in the range above $701 typically have financial aid for residents. CCRCs with monthly fees in the $601–$700 range are less likely to have financial aid than are those with monthly fees at the low end of the scale, implying that they have higher financial requirements at admission and/ or that they are relatively new and their residents have not yet experienced financial problems.

REFUNDS

The subject of entry fee refunds paid by continuing care retirement communities is one which has been debated and studied for many years. Some community organizations believe there is a moral commitment to return any unused fees to a person or the estate, while others return very little money, if any, basing their policy on the belief that residents accept the insurance, or "pooled risk," concept underlying continuing care. Several questions were asked in the empirical survey to identify trends among CCRCs with respect to refunding policies. Three areas were addressed: refunds upon death, refunds upon withdrawal, and refunds made when the community terminates a contract.

Refunds upon Death

Communities are divided evenly on the policy of providing entry fee refunds upon the death of a resident: 48.8 percent give refunds; 46.9

percent do not (2.4 percent = not applicable; 1.9 percent = no response). Of the CCRCs that do give refunds, most (78.2 percent) base the refund on the death of the second member of a couple, and only 8.9 percent base it on the death of the first member (1.0 percent base it on the death of both, and 11.9 percent did not respond).

Among the communities following a policy of refunds upon death, there is little agreement on the period after which the refund is not provided, as the following data illustrate:

Length of death refund provision (after which there is no refund)
(n = 101)

1–90 days	20.9%
91–180 days	10.9
181–270 days	0.0
271–365 days	19.8
1 year, 1 day–2 years	9.9
2 years, 1 day–3 years	9.9
3 years, 1 day–4 years	3.0
4 years, 1 day–5 years	9.8
Over 5 years	6.9
No response	8.9

Newer communities, particularly those built since 1980, tend to provide refunds upon the death of a resident, but these communities make the refund contingent upon reoccupancy of the living unit. Table 2–9 shows the progression of this trend over time.

Regional differences exist with respect to policies on refunds made to a resident's estate; CCRCs in the Northeast are most likely and those in the West are least likely to offer refunds upon death. Policies on death refunds are not related to the level of fees charged by CCRCs.

The refund policies described by communities on the survey questionnaire are so heterogeneous that they almost defy categorization, though it can be stated that a majority follow a prorated schedule over the refund period. A sample of these policies is presented to illustrate this point:

"100 percent of total entry fee upon death."

"Community retains 1/12 of fee per month of occupancy."

"First year 75 percent; second year 50 percent; third year 25 percent."

"All but 10 percent is refunded."

"One third is refunded."

"Prorated based on 5½-year refund schedule."

"80 percent less sum used for skilled nursing care is refunded."

"4 percent deducted for first and second months; 2 percent a month thereafter."

"50 percent refunded."

BIERLEY

TABLE 2-9
Summary: Refund Provisions

Refund type and condition	Community age					Region			
	Total	Pre-1960	1960-1969	1970-1979	1980-post	NE	NC	S	W
Upon death	48.8%	38.7%	42.1%	59.7%	78.6%	73.3%	55.8%	56.3%	20.9%
Contingent upon reoccupancy*	37.6	10.0	20.9	34.9	46.2	47.7	26.0	28.1	8.7
Upon withdrawal	89.0	87.1	96.1	92.5	85.7	96.7	87.0	93.8	100.0
Contingent upon reoccupancy*	44.8	22.2	40.8	54.8	64.3	53.3	49.2	46.7	30.2
Upon termination									
Contingent upon reoccupancy†	23.2	14.8	16.7	47.4	28.6	39.3	35.0	28.6	9.8

* The values in these rows are based on the number of CCRCs that responded positively to refund condition. For example, 18.3 percent (0.488 × 0.376) of all CCRCs (n = 207) hold entry fee refunds in the event of death until the unit is reoccupied.
† These percentages are based on n = 207.

"First two months, full refund; thereafter, 10 percent a month is deducted."

"2 percent a month is deducted."

"1/60 per month deducted until year 2."

"1/180 per month with a minimum of 36/180 deducted."

"Prorated over 10-year period" and so on.

"4 percent of fee plus 1 percent per year per person plus 2 percent per month."

"8 1/3 percent per month."

"1 2/3 percent per month for period not used."

Refunds upon Termination by Community

Most communities (70 percent) apply the same or similar provisions to refunds upon withdrawal as are applied to refunds when the community terminates a continuing care contract. But some communities (12.6 percent) follow yet another refund schedule; 3.9 percent apply the "refund upon death" provision; 2.9 percent base their refunds on state requirements; and 10.6 percent did not respond.

One of the ways a community can reduce its exposure or risk in refunding entry fees, or portions thereof, is to make the refund contingent upon reoccupancy of the independent living unit by a new resident. Indeed, there is a trend among newer communities to follow such a policy. The data presented in Table 2–9 show that approximately 45 percent of CCRCs opened since 1970 currently have such a requirement. ■

Chapter Three

An Empirical Survey of CCRCs II

RESIDENT POPULATION

Individuals who are attracted to, and become residents of, continuing care retirement communities have not yet been studied. Information collected through the survey questionnaire, however, sheds some light on demographic characteristics of CCRC resident populations, such as size and average age.

Each community was asked to provide its census of residents holding continuing care contracts and the total resident census for each level of care or service available in the community. These census figures, presented in Table 3–1, represent about half of the total number of continuing care retirement community residents in the country today.

Planners and developers of continuing care retirement communities, as well as many others, have wondered whether there is an optimum resident population size. There appears to be little consensus on this question. The distribution of CCRCs by resident population is relatively flat, as seen in Figure 3–1. The median continuing care resident population is 218; for all residents, the median is 245.

Communities have been getting larger over time. The data in Table 3–2 show a strong trend toward larger resident populations in newer communities.

One of the intriguing issues in continuing care is whether residents live longer because of the continuing care environment or because continuing care communities attract a population predisposed to good health and longevity. This question is beyond the range of this report.

TABLE 3–1
Resident Census by Level of Care

Living status	Continuing care contractholders		Total residents	
ILU	39,907	(n = 188)	40,827	(n = 191)
PCF	2,338	(n = 76)	2,954	(n = 81)
ICF	2,735	(n = 93)	4,118	(n = 99)
SNF	4,396	(n = 132)	6,810	(n = 144)
Other	538	(n = 12)	736	(n = 15)
Total	49,914		55,445	

FIGURE 3–1
Distribution by Total Number of Residents

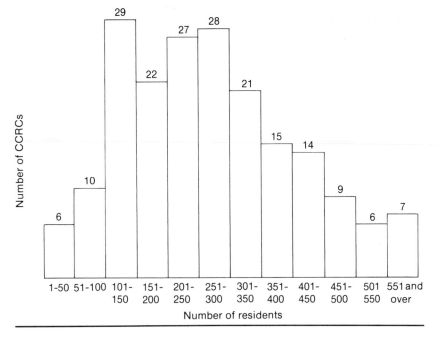

TABLE 3–2
Size of Resident Population by Age of Community

Size	All CCRCs	Pre-1960	1960–1969	1970–1979
100 and less	11.1%	13.9%	6.6%	11.9%
101–200	27.5	41.7	31.6	17.9
201–300	22.2	16.7	32.9	19.4
301 and more	30.9	25.0	26.3	46.3
No response	8.3	2.7	2.6	4.5
	100.0%	100.0%	100.0%	100.0%
Median size	245 res.	219 res.	250 res.	305 res.

Baseline data analyses indicate, however, that residents of continuing care retirement communities are among the "old-old" of the elderly population. More than half of CCRCs (52 percent) have an average resident age of 80 to 82 years or higher. Considering each level of service individually, average ages range up to over 85 for residents of intermediate nursing care.

Residents of:	Average age
Independent living units (n = 173)	80.2 years
Personal or domiciliary (n = 70)	84.2
Intermediate nursing care (n = 78)	85.4
Skilled nursing care (n = 115)	84.7

As one might expect, average resident age increases in a direct relationship to a community's age since a large majority of the first cohort of residents enter in their early to middle 70s and continue to live and age in the community for more than 10 years. There is a relationship between regions and community ages; thus, it is not surprising that the average resident age varies by region as well (see Table 3–3).

TABLE 3–3
Average Resident Age by Community Age and Geographic Region

	Community age				Region			
Average age	Total	Pre-1960	1960–1969	1970–1979	NE	NC	S	W
74 and below	7.8%	2.9%	5.5%	14.1%	3.7%	12.9%	23.5%	4.5%
74–77	8.2	0.0	1.4	20.3	11.1	11.4	7.8	0.0
78–81	36.2	14.7	35.6	45.3	55.6	31.4	29.5	31.8
82–85	40.7	61.8	50.7	18.8	25.9	32.9	39.2	54.5
86 and over	7.1	20.6	6.8	1.5	3.7	11.4	0.0	9.2
	100.0%	100.0%	100.0%	100.0%	100.0%	100.0%	100.0%	100.0%

HEALTH CARE UTILIZATION

The most essential and expensive aspect of the package of services provided by continuing care retirement communities is health care. In order to study health care utilization among residents of CCRCs, two ratios were calculated for each community: health care ratio and nursing care ratio.

Definitions

Nursing care ratio: The number of residents receiving intermediate and skilled nursing care divided by the total number of residents, where resident is defined as an individual holding a continuing care contract.

Health care ratio: The number of residents receiving personal care, intermediate nursing care, and skilled nursing care divided by the total number of residents.

Nursing Care and Health Care Ratios

In general, when a community is newly opened, its resident population is relatively young and healthy. Over the years, this initial cohort of residents ages and grows increasingly frail, calling upon the various health care and health-related services provided by a continuing care retirement community. This relationship between health/nursing ratios and community age should be kept in mind for the following discussion.

Overall, the distribution of CCRCs' health care and nursing care ratios is as follows:

Ratio	Nursing care ratio	Health care ratio
0% and N/R	12.3%	15.4%
1–5%	8.7	6.6
6–10%	16.3	13.3
11–15%	21.9	16.8
16–20%	13.8	17.3
21% and over	27.0	30.6
	100.0%	100.0%

Communities with higher ratios—for both health care and nursing care—are located predominantly in the North Central and Western regions. Since higher ratios are found in older communities and these two regions have relatively large, and equal, numbers of older communities, this finding is not surprising. A closer inspection shows that ratios are quite high among CCRCs in the North Central region and in the upper-middle range for Western region CCRCs.

Conversely, communities with lower ratios are clustered in the Southern region—where most of the new communities are being built—and in the Northeastern region, for a reason other than community age, since CCRCs in that region are evenly distributed with respect to community age. To analyze further the relationship between these ratios and various factors such as geographic region and management policy, the community age factor should be controlled; this analysis remains for future research.

Communities with extensive health care guarantees have lower nursing and health care ratios than communities with limited health care guarantees (see Table 3–4). Perhaps this finding indicates a successful effort on the part of CCRCs with extensive health care guarantees, responsible for a larger portion of residents' health care costs, to give residents appropriate and cost-effective care. These communities

TABLE 3–4
Nursing Care Ratio and Health Care Ratio by
Health Care Guarantee

Median ratio	Health care guarantee		
	Extensive	Limited	All CCRCs
Nursing care	13.1%	22.3%	17.4%
Health care	15.6	25.8	20.2

have a financial incentive to monitor nursing care utilization carefully, while communities lacking this financial incentive have a higher proportion of residents receiving nursing care and health care.

The size of a community's resident population is also significantly related to the health care ratio: larger CCRCs have lower ratios, and smaller CCRCs have higher ratios. Since newer communities tend to be larger than older ones, this finding may be related to community age.

Policy on Moving Residents to Health Care

Overall, 45.4 percent of all communities have a management policy or contractual statement that specifies whether or not, and when, a resident must relinquish his or her apartment and move permanently to the health care facility; 52.2 percent do not have such a policy (2.4 percent = no response).

Among these communities (n = 94), most specify a certain time period or schedule for such a move, while other communities make these decisions on an informal, individual, or unspecified basis, as the data below show:[1]

After what period of time in HCC must a resident give up his/her ILU? (n = 94)

1–30 days	7.4%
31–60 days	20.2
61–90 days	36.2
91–120 days	23.4
Over 120 days	2.2
No response	10.6

The existence of such a policy in a community is unrelated to the proportion of residents receiving health or nursing care. This finding is surprising, since a community with a low number of residents in its

---

[1] Responses include answers based on informal policies but not necessarily contractual provisions.

health care facility might be expected to have a policy encouraging residents to fill empty beds, while a community with a higher ratio—and therefore fewer beds available—might be expected to have a policy that discourages such moves. It is possible that this is, in fact, what occurs, but if so, it is done on an informal, selective basis. These figures show no difference in policy among CCRCs by health care ratio.

A definite trend is emerging among newer communities not to have a policy regarding permanent moves to a health care facility. Two thirds of CCRCs built prior to 1970 have such a policy, while only one third of those built since 1970 have one.

Outside Admission to Health Care

Continuing care retirement communities accept new residents at the personal care and nursing care levels as well as into their independent living units. Some of these outside admissions pay a per diem rate, while others are covered by a continuing care contract that lasts for more than one year.

Three quarters (75.4 percent) of CCRCs admit individuals from the outside community directly into their health care facility; 36.2 percent admit outside individuals into their personal care facility (only 40 percent of CCRCs have personal care facilities). Communities are much more likely to offer contracts that last for more than one year to persons becoming residents of personal care than to those admitted directly to health care, as these figures show:

Offer contract that lasts for more than one year for direct admissions to outside individuals to:

Personal care facility	Yes	80.0%
(n = 75)	No or N/A	20.0
Health care center	Yes	44.9%
(n = 156)	No or N/A	55.1

Nursing Care Certification by Medicare and Medicaid

All CCRCs participate in the Medicare program in terms of their residents being protected against hospital costs, and most CCRCs require their residents to subscribe to Part B to cover physicians' costs. Medicare coverage of skilled nursing is extremely limited, however, and requirements for the facility are high, while Medicaid covers most long-term nursing care costs. CCRCs participate in the Medicare and Medicaid programs in about equal numbers: 54.6 percent are certified by Medicare, and 48.8 percent are certified by Medicaid (in both cases, nonresponse = 5.5 percent). Yet the profiles of CCRCs participating in each of these programs are different, as shown in Table 3–5.

Communities participating in Medicare certification tend to have larger resident populations, are predominantly in the Northeastern re-

TABLE 3–5
Medicare and Medicaid Certification by Size, Region, Guarantee, and Age

	Percent CCRCs certified by Medicare	Percent CCRCs certified by Medicaid
All communities	54.6%	48.8%
Size		
100 and less	45.0	55.0
101–200	34.5	56.4
201–300	58.7	50.0
301–400	81.1	47.2
401 and over	80.0	52.0
Region		
Northeast	87.5	50.0
North Central	44.9	65.4
South	49.0	34.7
West	65.0	42.5
Health care guarantee		
Extensive	65.4	40.6
Limited	50.0	65.1
Age		
Before 1970	47.7	50.5
Since 1970	67.5	49.4

gion, offer extensive health care guarantees, are newer (built since 1970), have higher fees (total expected fees and entry fees), and have lower nursing and health care ratios. All of these factors are statistically significant.

In contrast, most of these same factors are significantly related, but in the opposite direction, to communities certified by the Medicaid program. Since the Medicaid program is administered at the state level, it is not surprising that regional variation appears. More of the communities in the North Central region are certified by Medicaid (65.4 percent) than of the communities in other regions, particularly in the South, where only 34.7 percent participate in the program. Medicaid certification does not vary by community age, so the difference between regions is probably due to interstate differences in Medicaid payment levels and certification procedures.

The fact that communities offering limited health care guarantees are more likely to be certified by the Medicaid program than are communities with extensive health care guarantees supports the observation that residents of CCRCs with limited guarantees experience greater risk and health care cost, causing them to "spend down" their assets. Thus, these communities are likely to utilize the Medicaid program to a greater extent than the communities with extensive guarantees.

SERVICES AND SPECIAL FEATURES

A CCRC is a microcosm of a larger community, with most of the services needed for its residents' daily living provided on-site.

The survey instrument contained a list of the services that a CCRC might provide. However, it did not include questions to differentiate the extent of specific services (such as home health care, occupational therapy, physical exams, physical therapy, and prescription drug service) among communities. This type of analysis is necessary to compare health care delivery systems fairly and is an important area for future research. Questionnaire respondents were asked to check each item, indicating whether or not it was included in the basic fees and contract.[2] The information collected in this manner is presented in this section, together with the results from a smaller but similar list of special features. It is interesting to note that most services are either quite prevalent or rather unpopular, an indication of broad similarity among CCRCs, at least with respect to the selection of necessary and desirable services.

Services included in the basic contract and fees of at least 80 percent of CCRCs are: utilities, special diet, apartment cleaning, parking, kitchen appliances, replacement of apartment equipment, storage, emergency call system, and social services.

Conversely, 80 percent or more of CCRCs do not include in their contracts and fees services such as prescription drugs, therapy for psychiatric disorders, special duty nurses, dental care, podiatry, hearing aids, or membership in a health maintenance organization.

Table 3–6 summarizes 34 services in alphabetical order and shows percentages for each by several key factors: health care guarantee, region, and community age.

Categorized Services

The services listed in Table 3–6 were divided into three groups or types: medical, support/preventive health care, and services related to

---

[2] It should be noted that even though a service is not included in basic fees, it may be available from a community for an additional charge.

TABLE 3–6
Summary of Services: Percent of CCRCs Including Service in Fees

Services	All CCRCs	Guarantee Ext.	Guarantee Ltd.
Apartment cleaning	83.1%	91.6%	83.5%
Bed and bath linen	71.0	81.0	67.8
Community's own physician	32.4	45.9	17.6
Dental care	6.8	6.4	4.3
Emergency call system	88.9	94.5	90.7
Garages/carports	25.6	24.8	27.2
Health maintenance organization	4.3	5.5	2.2
Hearing aids	3.4	2.7	1.1
Home health care	28.5	41.1	16.3
Hospitalization	25.6	39.8	9.3
Illness or accident away from community	20.3	34.3	4.7
Kitchen appliances	84.1	88.1	79.3
Occupational therapy	36.3	50.0	23.0
Parking	85.5	84.4	85.9
Personal laundry facilities	78.7	85.3	79.1
Physical exams	26.1	38.5	10.1
Physical therapy	35.3	48.1	21.6
Podiatry	10.6	7.3	4.3
Prescription drugs	15.9	28.7	3.4
Private room in nursing care center	25.1	20.2	16.3
Recreational therapy	72.0	84.4	61.8
Referred specialist	23.7	30.3	9.8
Replacement of apartment equipment	86.0	88.9	80.4
Resident's physician	22.2	22.1	26.2
Social services	83.6	89.0	85.1
Special diet	83.6	92.5	81.6
Special duty nurses	9.2	11.9	5.4
Storage	81.5	87.1	72.3
Telephone	32.4	42.2	16.3
Therapy for psychiatric disorders	15.5	25.5	2.3
Tray service	56.5	73.3	43.2
Treatment for preexisting conditions	29.5	35.3	25.6
Transportation	72.5	84.9	57.4
Utilities	91.3	95.3	96.6

the physical plant or nonmedical. The breakdown for each category follows:

Medical	Supportive/preventive	Physical plant
Community's physician	Emergency call system	Utilities
Treatment for preexisting conditions	Special diet	Replacement of apartment equipment
Physical exams	Social services	Parking
Hospitalization	Transportation	Kitchen appliances
Referred specialist	Recreational therapy	Apartment cleaning
Resident's physician	Tray service	Storage
	Occupational therapy	

	Region			Community age			
NE	NC	S	W	Pre-1960	1960–1969	1970–1979	1980–post
92.9%	82.9%	85.7%	97.9%	82.9%	97.2%	84.6%	80.0%
85.7	72.0	70.0	81.0	85.3	80.3	67.2	66.7
43.3	25.3	28.0	50.0	40.0	37.0	30.8	20.0
0.0	8.1	8.0	4.8	16.7	14.6	4.2	0.0
93.1	89.3	94.0	97.7	85.3	93.2	94.0	100.0
37.0	20.6	22.7	47.4	30.9	27.6	22.4	33.3
4.0	5.7	4.2	2.5	—	—	—	—
—	—	—	—				
50.0	17.3	34.0	34.9	19.4	30.1	39.1	13.3
50.0	11.8	18.8	46.5	33.3	24.3	29.9	21.4
34.5	8.0	20.4	38.1	23.5	23.6	20.0	20.0
92.9	90.1	91.5	92.5	76.2	77.6	95.5	100.0
66.7	29.3	36.7	34.1	34.3	37.8	45.5	28.6
100.0	93.0	92.0	82.5	94.7	85.9	95.4	100.0
86.7	82.9	75.5	86.0	85.3	76.7	88.1	86.7
53.3	18.2	18.0	34.1	41.7	23.0	25.4	20.0
50.0	27.6	38.8	40.9	42.9	28.4	45.5	40.0
4.0	6.9	13.0	5.0	13.5	4.2	7.8	0.0
50.0	10.5	12.2	16.7	25.7	8.3	26.7	6.7
29.2	30.0	26.1	20.0	60.9	21.1	19.6	0.0
86.7	72.7	78.0	63.6	66.7	74.3	77.6	73.3
43.5	11.9	20.9	47.2	32.3	29.0	24.1	0.0
96.3	91.3	93.9	90.0	76.2	85.5	88.1	100.0
17.9	27.0	12.8	35.7	33.3	25.0	21.2	21.4
96.6	85.7	90.0	79.1	86.1	86.3	87.9	86.7
89.3	88.2	92.0	81.4	79.4	90.4	88.1	100.0
7.7	9.6	2.0	18.6	9.5	9.2	8.9	0.0
77.7	83.3	88.0	92.9	80.9	73.7	88.1	100.0
27.6	24.7	38.0	40.5	21.4	36.3	29.9	66.5
41.4	9.3	10.4	18.2	22.9	12.2	21.9	0.0
86.2	43.4	58.3	72.1	58.8	54.8	66.7	64.3
33.3	28.8	35.4	32.6	36.4	33.3	31.7	26.7
89.3	72.6	84.0	68.2	65.6	64.4	93.9	93.3
96.9	97.3	90.0	100.0	94.3	97.2	97.0	93.3

Medical	Supportive/preventive	Physical plant
Illness or accident away from community	Physical therapy	Personal laundry facilities
Prescription drugs	Home health care	Bed and bath linen
Therapy for psychiatric disorders	Health maintenance organization*	Telephone
Podiatry*	Hearing aids*	Garages/carports
Special duty nurses*		Private room in nursing care center
Dental care*		

* Included in basic fees for less than 10 percent of cases and therefore not included in the percentage totals and averages tabulated.

Health Care Guarantee/Service Analysis

One of the hypotheses tested by this preliminary analysis is that CCRCs offering extensive health care guarantees are more likely than those with limited guarantees to provide supportive/preventive health care–related services to residents of independent living units, thereby reducing health care utilization. While by no means conclusive, and offered in this report primarily as a basis for future research, a review of the data presented in Table 3–7 indicates that the hypothesis is

TABLE 3–7
Type of Services by Health Care Guarantee

Service type	Average percent of CCRCs		
	Extensive	Limited	Differential
Medical	33.4%	12.1%	21.3%
Supportive/preventive	73.0	54.5	18.5
Physical plant	71.7	64.1	7.6

correct. Overall, an average of 73.0 percent of CCRCs with extensive health care guarantees have supportive/preventive services, compared to an average of 54.5 percent of CCRCs with limited health care guarantees. This differential is particularly strong in comparisons with the services of tray service, occupational therapy, physical therapy, and home health care.

The difference between the two groups of CCRCs with respect to medical services was expected since, by definition, medical and health care is included in contracts offering extensive health care and is generally not included in contracts providing limited health care.

The relative similarity between the two groups of CCRCs on physical plant and facilities provided indicates that, except for the extent to which communities cover the cost of health care incurred by residents holding continuing care contracts, continuing care retirement communities constitute a unique and discrete group and provide a standard package of services.

Regional Variation in Services Offered

Overall, communities in the Northeastern and Western regions include more services as part of their basic fees; CCRCs in the Northeast are particularly high in providing services categorized as supportive, while CCRCs in the West are slightly higher in providing medical services. Communities in the North Central region generally have the same physical plant services that other communities have but are underrepresented on services classified as supportive and medical. CCRCs in the Southern region are low in providing physical plant services, most notably personal laundry facilities and bed and bath linen, and in covering the cost of a resident's own physician. These differences are shown in Table 3–8.

TABLE 3-8
Type of Services by Region

Service type	Northeast	North Central	South	West
Medical	40.8%	16.8%	19.7%	35.5%
Supportive/preventive	78.7	58.5	67.3	63.6
Physical plant	74.8	70.7	70.3	75.5

Markets in each region influence to some extent what services are expected and provided in CCRCs, and this is reflected in the data presented. Furthermore, to the extent that regions are related to community age, regional variations reflect differences in the cost of construction and capital over time.

Community Age/Service Analysis

Based on the data presented in Table 3–6, some services are becoming more prevalent, whereas others are diminishing and are not as likely to be included in contracts and fees offered by new communities. Among the services declining in coverage are bed and bath linen, apartment cleaning, community's or resident's physician, referred specialist, treatment for preexisting conditions, and special duty nurses (the last four of which are costly medical or medical-related services). Services that have been added by newer communities are parking facilities, kitchen appliances, replacement of apartment equipment, storage, and emergency call system.

The picture drawn by these data forms a *W* or up-and-down line rather than a smooth slope. Communities in the pre-1960 group are nonstandard and have a multitude of backgrounds, histories, and patterns of services. CCRCs built in the early 1960s, without the benefit of Medicare, individually covered many of the items later covered by that program. Communities built in the late 1960s and early 1970s often structured their service package around the Medicare program and, therefore, are more likely to include many of the listed services in their fees and contracts. Communities built since 1975 have had to deal with higher construction and health care costs. More important, those built since 1980 or currently under construction are facing the possibility of cutbacks in Medicare and other programs in addition to higher costs and have reduced the range of services provided by continuing care contracts (more services are provided on an "a la carte" basis).

Fees and Service Package

An index, called the *total expected fee index,* was developed to more fairly compare fees among CCRCs which vary their combination of monthly and entry fees. This index is a present value combination of the total anticipated entry fee and monthly fees to be paid by an individual resident in his or her lifetime.[3]

Total Expected Fee Definition

Total expected fee is the total anticipated dollars to be paid by an average resident. The index is equal to the entry fee paid by the resident plus 12 times the monthly fee times the resident's expected lifetime.

TEF = Entry fee
+ 12 times ILU monthly fee times resident's life expectancy

In the following analysis, one-bedroom fees are used; however, fees and fee plans of continuing care retirement communities are presented in detail in the *1982 Reference Directory of Continuing Care Retirement Communities.*[4]

Using the "total expected fees" variable as a measure of a community's relative fee structure, each of the services was analyzed to determine which services are related to fees, or which services are added when fees are higher. Not unexpectedly, the services classified as "medical" are marginally related, as are three services from the other two categories. Services related to higher fees—both entry and monthly—are: tray service, bed and bath linen, physical exams, hospitalization, illness away from the community, physical therapy, therapy for psychiatric disorders, and the community's physician. A few services are related to either high entry fees or high monthly fees but not both. For example, personal laundry facilities are related to entry fees since they are a capital expenditure, whereas apartment cleaning, prescription drugs, and occupational therapy are significant only with respect to the level of monthly fees. Several services, for example, trans-

---

[3] It should be noted that the version of the TEF index used in this report is biased toward limited health care guarantees since it is based on apartment monthly fees and does not reflect changes in monthly fees after transfer to the health care center. Hence, TEF indices for limited-guarantee contracts that charge lower apartment monthly fees will typically be lower than the indices for extensive guarantees.

[4] Howard E. Winklevoss and Alwyn V. Powell, *1982 Reference Directory of Continuing Care Retirement Communities* (Philadelphia: Human Services Research, Inc., 1982). This report provides a brief overview of data collected on fees charged by CCRCs in the aggregate.

portation and emergency call system, are more likely to be included in contract fees by CCRCs with fees in the middle range.

Number of Meals

Although all communities serve meals to residents, usually in one or more central dining rooms, CCRCs are divided into two essentially equal groups with respect to the number of meals that are included in standard fees:

**Number of meals included in
standard fee schedule**

Three meals a day	50.3%
One meal per day	27.1
Two meals per day	5.3

Table 3–9 presents the results of three cross-tabulations performed to determine whether communities including three meals differ from

TABLE 3–9 _____
Number of Meals by Community Age, Size, and Guarantee

Percent of CCRCs/Number of meals included

	All CCRCs	One meal (n = 55)	Two meals (n = 10)	Three meals (n = 102)
Community age				
Before 1970	57%	31%	30%	77%
Since 1970	34	62	70	15
No response	9	7	0	8
	100%	100%	100%	100%
Resident population				
Less than 200	38%	33%	30%	43%
201–400	39	38	30	44
401 and over	12	13	40	9
No response	11	16	0	4
	100%	100%	100%	100%
Health care guarantee				
Extensive	53%	54%	70%	53%
Limited	45	46	30	45
No response	2	0	0	2
	100%	100%	100%	100%

those including just one meal a day with regard to the factors of community age, resident population size, and health care guarantee. The factors of resident population size and health care guarantee do not differentiate among communities on the number of meals included in fees. However, the factor of community age shows a strong trend away from three meals a day among newer communities. In many communities, residents can choose from among several meal plans or options, and fees are adjusted accordingly.

Special Features

Some of the special features and amenities that continuing care retirement communities were hypothesized to have were listed in the survey instrument, and respondents were asked to check whether or not their community had them. These responses are presented in Table 3–10.

TABLE 3–10
Special Features

Feature on premises	Percent CCRC with feature
Religious services	95.2%
Beauty salon	94.7
Garden space	90.8
Residents' association	89.4
Master TV antenna	88.9
Barber	78.3
Guest facilities	73.4
Hiking trails	42.0
Fireplaces	38.2
Bank	19.3
Swimming pool	16.4
Pharmacy	15.5

No further analysis was done to determine what kinds of CCRCs tend to have certain features; this remains for future research. There is consensus on most of the items, with two exceptions—hiking trails and fireplaces, both of which are tied to a community's setting and type of construction. Although these were not listed as special features, it is known that many CCRCs have a gift shop and/or a convenience store where residents can purchase food and household items. Other features common to most CCRCs may also be missing from the list.

MANAGEMENT AND FINANCIAL POLICIES

The process of managing a continuing care retirement community is complex, challenging, and becoming increasingly sophisticated. This section does not purport to cover the multitude of issues, policies, and concerns that properly come under the heading "Management." Several specific topics were targeted in the survey questionnaire, and the results are presented in this section. These topics are: purchased management services, aggregate expenses, financial statements, admission policies, and residents' role in decision making.

Purchased Management Services

In response to the explosive growth and the increased complexity of the continuing care industry, companies have been formed to provide services to CCRCs. Of particular interest was the purchase of management services by communities: how many and what kinds of CCRCs purchase such services? The survey data show that about one third (36.3 percent) of communities purchase management services (including health care management) from another organization;[5] 61.8 percent of CCRCs do not and are, presumably, self-managed (1.9 percent = no response/not applicable).

More than half (56 percent) of communities purchasing management services (n = 75) do so from a proprietary or for-profit corporation; 42.7 percent purchase such services from nonprofit organizations (1.3 percent = not applicable). Thus, approximately 40 nonprofit CCRCs, or one fifth of the total CCRCs surveyed (n = 207), are managed by a proprietary firm. Communities with a lower percentage of residents receiving health care, in the middle range of fees, with larger resident populations, and/or built before 1970 are representative of the group that purchases management services. These CCRCs also are less likely to offer extensive health care guarantees.

Aggregate Expenses

Detailed financial information was not collected from communities, but most communities responded to a question regarding expenses, as follows.

Aggregate expense values	Average		Per capita	
Departmental expenses	$2,171,710	(n = 151)	$7,929	(n = 147)
Depreciation expense	297,204	(n = 149)	1,038	(n = 145)
Interest expense*	361,436	(n = 136)	1,425	(n = 133)
Mortgage reduction	146,897	(n = 108)	560	(n = 105)
Capital expenditures	170,255	(n = 125)	751	(n = 125)

* In some cases, this value was not listed separately but was included with depreciation expense.

Financial Statements

Virtually all communities (93.7 percent) have external financial statements prepared by independent certified public accountants (CPAs); the remaining 6.3 percent either gave no response or considered the question not applicable.

Slightly more than one third (37.2 percent) of communities prepare and use internal management statements that differ from external fi-

---

[5] It could not be determined whether communities managed by their sponsoring/affiliated body are counted among those that purchase management services. We assume they are included if a management fee is paid to the sponsoring organization.

nancial statements; in 54.6 percent of CCRCs these statements are the same (6.3 percent = no response; 1.9 percent = not applicable).

Communities differ on the question of whether to use external or internal statements in determining fee increases, and some use another method entirely, as the following figures indicate.[6]

What financial statements are used to determine fee increases?

External statements	42.0%
Internal statements	57.0
None used	1.9
Other	15.0

Admission Policies

Over the years, communities have developed fairly standard admission policies for new entrants. Most communities (90.8 percent and 94.2 percent, respectively) require potential residents to have a physical examination and to be of certain minimum age, usually 65 years. A large number (70 percent) require minimum levels of assets; two thirds (65.7 percent) require a minimum monthly income; and more than half (57.5 percent) require medical insurance coverage. Neither a religious requirement nor a maximum age requirement is imposed by most communities (87 percent and 89.4 percent, respectively, do not impose these requirements). Since individuals generally enter communities at the independent living unit level, it is not surprising that most communities (81.6 percent) impose health requirements.

Communities requiring minimum monthly income and minimum assets have similar characteristics. These communities tend to have been built during the period 1970 to 1979 and are perhaps more wary of inflation. In spite of this, the fee variable (total expected fees) is not related significantly to communities having these financial requirements.

Communities that require medical insurance coverage upon admission are larger, have higher fees, and offer extensive health care guarantees (as shown in Table 3–11). Their health care ratios are in the middle range. The medical insurance requirement does not vary by community age.

Outside Admission to Nursing Care

Among the communities studied, 75.4 percent admit patients other than those holding continuing care contracts to their nursing care facilities. Such outside admissions are hypothesized to be influenced by two related factors: (1) the nursing care ratio and (2) the number of years a community has been open (community age). Older communities have

---

[6] More than one response was recorded for this question in some cases.

TABLE 3–11 _____
**Medical Insurance Requirement by
Health Care Guarantee
(supplementary to Medicare)**

Medical insurance required	Health care guarantee	
	Extensive	Limited
Yes	76.0%	44.2%
No	24.0	55.8

higher nursing care ratios because their resident populations have aged, while newer communities have healthier resident populations and lower nursing care ratios. These newer communities generate additional income by taking outside admissions into their new, largely unfilled, nursing care facilities.[7]

The data in Table 3–12 support this conclusion. Communities built before 1970 are less likely to admit outside residents, while all new

TABLE 3–12 _____
Outside Admissions by Community Age

Percent outside admissions to total census	Pre-1960	1960–1969	1970–1979	1980–post
0%	54.3%	59.5%	26.2%	54.5%
1–20%	28.6	32.4	58.5	0.0
21–40%	5.7	5.4	7.7	27.3
41–60%	5.7	2.7	1.5	9.1
61% and over	5.7	0.0	6.1	9.1

communities have outside admissions to their nursing facilities. A regional variation exists with respect to outside admissions: CCRCs in the Northeast are more likely, those in the West much less likely, to have them.

More surprising is the finding that the size of a community is not related to its policy or practice on taking outside admissions. This may imply that communities are building the correct number of nursing beds for their resident populations.

Residents' Role in Decision Making

Residents of continuing care retirement communities participate in decision-making processes in both formal and informal ways. Resident

_____

[7] This change over time often poses a problem to CCRC developers in obtaining a certificate of need for nursing care beds when one must show that the surrounding geographic area (usually the Health Services Area) can support the additional beds.

associations are active in 89.4 percent of CCRCs, and in almost 20 percent at least one resident serves as a member of the board of directors.

Most resident associations are fairly well organized and sophisticated, reflecting the generally higher levels of education and socioeconomic status among continuing care residents. A resident association usually has an executive committee or a representative council and many standing committees that meet more frequently to carry out much of the work of the association. With such broad-based participation, it is not unusual to find that over half of all the residents in a community are involved in the decision making at some level.

Resident associations are somewhat less prevalent among communities built prior to 1960. In the past two decades, there has been a trend toward and a demand for greater resident participation and accountability. This trend is evident among the younger residents of newer communities.

Residents' access to financial statements, in connection with their role as investors/consumers, is an issue within the continuing care field. Consequently, questions regarding this topic were included in the survey instrument. Residents have access to external financial statements in 82.6 percent of CCRCs; they have access to internal management statements in 45.9 percent of CCRCs. Residents in communities built before 1970 are less likely to have such access, perhaps because they lack a resident association or other formal organization to work with community managers.

CAPITAL FINANCING

Continuing care retirement communities have obtained construction financing in different ways and through various sources. Responses to a fixed-choice question regarding financing methods show that CCRCs primarily have used conventional mortgages, entry fees, charitable gifts and donations, FHA-insured mortgages, and tax-exempt revenue bonds.

What financing methods were used for construction:*

Conventional mortgage	54.1%
FHA-insured mortgage	14.5
Private taxable bonds	4.8
Tax-exempt revenue bonds	15.5
Public taxable bonds	1.9
Gifts and donations	30.4
Entry fees	33.8
Other	11.6

* These values double-count instances in which the stated method is used in combination with another method.

Obviously, as the economic climate and mortgage markets have changed over the years, the sources of construction financing have also changed. It is not surprising, therefore, to learn that communities built since 1980 have turned away from a heavy dependence on conventional mortgages and entry fees and toward tax-exempt revenue bonds.

Changes in federal laws have also affected construction financing methods. In 1959, Congress enacted the National Housing Act, which established the Section 231 program of FHA-insured mortgages for housing for the elderly. Thus, many communities built in the early 1960s have FHA-insured mortgages. In 1964, however, new regulations were written which excluded the use of Section 231 in conjunction with accommodation or entrance fees, and consequently none of the communities built after that year have FHA-insured mortgages. These communities turned to the conventional mortgage lenders in large numbers for construction monies.

Communities built prior to 1960 are much more likely to have used only entry fees to construct their facilities. Older CCRCs used conventional mortgage money in combination with other funds, primarily entry fees or gifts and donations. Many of the older CCRCs evolved from homes established during the late 19th century and the early 20th century by individuals leaving property and bequests to private foundations expressly for the purpose of caring for and housing indigent, aged people, usually women. These endowments were often used as seed money for the new facilities which became continuing care retirement communities in the 1960s.

The type of construction financing varies by geographic region. In part, this is related to the ages of communities, but some other interesting findings emerge as well. For example, CCRCs in the Western region are much more likely to have used FHA-insured mortgages or entry fees (alone) because many of these communities were built and opened in the early 1960s, when these sources were available and it was practical to use them. The Northeastern and North Central regions have similar patterns of growth through the 1960s and 1970s, but very few, if any, CCRCs in the Northeast obtained FHA-insured mortgages, preferring conventional mortgage money instead, whereas CCRCs in the North Central region used both conventional mortgages and FHA-insured mortgages in combination with other financing and shunned the use of conventional mortgages alone. The Southern region, the location of most communities built in the past two years or currently under construction, is associated with a high use of tax-exempt revenue bonds, both as a sole funding source and in combination with other sources. Tables 3–13 and 3–14 present the data illustrating these trends. (The values in these tables are the number of CCRCs using a specific financing method.)

TABLE 3–13 ——————————————————————————————
Construction Financing by Community Age

		Year contract first offered			
Financing method	Total	Pre-1960	1960–1969	1970–1979	1980–post
Conventional mortgage					
Alone	46	3	18	25	0
In combination	66	12	30	20	4
FHA-insured mortgage					
Alone	18	2	13	2	1
In combination	13	2	6	5	0
Tax-exempt revenue bonds					
Alone	10	1	6	4	5
In combination	20	2	7	8	3
Entry fees					
Alone	4	2	1	1	0
In combination	62	9	26	20	7

TABLE 3–14 ——————————————————————————————
Construction Financing by Regional Location

	Region			
Financing method	Northeast	North Central	South	West
Conventional mortgage				
Alone	12	12	13	9
In combination	9	34	11	16
FHA-insured mortgage				
Alone	0	5	4	10
In combination	1	7	2	4
Tax-exempt revenue bonds				
Alone	2	5	4	0
In combination	1	10	8	2
Entry fees				
Alone	0	2	1	2
In combination	9	28	15	13

Regionally and over time, the data show a steady use of entry fees in whole or in combination with other sources of construction financing. Generally, lenders require developing CCRCs to secure a certain percentage of entrance fee commitments so as to demonstrate the community's feasibility; typically, 30–50 percent of all units are required. Total reliance upon entry fees for construction funding, however, has decreased steadily in the past decade.

RESERVES

Data provided by CCRCs on the types of reserves they hold and preliminary analyses of these data by several factors—community age,
geographic location, type of health care guarantee, level of fees, and
source of initial capital—are presented in this section. Five types of
reserves are discussed: debt service, equipment replacement, health
care, financial aid, and contingency funds.

Debt Service Reserve

About half (49.3 percent, n = 207) of the CCRCs surveyed hold reserves for debt service, making this the most frequently held reserve.
Generally, these debt service reserves are required by loan covenants
and management policy; in some states, they are required by regulation
or statute.

Whether a community is likely to hold debt service reserves is related to the community's age and to its source of construction financing, as one might expect (see Table 3–15). It is not related to geographic region or health care guarantee.

TABLE 3–15
Debt Service Reserve by Community Age and Source of Capital

Debt service reserve	Community age				Primary source of capital		
	Pre-1960	1960–1969	1970–1979	1980–post	Conventional mortgage	FHA-insured mortgage	Tax-exempt revenue bond
Yes	32%	64%	73%	92%	64%	55%	97%
No	68	36	27	8	36	44	3

Equipment Replacement Reserve

With respect to the factors of community age, health care guarantee,
and capital financing, there is no significant difference between CCRCs
with building and equipment replacement reserves and those without
such reserves. A geographic variation exists, however, with CCRCs in
the Western region more likely, communities in the North Central
region less likely, to have a reserve for equipment replacement. Communities with fees in the middle range are more likely to have reserves
for equipment replacement than are communities with either high or
low fees. (See Table 3–16.)

TABLE 3–16 Equipment Replacement Reserve by Region				
Equipment reserve	NE	NC	S	W
Yes	54%	42%	62%	74%
No	46	58	38	26

Health Care Reserve

The need to establish health care reserves to fund the liability of future health care costs for current residents is a recent development in the continuing care field and remains an open question. Of the seven types of reserves included in the survey instrument, communities are least likely to have a health care reserve; 18.4 percent responded affirmatively (n = 38). Three quarters of these do so as a result of management or board policy; one tenth do so in accordance with state regulations. California, Colorado, Florida, Arizona, and Minnesota have some form of reserve requirement in their legislation or regulations regarding CCRCs.

One might assume that communities offering extensive health care guarantees would be more likely to establish health care reserves since they pay a larger share of residents' future medical costs and assume greater risk. It is surprising, therefore, to learn that not only is the relationship between these factors statistically insignificant but that the actual percentages show a tendency toward the opposite relationship (see Table 3–17).

TABLE 3–17 Health Care Reserve by Health Care Guarantee		
Health care reserve	Extensive	Limited
Yes	30%	25%
No	70	75

A geographic difference exists among CCRCs on this issue as well.[8] Among the communities (n = 38) with health care reserves, 39.5 percent are in the Western region, 28.9 percent in the North Central region, 18.4 percent in the South, and 13.2 percent in the Northeastern region.

---

[8] Related to California, requirements for reserves under which state-approved mortality tables must be used to calculate a CCRC's health care liability.

TABLE 3–18 ───────────────────────────────
Health Care Reserve by Community Age

Health care reserve	Pre-1960	1960–1970	1970–1980	1980–post
Yes	8%	28%	34%	12%
No	92	72	66	88

As Table 3–18 shows, communities opened between 1960 and 1980 are more likely to have health care reserves than are those built either before 1960 or, more important, since 1980 (though this group includes CCRCs under construction which have not yet had the opportunity to establish such a reserve). These figures indicate a trend toward health care reserves.

Financial Aid Reserve

Of the communities surveyed, 44 percent (n = 91) hold reserve funds for financial aid to residents who become unable to pay some or all of the fees charged, a practice almost wholly due to management and/or board policy.

Residents of communities offering limited health care guarantees are more exposed financially and, presumably, more likely to need assistance over the long term. However, these communities are not more likely than other CCRCs to hold reserves for financial aid to residents (see Table 3–19).

TABLE 3–19 ─────────────────────
Financial Aid Reserve by Health Care Guarantee

Financial aid reserve	Extensive	Limited
Yes	62%	58%
No	38	42

The factors of community age, type of capital financing, and geographic location are not related to financial aid reserves. CCRCs with higher health care ratios tend to have reserves for financial aid, as do CCRCs with fees at either the high or low ends of the scale. Those with fees in the middle range are less likely to have assistance reserves.

Contingency Reserve

Seventy-nine communities (or 38.2 percent of all the CCRCs studied) hold a reserve fund for contingencies as a matter of management or board policy. Some of these communities (7.6 percent) stated that state regulation was their reason for holding a reserve for contingencies. As might be expected, CCRCs with fees at the low end of the scale hold reserves for contingencies.

Summary of Reserves

The five states that have regulations regarding CCRC reserves, particularly California and Colorado, require reserves in specified amounts. These regulations could be construed to cover several of the areas discussed in this section. More detailed information must be collected and analyzed before conclusions can be drawn regarding the types and amounts of reserves that CCRCs hold. However, some research questions for future study are raised by these preliminary findings. For example, why are communities with contracts offering extensive health care guarantees not holding reserves, especially health care reserves, in larger numbers? Should more communities with limited health care guarantees establish financial aid reserves? What other funding mechanisms are in place to meet the financial needs of residents who outlive their assets?

SUMMARY PROFILE AND TRENDS

No prototype of a continuing care retirement community exists. The heterogeneity among communities, documented in this book, results from the efforts of continuing care providers to create alternative styles and combinations of housing and services for older people to choose from. However, a fairly consistent, recognizable, and commercially viable "product" has emerged from the convergence of the ideas and practices of many independent sources and from the numerous trials, errors, and successes of many dedicated individuals and organizations. The following discussion summarizes the characteristics unique to continuing care retirement communities.

Organization and Physical Plant

Almost all CCRCs are owned and operated by nonprofit organizations, and many are sponsored by or affiliated with a religious organization or body. The median age of all identified CCRCs is 14 years, where age means the number of years since the community first offered a continuing care contract to a resident. Most of the older communities are located in the Western (primarily California) and the North Central regions of the United States, while the Sun Belt, or Southern region, is the location of many communities recently opened or under construction.

Communities have an average of 165 independent living units (ILUs) and have two or three levels of care on-site in addition to the ILUs: personal care, intermediate nursing care, and/or skilled nursing care. There are two styles of communities: campus and high-rise.

Contracts and Fees

Two kinds of payments are made by residents of CCRCs: entry fees and monthly fees. Entry fees are set according to the type and size of living unit. Throughout the past 25 years, part or all of the entry fees have been used to finance construction of the physical plant. Increases in entry fees have kept pace with recent inflation; the average increase for the period June 30, 1980, to July 2, 1981, was 12 percent.

Most communities have no limits on the monthly fees they can charge, and these fees, too, have risen with inflation; for the same 1980–81 period, the average increase was 10.4 percent. Financial aid is available in most communities to assist residents who outlive their assets. Communities with lower monthly fees (presumably including those with limits on rate increases) are more likely to participate in the Medicaid program than are communities with higher monthly fees. Communities that offer a limited health care guarantee to residents (causing residents to assume more of the financial burden and risk) are also more likely to participate in the Medicaid program. Very few, if any, residents have been asked to leave a community because of depletion of funds.

Contracts are generally mutually terminable by either the resident or the community, and refunds on entry fees, usually prorated, are given upon death or voluntary withdrawal. No consensus exists among CCRCs, however, on refund schedules of payment.

Residents

Typically, 90–100 percent of the residents in any particular community hold continuing care contracts. Communities (primarily new ones) also admit individuals without contracts directly into the health care facility, and some offer continuing care contracts to individuals entering personal care units.

The median number of continuing care contractholders in a CCRC is 218; the median total resident population is 245. Communities serve the relatively healthy "old-old"; the average of residents in independent living units is 80.2 years, and that of residents of intermediate nursing care units is 85.4 years. Board-based resident associations are active in most CCRCs.

Services Included in Fees

Communities in the Northeastern and Western regions include larger packages of services than do CCRCs in other locations. Three types of services were analyzed: services having to do with the physical plant or daily living, supportive or preventive health care services, and medical or medical-related services. Communities are fairly consistent in offering physical plant services but differ in the latter two categories depending on the health care guarantee of the continuing care contract offered. Communities offering extensive health care guarantees, and therefore assuming more of the risk and cost of medical care, are more likely to include and provide supportive/preventive services as part of the basic fee.

Services included in the fees of a typical continuing care retirement community are: utilities, special diet, apartment cleaning, parking, kitchen appliances, replacement of apartment equipment, storage, emergency call system, and social services.

Services not included in the fees of most communities are: prescription drugs, therapy for psychiatric disorders, special duty nurses, dental care, podiatry, and hearing aids.

Reserves

With the exception of debt service reserves, which are usually required by lenders through loan covenants, reserves, if held at all, are generally held as a result of management and/or board policy.

Trends

Continuing care retirement communities are constantly evolving in response to new markets (i.e., younger, consumer-oriented, and more educated residents), new economic climates as reflected in increased capital costs and new financing mechanisms, changes in public program appropriations and regulations, the long-term experience of continuing care providers, and the application of new technology. Some of the key trends emerging from the survey data are:

A move toward larger resident populations and communities.

Growth within the industry; new communities are under construction, particularly in the Sun Belt areas, and more than a third of the existing communities plan additions to their physical plants in the next two years.

Tax-exempt revenue bonds have replaced conventional mortgages and other sources of construction financing as the primary source of capital for CCRCs, but this could change if Congress changes the law regarding industrial bonds or if mortgage market interest rates decline.

Continuing care contracts are becoming more carefully defined and mutually terminable. There is a trend toward extending the period for refunds upon death but making them contingent upon reoccupation of the unit, and there is a trend away from allowing a probationary period in the contract.

Admission policies are becoming more standardized and include a physical examination, minimum age requirements, and minimum assets and income.

A trend exists toward holding reserves in accordance with management policies, particularly debt service and health care reserves.

Several trends indicate support for the hypothesis that continuing care retirement communities reduce health care utilization. Communities with extensive health care guarantees have lower health care and nursing care ratios, while communities with limited health care guarantees have higher ratios. Among newer communities, there is a trend away from having a set policy regarding a resident's permanent move to the health care facility, enabling these communities to make such decisions on a case-by-case basis and thus to maintain each person at the most appropriate, cost-effective, and independent level of care. CCRCs with extensive health care guarantees (and lower health care ratios) do not hold reserves for health care in greater proportion than CCRCs with limited guarantees and higher health care ratios, perhaps signaling the success of the extensive guarantees in keeping the lid on health care utilization and costs.

Communities are moving away from including three meals a day in their fees and toward including one meal a day, an example of a general shift toward greater flexibility and choice for residents.

Newer communities are dropping some services and picking up others in greater number than older communities. Among the services not included by newer communities in their basic fees and contracts are: bed and bath linen, apartment cleaning, community's or resident's own physician, referred specialists, treatment for preexisting conditions, and special duty nurses. Services being included in basic fees by newer communities are typically those related to the physical plant, such as parking, kitchen appliances, storage, emergency call system, and replacing apartment equipment. ■

Part Two

Financial Analysis

Chapter Four

Financial Management of CCRCs

■ In terms of financial management, a CCRC is analogous to a pension plan in several respects. In both CCRCs and pension plans, revenues are received in advance of the cash payments required for meeting promised benefits. For a pension plan, funds are accumulated during a participant's working years in order to pay for benefits after retirement. Similarly, the payment of a CCRC entry fee plus recurring monthly fees is designed to advance-fund the cost of future health care for a CCRC resident.

There is a tontine element in the operation of both pension plans and CCRCs. For a pension plan, funds are set aside in respect of a participant for each year of service the participant renders to the plan sponsor; however, only those participants meeting certain eligibility requirements will receive benefits. A participant who works only a few years and then terminates employment may never receive benefits from the plan. The same phenomenon exists with respect to a CCRC in that all individuals contribute an entry fee plus monthly fees to fund the high costs of extended health care, even though only those who become ill benefit financially from such advance funding.

There are many ways to fund a pension plan, but one acceptable approach is to set employer contributions equal to a level percentage of payroll each year. In other words, the dollar costs of the plan will increase, but only by an amount equal to the increase in payroll, which typically equals the inflation exposure of the plan sponsor. Similarly, the monthly fees of a CCRC can, and should, be designed to increase by the inflation to which the community is exposed (not necessarily equal to published indices such as the CPI). In order to accomplish this, a new CCRC *must* charge fees that will advance-fund the increase in health care costs that will occur during the first 10 to 15 years of its operation. If fees are established on a strict real estate approach, the effects of inflation plus the increased cost of higher health care utilization will almost assuredly force fees to be increased by more than inflation alone in order to maintain financial soundness.

In estimating the contributions needed to meet the obligations of a pension plan, the plan's actuary must make assumptions about the plan's experience for many years into the future—in some cases 20 to 40 years or more. Since the experience of the plan will inevitably deviate from these assumptions, the actuary calculates the financial consequences of such deviations and adjusts contributions accordingly. The same problem exists with CCRCs. Each year the experience of the community should be checked against the assumptions used to set fees, with the deviations being factored into the following year's fee adjustments. This is particularly important when dealing with small pension plans and, of course, with CCRCs, whose resident population typically totals only a few hundred individuals.

One of the ways in which a CCRC differs from a pension plan, however, is in the physical plant, or real estate, aspect. A CCRC must anticipate, financially, the cost of refurbishing its facility (and eventually replacing or making major renovation in the facility) and replacing other fixed assets. These items must be factored into the pricing structure of a CCRC. If they are not advance-funded in a manner similar to the advance funding of future health care costs, then there is little hope that the community's fee increases can be held down to the rate of inflation.

The real estate aspect of CCRCs complicates the financial arrangement and leads some managements to price (and market to prospective residents) the CCRC concept on the basis that entry fees are designed to cover the cost associated with the real estate portion of the transaction, while monthly fees (from all residents) are set to cover operating costs. Although this pricing approach may in fact be adequate, it is an oversimplification of the true nature of a CCRC and its financial obligation to residents.

There is a well-defined scientific approach to funding a pension system, based on actuarial mathematics, and this approach can, and should, be applied to establishing fees for a CCRC. Whereas the real estate approach may, by chance, establish fees that will maintain the long-term financial solvency of a CCRC, the actuarial approach attempts to achieve this goal by design.

Actuarial science, which has been applied to pension plans for many decades and is now required by law to be applied to most private pension plans, has seldom been applied to CCRCs. The purpose of the next several chapters is to set forth the fundamentals of actuarial science as applied to CCRCs so that both the actuarial community and the CCRC industry have a common basis to begin working together to help ensure the long-term financial viability of individual communities and the industry in general.

CURRENT PRACTICE

It is a common belief within the CCRC industry that, although the goals and characteristics of a CCRC pricing structure are complex, the financial soundness of a given pricing policy can be adequately addressed by projecting the community's cash flow over a period of years. This belief hinges on the assumption that so long as fees generate revenues sufficient to service the community's debt and to cover operating expenses and so long as depreciation is funded, the community is financially sound. Communities employing this approach, particularly new communities, have not addressed some of the most important financial issues involved with CCRCs, such as assessing and funding the future health care obligation of current residents or defining reserve-level targets and setting fees that will generate liquid assets to meet such targets. In fact, cash flow analyses can promote a false sense of security inasmuch as they can mask serious long-term financial problems, whereas the actuarial methodology described in later chapters is designed to uncover such problems.

To illustrate the dangers of relying on cash flow analyses, four hypothetical cases have been constructed to represent different pricing policies that CCRCs might adopt. All four communities are assumed to be new, identical in size and construction costs, offer the same contracts (extensive health care guarantees), and have the same expense and health care utilization experience. The only difference among the communities is the initial (and subsequent) fees, and the first case is assumed to have a smaller debt ($12 million versus $15 million) since a larger portion of its entry fees were applied to construction costs.

The first-year fees for one-bedroom apartments for each case are given in Table 4–1. The fees for Case 1 were established so that ex-

TABLE 4–1 _____
Base Year One-Bedroom
Fees for a Single Entrant

Case	Monthly fee	Entry fee
1	$468	$39,097
2	684	46,916
3	684	52,129
4	720	52,129

pected cash receipts would match expected cash disbursements. This implies, of course, that monthly fees must increase faster than the community's inflation rate in order to keep pace with expenses that are additionally affected by the increased health care utilization during the community's maturation.

The fees for Cases 2 through 4 were based on the policy that a significant portion of the initial entry fees for the first generation of residents would be held in reserve (the amount of the first-year reserve is the same in all cases). The fees for Case 2 were based on what appeared to be a favorable five-year cash flow projection. The Case 3 fees were based on the goal of maintaining a positive cash flow over 20 years. The Case 3 monthly fees are the same as the monthly fees for Case 2; however, the Case 3 entry fees are approximately 11 percent higher. The fees for Case 4 are actuarially based, with the monthly fees approximately 5 percent higher than those for Cases 2 and 3 and the entry fees approximately 11 percent higher than those for Case 2 (i.e., the same as those for Case 3). In all three cases, both monthly fees and entry fees are assumed to increase for inflation.[1]

The expected end-of-year cash balance for each pricing policy is presented in Figure 4–1.[2] Case 1 has a relatively small cash balance

FIGURE 4–1
Expected End-of-Year Cash Balances under Four Pricing Policies

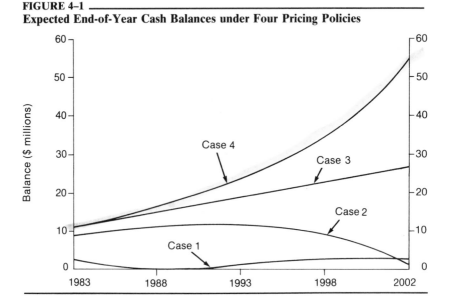

---

[1] This rate varies, depending on the expenses that monthly fees and entry fees are designated to cover. The long-term inflation rate is assumed to be 10 percent for illustrative purposes.

[2] The methodology for developing revenues, expenses, apartment turnover, and health care utilization is discussed in subsequent chapters.

throughout the forecast. At the end of the first five years, Cases 2 through 4 hold $11 million to $16 million in cash. However, extending the projection for another 15 years shows that the pricing policy underlying Case 2 is seriously inadequate. Its cash balance increases for the next four years and then decreases to under $1 million by the end of 20 years (in today's dollars, adjusting for inflation, the cash balance declines continuously from $9,069,000 to $136,009). Although management may not continue the same underpricing policy in light of declining cash balances, this example illustrates the potential problems of using short-term cash flow analyses.[3]

Even if a long-term cash flow projection is made, management may still not have enough information to select among competing pricing policies. For example, consider the expected cash flows associated with Cases 3 and 4. Although both cases generate large cash balances by the end of 20 years, a cash flow analysis itself does not provide a justification for the $54 million ($8 million in today's dollars) accumulated under the so-called actuarial policy. Nor does it provide a justification for the accumulation of $27 million ($4 million in today's dollars) associated with Case 3. Such justifications, however, can be provided by additional actuarial analyses described in later chapters.

Another deficiency of using projected cash flows alone for management decision making is that a long-term projection might show positive *expected* cash balances, while the probability of a negative cash balance due to random deviations from the underlying assumptions might be extremely high. Table 4–2 shows the implications of random deviations in two key assumptions used to project future cash flows: apartment turnover and health care utilization. The pricing policy selected by management should minimize the probability of having to borrow money to cover negative cash balances. Case 1 shows a high probability of a negative cash balance, ranging from 15 percent to 45 percent after the third year. Case 2 also shows a positive probability of a negative cash balance after 16 years. The probability of a negative cash balance due to random deviations is zero for Cases 3 and 4. This table illustrates a flaw in the use of cash flow analysis based on expected values, since management does not have information on the risks associated with random deviations.

Even if a cash flow analysis involves a long-term projection (20 years or more) and generates information on the risks associated with random deviations, it is still not a sufficient tool to help management select among various pricing policies. In order to select a prudent pricing policy for a CCRC, management must not only look at cash flows, and at the potential variability in cash flows, but must also

---

[3] Although the values projected 20 years from now are different from the ones that will actually occur, long-term projections serve the purpose of providing the community with ample time to make modest fee adjustments currently in order to avoid undesirable trends instead of having to make more severe adjustments at as later point.

TABLE 4-2 _____
**Probability of Short-Term Cash Deficits
Due to Random Deviations under Four
Pricing Policies**

Fiscal year	Pricing policy			
	Case 1	Case 2	Case 3	Case 4
1983	0%	0%	0%	0%
1984	0	0	0	0
1985	0	0	0	0
1986	15	0	0	0
1987	45	0	0	0
1988	40	0	0	0
1989	30	0	0	0
1990	25	0	0	0
1991	20	0	0	0
1992	20	0	0	0
1993	15	0	0	0
1994	15	0	0	0
1995	20	0	0	0
1996	30	0	0	0
1997	30	0	0	0
1998	30	0	0	0
1999	30	15	0	0
2000	30	20	0	0
2001	35	30	0	0
2002	45	40	0	0

identify the size of the deferred obligations to continuing care contract-holders and establish a pricing policy to fund those obligations (or some financially acceptable portion thereof).

Unfortunately, the existing literature on CCRCs does not contain a set of financial guidelines, or a pricing and financial evaluation methodology, that allows management to address these pertinent issues. Such a methodology will be developed in subsequent chapters.

OBJECTIVES OF PRICING METHODOLOGY

As noted in the empirical analysis presented in Chapters 2 and 3, there is considerable variability among CCRCs. Communities do not fit one mold but retain their individual identity by offering variations that embody their own philosophy on serving the elderly. Just as each community's management has its own ideas about the services it should provide to residents and about the structuring of the physical plant, community managements also vary in their ideas for setting fees. At one extreme, management could set actuarially adequate fees, following a pure actuarial approach in which fees vary according to the resident's entry age, sex, apartment type, health status at entry, and so forth. At the other extreme, all residents could be charged the same fees.

Typically, the fees for CCRCs fall between these extremes. For example, fees tend to vary by the apartment type and by the number of apartment occupants. Some communities allow residents who have permanently transferred to the health care center to pay the same fees they did before permanent transfer. Other communities require that all health care residents pay a uniform fee. All of these variations in pricing structures are based on management's objectives. Therefore, one goal of the pricing methodology should be that the methodology not dictate such objectives but rather inform management whether or not its pricing structure as a whole, or in aggregate, is financially sound, leaving to management discretion decisions regarding equity among current residents and among successive generations of residents.

In the preceding section, the cash balances associated with the two acceptable pricing policies (Cases 3 and 4) might seem extremely large for a nonprofit operation. This could make it difficult to extract fee increases from residents, who might feel that such balances are unnecessary and inappropriate "profits." Therefore, a second objective of pricing methodology is that it provide a basis for justifying both to management and to residents the size of a community's assets and continued fee increases. This objective is closely related to the types of financial statements (both internal and external) that are developed by the community. Most communities prepare such statements according to generally accepted accounting principles (GAAP). As discussed more fully in later chapters, statements prepared in this way must be modified to present a financial picture consistent with the community's actuarial position, and the pricing methodology should provide guidance for such modifications.

Finally, any organization that offers a continuing care contract is committing itself to a long-term venture. Even though the typical resident is expected, on average, to survive 12 to 14 years in the community, a certain percentage will survive 20 years or more. This means that the methodology used to set fees must determine whether the fees set will support current residents over their potential (not just expected) lifetimes in the community. Moreover, the methodology should require that management establish policies to help ensure the continued operation of the community, such as setting aside funds to replace equipment and furnishings and to eventually replace the facility. Since new entrants are an important component of the success of the ongoing community, management will also need to set aside reserves for future refurbishment and/or modernization to maintain the facility's attractiveness to prospective residents.

ALTERNATIVE PRICING METHODOLOGIES

Three generic pricing methodologies used by actuaries in connection with pension plans are: (1) pay-as-you-go, (2) open-group, and (3) closed-group. These three methodologies, in fact, were used in the cash flow projections for Cases 1, 3, and 4, respectively. The pay-as-you-go method looks at one year at a time, setting current fees at a level sufficient to cover current expenses. The open-group method examines a fixed period of years, such as 20 years, and determines current and projected fees such that their present value equals the present value of current and projected expenses for *all* residents (current plus new entrants) during the period. Under this approach, current fees will generally be higher than current expenses in anticipation of increased health care utilization and future fixed-asset expenditures. The closed-group method is based on the goal of setting fees for a cohort group of residents (typically each group of new entrants) to cover their anticipated expenses over their remaining lifetimes in the community. This method differs from the open-group method since it examines each cohort separately and requires that fees be self-supporting without the benefit of new entrants' fees.

A comparison of the three pricing methodologies is given in Table 4–3, based on five characteristics: (1) relative fee levels, (2) simplicity of determining annual fees, (3) ability to maintain inflation-constrained increases in monthly fees, (4) ability to achieve group equity, and (5) size of contract termination reserves. The comparisons are presented for both a new (or maturing) community and a mature community.

Fee Levels

Since most communities are nonprofit, a common goal is to offer the maximum service at the lowest possible cost to residents. A constraint on this policy is that communities do not wish to set fees so low that their financial stability is jeopardized.

For a new community, the pay-as-you-go method requires the lowest fees, while the closed-group method generates the highest. However, if a community adheres to these policies to maturity, the pay-as-you-go method will have the highest fees, while the closed-group method will have the lowest. The reason for this difference is that under the closed-group method, the initial fees will be higher than the initial expenses, generating reserves that produce interest income in later years. The interest income, in turn, covers a portion of the expenses and thus allows fees to be lower than the fees required by the pay-as-you-go method. This phenomenon also occurs with the open-group method, but generally to a lesser extent than with the closed-group method.

TABLE 4-3
Comparison of Alternative Pricing Methodologies

Community age	Pricing method	Characteristics				
		Fee levels	Simplicity of fees	Maintenance of inflation-constrained monthly fees	Group equity	Contract termination reserve
Maturing	Pay-as-you-go	Lowest	Easy	Difficult	Difficult	None
	Open-group	Intermediate	Complex	Possible	Possible	Partial to full funding
	Closed-group	Highest	Complex	By definition	By definition	Full funding
Mature	Pay-as-you-go	Highest	Easy	Difficult	Difficult	None
	Open-group	Intermediate	Complex	Possible	Possible	Partial to full funding
	Closed-group	Lowest	Complex	By definition	By definition	Full funding

Simplicity of Preparing Financial Projections

The second characteristic in Table 4–3 refers to the difficulty of developing projections to determine annual changes in fees. Pay-as-you-go is the easiest method to employ, since it requires that revenues equal expenses for only a one-year projection. Both the closed-group and the open-group approach are more complex, as explained in later chapters.

Maintenance of Inflation-Constrained Monthly Fees

Limiting increases in monthly fees to the internal inflation rate of the community is a desirable goal for a CCRC. The closed-group method, by definition, establishes fees to meet this objective. It is also possible to achieve this goal with open-group pricing. Fee increases under the pay-as-you-go method depend on the rate of increase in expenses, which typically increase by more than inflation because of increased health care costs.

Group Equity

Group equity, another desirable goal for CCRCs, implies that the fees for a cohort group of residents (typically a new entrant cohort) are set such that they cover all future expenses allocated to that group. Thus, the fees for each cohort are self-supporting and require no intergenerational transfer of funds. The only method that accomplishes this goal by definition is the closed-group approach. This objective is virtually impossible to achieve using pay-as-you-go and is difficult to achieve under the open-group approach, since these methods do not set fees to be adequate for a cohort group; instead, they rely on new entrants to maintain the community's financial soundness.

Contract Termination Reserves

Many communities state that it is their policy to offer continuing care contracts for the foreseeable future. However, recent experience shows that this has not been possible for some communities, even though they may have wished to continue doing so. Some of the discontinuations have been caused by fluctuations in the marketplace, and others have been caused by failure to set fees properly during the earlier years after start-up.

The contract termination reserves refer to the ability of the community to cover its future liabilities for continuing care contractholders in the event that the community decides to no longer offer such contracts.[4] Fees under the closed-group method will generate sufficient

---

[4] Alternatively, it can be viewed as the strength of the pricing methodology to withstand financial variations that might otherwise cause the community to change the contractual guarantee offered to prospective residents.

reserves to liquidate (close out) the liabilities associated with current residents while maintaining inflation-constrained monthly fees. The open-group method partially funds such reserves, and in some cases may result in full funding. The pay-as-you-go approach does no funding in this regard. Thus, if continuing care contracts were no longer offered to new entrants, management would have to increase the surviving continuing care contractholders' fees by more than inflation and/or subsidize a portion of the liability from other sources.

Summary

The pay-as-you-go method is an extremely risky approach for a new community, especially in an inflationary environment. Existing communities that have already reached a mature state may find this approach to be satisfactory; however, it does not provide the financial security that the authors believe is appropriate for CCRC residents.

The open-group method can provide a satisfactory approach to pricing a CCRC, but there may be a temptation to select a planning horizon and assumptions that postpone too large a portion of current expenses to future periods.

The closed-group method does not suffer from the above problems, but it may generate fees for some existing CCRCs that are simply too large to implement, in which case the open-group method would have to be employed. Because of the strengths of the closed-group method, the remaining chapters will describe this approach. However, many of the principles set forth apply to the open-group method as well. ■

Chapter Five
Actuarial Assumptions Required for Financial Projections

■ The actuarial assumptions required to evaluate the long-term financial status of CCRCs are discussed in this chapter. They may be separated into three categories: (1) decrement assumptions, (2) new entrant assumptions, and (3) economic assumptions. Decrement assumptions are used to estimate the survival of CCRC residents, as well as their future living status, over time. These assumptions include mortality rates, morbidity rates (i.e., rates of health care utilization), transfer rates between different apartment units, and withdrawal rates. New entrant assumptions are used to estimate the characteristics of future entrants to the community. They include the distribution of entry ages, the probability that specific units will become occupied by a single resident versus two or more residents, and the sex of single and paired residents. Economic assumptions are used to estimate the community's future expenses and revenues, including the interest earnings on any invested funds.

DECREMENT ASSUMPTIONS

Mortality Rates

Mortality rates specify the probabilities of death for residents of CCRCs. Although they can be used to calculate life expectancies, which are useful for comparing mortality rate tables, such statistics are not particularly useful for performing financial analyses. Financial projections require assumptions about the probability of residents living to future years, not simply the average length of time a group of residents will live in a CCRC.

Mortality rates must have various characteristics. First, they must be based on age and sex, since younger residents have lower mortality rates than older residents and females have lower rates than males. Second, they must be established for different living statuses, since apartment complex residents have lower mortality than health care center residents. Third, a select period is often appropriate. A select period refers to a table of rates in which the rates for a new entrant to the community are *less* than those for a long-term resident of the community at the same age. Finally, a mortality improvement factor should be included to reflect decreases in future mortality rates (i.e., a generation mortality table). This refinement is consistent with the current trends in mortality rates at all ages.

Morbidity Rates

Taken alone, mortality rates do not provide sufficient information for estimating future CCRC costs. To properly estimate these costs, it is necessary to project future health care utilization so that the higher costs of health care can be reflected in the financial analysis. Health care utilization assumptions are referred to as morbidity rates. There are two types of morbidity rates for CCRCs. One type defines the probabilities of *permanent* transfer between different levels of care. The other defines the average number of *temporary*[1] transfer days spent in the health care center annually.

Permanent transfer rates tend to vary significantly among CCRCs. One factor contributing to this variability is that management policies have an influence on these rates. Communities that actively strive to keep residents in their apartments will have lower permanent transfer rates relative to those of communities that move disabled residents into the health care center fairly quickly. This factor again points to the drawbacks in using life expectancies for financial analysis. Two communities could have identical life expectancies but different management policies, resulting in different permanent transfer rates and different health care expense projections.

Morbidity rates for *temporary* transfers, which specify the expected number of days for all short-term transfers to the health care center during the year, are also required in developing financial analyses because many continuing care contracts allow residents to use the health care center on a temporary basis with no additional charges even though they tie up two units (both their apartment unit and a health

---

[1] A temporary transfer is one in connection with which the resident is expected to return to his or her apartment after a stay in the health care center.

care unit).[2] Hence, temporary utilization can have important cost consequences.

Apartment Transfer Rates

Apartment transfer rates specify the probabilities of transfer from one apartment unit to another (typically transfer to a smaller apartment after a spouse's death or permanent transfer to the health care center). These rates are also influenced by management policy. Based on discussions with several CCRC managers, it would seem that transfer rates tend to be low despite management policies and/or financial incentives for single residents to move to smaller apartments after the death or permanent transfer of a spouse. The reason given is that such moves are generally considered too traumatic for the survivor. Nevertheless, if transfers of this kind do take place for a given community, then any financial analysis must take this factor into account.

Withdrawal Rates

Withdrawal rates specify the probability that a resident will voluntarily leave the community. The financial consequences of withdrawal depend on the contractual provisions of the community. The financial impact of withdrawal is of little consequence for many CCRCs that provide refunds for less than five years. However, if the refund provision is extensive and/or a high incidence of withdrawal is expected, then this factor must also be considered.

METHODOLOGY FOR DEVELOPING DECREMENT ASSUMPTIONS

Decrement assumptions for an existing CCRC can be derived from an "experience study" of the community's historical records. The primary consideration in developing any actuarial assumption is the size of the data base from which historical experience is examined. The data bases for CCRCs are relatively small, by actuarial standards, since most communities are relatively new and small (the median age and size for CCRCs are 14 years and 245 residents, respectively). The small size of CCRCs means that no one community will have sufficient data to develop mortality and morbidity rates from its experience alone.[3]

---

[2] The results of the empirical analysis indicates that 54 percent of the CCRCs did not charge residents additional fees (except for meals) for temporary utilization of the health care center.

[3] Most actuarial studies are based on thousands of lives. The "small group" problem associated with CCRCs also means that the methodology used to make population projections based on these assumptions should compensate for the possible misstatement of assumptions and the variability about the assumptions due to random deviations.

There are two ways of dealing with this data base problem: (1) combining the experience of several communities and applying actuarial techniques of mortality table construction to develop probabilities of decrement or (2) modifying a schedule of rates taken from a "base table" derived from a group of individuals likely to have characteristics similar to those of CCRC residents. The second approach is referred to as standardized mortality ratio method. Under either approach, a community should be monitored periodically in order to adjust the assumptions in light of its experience.[4]

The first approach has been used to develop mortality rates and life expectancies which serve as the basis for one state's (California) reserve calculation; however, this approach has limited application for CCRCs since admission policies vary greatly among them. Combining data from several communities assumes that the residents form a homogeneous group, which may be unlikely for different management groups and philosophies. It may be practical to combine communities under the same management that have similar admission standards, but for most CCRC experience studies, it is better that the community use its own data under the standardized mortality ratio approach.

The standardized mortality ratio approach, which is recommended for developing mortality rates for both apartment and health care residents and for developing permanent transfer morbidity rates, involves four steps. The first step is to select a set of rates appropriate for use as a base table. With regard to mortality rates, an insurance company annuitant mortality table is recommended as the base table. Rates in such a table are appropriate because both annuitants and continuing care contractholders are willing to make substantial up-front financial commitments to protect themselves from outliving their resources, and the members of both groups would be unlikely to purchase these contracts if they did not feel they were in good health. The two annuity tables used in such studies are the 1971 Individual Annuitant Mortality table (1971 IAM) and Table 1983a. Both tables are currently used as standards for determining reserves for individual annuity policies.

The base table to be used for permanent transfer morbidity rates is more problematic. Permanent transfer rates represent a type of disability status for continuing care residents. Insurance company disability tables are typically derived for the working population, and therefore standard tables do not exist for the elderly population (over age 65). Hence, the authors again recommend that the annuitant mortality tables be used as the base table. Although the overall level of rates will be adjusted substantially by the experience morbidity study, the mortality

---

[4] For a detailed explanation of mortality table construction, refer to Robert W. Batten, *Mortality Table Construction* (Englewood Cliffs, N.J.: Prentice-Hall, 1978). A discussion of the standardized mortality ratio method is contained in R. C. Elandt-Johnson and N. C. Johnson, *Survival Modes and Data Analysis* (New York: John Wiley and Sons, 1980), pages 22–24.

table should have approximately the same shape as the true morbidity table.

The second step is to select the length of the observation period over which data are to be collected. The longer this period is, the more data there are. However, a long observation period may have the drawback of including prior trends that may not be consistent with the more recent experience of the community.[5] The observation period should be at least five years to generate a reasonable amount of data. On the other hand, the observation period probably should not include more than 10 years in order to reflect the most recent trends in experience.

The third step in the standardized mortality ratio methodology is to determine the life years of exposure for all persons who are (or were) members of the community. The term *life year of exposure* means one resident living in the community for one year. In addition, each life year of exposure should be categorized according to the resident's age, sex, and length of residency in the community so that rates can be developed along these dimensions.

The fourth step is to multiply the exposure data by the rates of decrement suggested by the base table. This generates the *expected* decrements, which are then compared with the *actual* decrements, resulting in an actual-to-expected ratio. This ratio indicates the required modification to the base table rates that is needed to reflect the community's historical experience.

The standardized mortality ratio methodology generally cannot be applied to developing morbidity rates for temporary transfers, apartment transfer rates, and withdrawal rates, since these rates tend to be unstable. Rates for each of these decrements must be derived directly from the community's data by dividing the actual decrements by the life years of exposure. Temporary transfer rates are generally stated as the expected number of days per 100 residents, a value that combines the frequency of temporary transfers with the length of stay (severity). Apartment transfer and withdrawal rates are generally expressed in terms of a single rate for all residents, ignoring age or sex differences.

RESULTS OF MORTALITY AND MORBIDITY EXPERIENCE STUDIES

Seven communities contributed data for the mortality and morbidity experience studies presented in this section. The rate schedules developed from these data are used at a later point in this book to study

---

[5] Over the past 20 years, the life expectancies for age-75 females in the general population have increased on average 11 percent per decade. *Life Tables*, vol 2, sec. 5, *Vital Statistics of the United States, 1978*, DHHS Publication no. (PHS) 81–1104.

various financial aspects of each community. The experience studies revealed several interesting characteristics regarding actuarial data for CCRCs. These characteristics were the accessibility and completeness of historical records, the longevity of CCRC residents, and hospital utilization by continuing care residents. The findings on each characteristic are explained with the following discussion of the data analysis.

Data Base Description

Table 5–1 presents four summary statistics from the seven case studies: earliest date of data, life years of exposure, number of deaths, and number of permanent transfers to the health care center.[6] The size of the total data base is small compared to the volume that is normally used for actuarial experience studies. The total life years of exposure are slightly more than 25,000.[7] Nevertheless, it is possible to use an existing table of rates, appropriately modified as described in the preceding section, to develop mortality and morbidity rates from the data of this volume.

The observation period, which is determined from the earliest date of data through 1981, does not necessarily coincide with the opening of the community. In a few cases, it was difficult, if not impossible, for the community to reconstruct historical data because records either were not kept at that time or were no longer available. Record keeping is an area in which the entire CCRC industry could benefit from standardization.

Life Expectancies

Even though life expectancies have limited usefulness for financial projections, these statistics are useful for comparing the mortality tables developed from each community studied. Moreover, life expectancy statistics offer information on whether CCRC residents live longer than their counterparts in the general population. The first step in developing life expectancies was to calculate actual-to-expected mortality ratios. These ratios were calculated for each age and sex, with no distinction being made for the resident's living status (aggre-

---

[6] The health care center for Cases 3, 6, 7, and 8 includes both personal care and nursing care. The health care center for the other cases consists of nursing care only. Also, the numbering convention, which excludes 4, is used as a linkage to later analyses, which include a community numbered as "4" but exclude communities 7 and 8.

[7] This data base is relatively large for CCRC standards. The largest publicly available actuarial data base is the one used to develop the California Life Care Tables, and we estimate from data contained in the report that it was developed on slightly more than 45,000 life years of exposure. *Life Table Estimation and Financial Evaluation of California Life Care Homes,* Contract no. 77–60991.

TABLE 5-1
Size and Observation Period of Actuarial Data Base for Case Study CCRCs

Characteristics	Sex	Case 1	Case 2	Case 3	Case 5	Case 6	Case 7	Case 8	Combined cases
Date of earliest data	Combined	1974	1978	1975	1978	1971	1962	1962	
Life years of exposure	Female	2,435	1,361	2,157	696	2,786	3,985	6,632	20,052
	Male	422	238	678	259	1,131	941	1,385	5,054
	Combined	2,857	1,599	2,835	955	3,917	4,926	8,017	25,106
Deaths	Female	129	78	106	30	142	299	369	1,153
	Male	38	26	85	16	120	83	116	484
	Combined	167	104	191	46	262	382	485	1,637
Permanent transfers	Female	99	67	196	13	84	46	242	747
	Male	18	6	76	5	51	11	39	206
	Combined	117	73	272	18	135	57	281	953

gate rates). The base table for this comparison was a new mortality table used to calculate life insurance company reserves for individual annuities, referred to as Table 1983a. The actual-to-expected ratios are not shown; however, such ratios were used to generate the life expectancies presented in Table 5–2 along with the life expectancies for the general population (1978 U.S. Life Tables) and Table 1983a.

Table 5–2 shows that life expectancy for an age-75 female entrant is 14 years or more for five of the seven cases. Life expectancies for entrants to CCRCs are 3 to 26 percent longer than life expectancies for the general population. However, life expectancies for CCRC entrants are slightly less than life expectancies for their counterparts who purchase individual annuities (based on the 1983a Mortality Table). Male life expectancies tend to vary more than those of females, but this may be due in part to the smaller volume of male data. Life expectancies for age-75 male entrants range from 9.1 years to 11.7 years, values which are 6 to 36 percent greater than life expectancies for the general population.

The bottom section of Table 5–2 contains last survivor life expectancies for a female/male couple who are assumed to be the same age. The term *last survivor life expectancy* refers to the number of years that *at least one* member of the couple is expected to survive in the community. At entry age 75, the last survivor life expectancies for CCRC entrants are 14 to 25 percent higher than the corresponding single female life expectancies, and the differential increases with age. This observation supports the notion that there should be higher fees for a second person entering a CCRC unit.

Based solely on a review of life expectancies, CCRC entrants seem to live longer than the general population. This study does not address the question of whether this is due to a selection process (i.e., healthier persons moving into a CCRC) or is an effect that the retirement community environment has on residents. However, that question is an important area for further research.

Mortality Rates

Aggregate life expectancies are useful for comparing longevity among communities, but they are not sufficient for actuarial analyses. For financial analyses, it is necessary to define separate mortality rates according to the living status of the resident and to develop morbidity rates as well. Tables 5–3 and 5–4 show the results of such a mortality analysis. Table 5–3 contains "crude" death rates for apartment and health care residents, that is, rates derived by dividing the total number of deaths by the total number of life years of exposure. These represent a simple measure for comparing death rates among communities. For example, the combined (female and male) crude rates for apartment

TABLE 5–2
Life Expectancies for Entrants to Case Study CCRCs

Gender	Age	1978 U.S. Life Table	Table 1983a	Case 1	Case 2	Case 3	Case 5	Case 6	Case 7	Case 8
Female	65	18.4	23.7	22.6	22.7	19.8	21.9	22.7	22.8	23.1
	70	14.8	19.3	18.3	18.4	15.7	17.5	18.3	18.4	18.7
	75	11.5	15.0	14.0	14.1	11.8	13.4	14.0	14.2	14.5
	80	8.8	11.3	10.5	10.6	8.5	10.0	10.4	10.6	10.9
	85	6.7	8.2	7.5	7.6	5.9	7.0	7.5	7.6	7.8
Male	65	14.0	20.2	18.6	15.8	16.1	19.1	16.8	19.3	18.8
	70	11.1	16.1	14.7	12.2	12.5	15.2	13.1	15.3	14.9
	75	8.6	12.5	11.3	9.1	9.4	11.7	9.9	11.8	11.4
	80	6.7	9.5	8.4	6.6	6.8	8.8	7.3	8.9	8.6
	85	5.3	7.1	6.2	4.7	4.9	6.5	5.3	6.6	6.3
Last survivor*	65	—	27.9	26.4	25.3	23.2	26.1	25.6	26.8	26.8
	70	—	23.1	21.6	20.6	18.7	21.4	20.9	22.0	22.0
	75	—	18.3	17.0	16.1	14.3	16.8	16.3	17.4	17.4
	80	—	14.3	13.1	12.2	10.7	12.9	12.4	13.4	13.4
	85	—	10.7	9.7	8.9	7.6	9.5	9.1	10.0	10.0

* Both entrants (a female and a male) are assumed to be the same age.

TABLE 5–3
Crude Mortality Rates

Living status	Sex	Case 1	Case 2	Case 3	Case 5	Case 6	Case 7	Case 8
Apartment	Female	3.1%	3.4%	3.3%	3.6%	3.1%	5.1%	3.6%
	Male	6.1	11.3	3.0	5.5	7.3	8.1	6.6
	Combined	3.6	4.6	3.2	4.1	4.3	5.7	4.2
Health care	Female	26.8	25.3	26.2	27.3	29.3	27.8	17.0
	Male	46.7	6.2	41.6	50.0	51.8	30.0	26.2
	Combined	29.1	23.4	29.6	30.8	25.8	28.3	18.2

residents indicate that 3 to 6 of every 100 continuing care contract holders will die annually. The combined health care rates are 4 to 9 times higher, ranging from 18 to 36 deaths per 100 residents. In virtually every case, the crude rates for females are lower than those for males. The exceptions are probably due to the small size of the data base.

Crude rates are useful for rough comparisons, but they are not sufficient for developing mortality assumptions since they do not take age and sex differences among residents into account. A more sophisticated measure adjusts for the age and sex of residents. The results of this measure, based on Table 1983a, are presented in Table 5–4. By

TABLE 5–4
Age/Sex-Adjusted Actual-to-Expected Mortality Ratios
(based on Table 1983a)

Living status	Sex	Case 1	Case 2	Case 3	Case 5	Case 6	Case 7	Case 8
Apartment	Female	70.4%	73.0%	61.7%	104.0%	72.3%	101.3%	81.1%
	Male	85.7	173.8	42.4	100.2	102.5	102.3	96.7
	Combined	73.8	93.6	55.8	102.6	84.3	101.6	85.0
Health care	Female	368.9	270.3	350.6	487.4	433.2	258.9	179.6
	Male	349.1	69.7	428.3	682.1	533.0	301.1	247.8
	Combined	365.0	251.2	371.5	524.8	470.1	267.1	188.1

way of example, female apartment residents in Case 1 show an actual-to-expected ratio of 70.4 percent of the Table 1983a rates. If the death rate from that table for an age-75 female is 2.01 per 100, then the derived rate is 1.41 per 100 (2.01 × 0.704). This table shows that apartment resident mortality rates for most cases (five of seven) are less than that suggested by Table 1983a. Health care residents experience significantly higher mortality, ranging from 2 to 5 times that suggested by the annuity table.

Morbidity Rates

Also required for actuarial analyses are morbidity rates, or rates of health care utilization, which are needed to make the tie between apartment and health care mortality rates. Morbidity rates are categorized as permanent transfers, where the resident releases his or her apartment, and temporary transfers, where the resident retains the apartment unit.

Crude morbidity rates and age/sex-adjusted actual-to-expected ratios for permanent transfers are presented in Table 5–5. This table

TABLE 5–5
Crude Morbidity Rates* and Age/Sex-Adjusted Actual-to-Expected Morbidity Ratios *(based on Table 1983a)*

Ratio	Sex	Case 1	Case 2	Case 3	Case 5	Case 6	Case 7	Case 8
Crude	Female	4.4%	5.5%	11.8%	1.9%	3.3%	1.2%	4.2%
morbidity	Male	4.6	2.9	13.7	2.0	4.9	1.3	3.1
ratios	Combined	4.5	5.1	12.3	1.9	3.7	1.2	4.0
Actual-to-	Female	76.9	117.4	215.0	56.8	75.3	25.2	93.8
expected	Male	54.4	45.1	187.1	36.6	69.3	13.0	45.6
ratios	Combined	72.3	103.7	206.4	49.2	72.9	22.0	81.8

* Rate of permanent transfer to the health care center (either personal care or nursing care).

shows that female crude permanent transfer rates are approximately equal to those of males for five cases. This observation appears to be corroborated by the comparison of age/sex-adjusted ratios. Even though female ratios are consistently higher than male ratios, the permanent transfer rates derived from these ratios will be approximately equal since the underlying base rate for males is higher. However, female health care utilization is greater since they live longer after permanent transfer. It should be noted that this analysis shows considerably more variation than did the analysis of mortality rates, suggesting that it is not appropriate to combine the data from all communities to develop a single table because doing this would remove such variations.

Table 5–6 contains the results for temporary transfers. It shows the expected number of hospital days per year per 100 residents, the expected number of health care (both personal and nursing care) days per year per 100 residents, the probability of temporary transfer to the health care center, and the distribution of length of stay given that the resident temporarily transfers.

An interesting finding regarding temporary transfers is the expected length of stay in an acute-care hospital. There is a belief among some CCRC administrators that their residents, whose average age is approximately 80, utilize hospital services on a less frequent basis than do their counterparts in the general population. The first row of Table

TABLE 5–6
Hospital and Temporary Health Care Utilization by Residents of Case Study CCRCs

Statistic	Sex	Case 1	Case 2	Case 3	Case 5	Case 6	Case 7	Case 8
Expected number of hospital days per year per 100 residents	Combined	373 days	—	151 days	67 days	100 days	—	250 days
Expected number of health care days per year per 100 residents	Female	1,074	1,251	280	656	1,222	810	1,164
	Male	673	1,595	170	583	825	870	1,166
	Combined	1,014	1,302	230	638	1,114	821	1,164
Probability of temporary transfer	Combined	35%	37%	18%	12%	13%	22%	34%
Distribution of length of temporary stay	Combined							
1–14 days		59%	42%	71%	20%	43%	48%	65%
15–29 days		21	22	14	30	16	16	14
30–59 days		14	22	9	20	14	16	10
60–179 days		4	14	5	27	14	17	9
180 days and over		2	0	1	3	13	3	2
		100%	100%	100%	100%	100%	100%	100%

5–6 shows that the expected number of hospital days per 100 residents[8] ranges from 67 to 373 days. The upper value of this range is slightly less than the national average of 380 days for Medicare patients over age 65.[9] However, the data from which these statistics are derived are fairly thin. This is an area worthy of additional investigation with the goal of determining whether potential cost savings may be associated with the care provided in CCRCs.

Table 5–6 shows a large range in the expected number of temporary health care days per 100 residents, from a low of 230 days to a high of 1,595 days. Removing the outlier of 230 days for the second oldest community, there appears to be a slight association between the expected number of days and the age of the community (younger communities showing lower averages). The probability of transfer during the year also varies significantly among the communities. The highest probability, for Case 2, is 37 percent, and this case also has the highest expected number of temporary days. The distribution of the length of a temporary stay is skewed toward the lower end, with 50–80 percent of the transfers lasting less than 30 days for all cases.

Observations from Experience Studies on Decrement Assumptions

One of the primary findings of the mortality and morbidity case study investigations is that the historical records of the case study CCRCs were reasonably complete. Those communities that had good records put forth a substantial effort to maintain them. The second finding was a conformation of the view that residents of CCRCs tend to live longer than their counterparts in the general population. No explanation can be advanced from this finding, but this is an area that merits more research. Finally, it appears that CCRC residents tend to have lower hospital utilization than the general population.

NEW ENTRANT ASSUMPTIONS

New entrant assumptions are used to specify the characteristics of replacements for apartment residents who either die or permanently transfer to the health care center. These assumptions are required in projecting future population flows since differences in entry ages and in the number of coupled entrants will affect the community's apartment turnover and health care utilization.

---

[8] This statistic combines frequency of transfer with the average length of stay given that the resident transfers.

[9] David Rothberg, ed., *Regional Variations in Hospital Use* (Lexington, Mass.: Lexington Books, 1982).

Entry Age Distribution

The entry age assumption has a significant impact on future population flows and, in turn, on the financial aspects of a CCRC. Many forecasts use an average entry age assumption; however, this simplification could lead to errors in financial planning since health care utilization and the expected number of years a resident will occupy an apartment vary according to entry age. More accurate financial forecasts will result in the use of entry age distributions that specify the percentages of residents that enter from a range of ages, typically 65 to 90.

Table 5-7 shows the entry age distribution for the seven case studies. The average entry age is consistent for all cases, even though there are wide geographic and age variations in the communities. For both females and males, it is 76 or 77. However, there is variation in the actual distribution of ages. This variation should be reflected in assumptions used to project future populations and to determine weightings for fees that do not reflect cost differences associated with entry age.

Gender Distribution for Entrants

This assumption refers to the percentage of single entrants who are female and to the sex of members of double occupancies (i.e., the number of paired entrants who are of the same sex versus the number who are of the opposite sex). This distribution is needed because females are expected to live longer than males, and possibly use the health care center more, a factor that affects the financial aspects of the community.

Double-Occupancy Percentage for Entrants

This assumption reflects the probability that new entrants to an apartment unit will consist of two persons. This probability varies according to the size of the unit and may also be affected by management policies (e.g., a policy to sell certain units only to couples). The double-occupancy percentage is used to project the financial consequences of having two persons live in an apartment.

ECONOMIC ASSUMPTIONS

Inflation Rates

An estimate of future inflation is required for forecasting the increases in various expenses associated with operating the community and the expected increases in various revenue sources, primarily monthly fees

TABLE 5–7
Entry Age Distributions for Entrants to Case Study CCRCs

Sex	Age range	Case 1	Case 2	Case 3	Case 5	Case 6	Case 7	Case 8
Female	64 and younger	1%	2%	5%	3%	5%	2%	4%
	65–74	36	34	30	43	35	42	42
	75–84	56	54	50	44	52	54	51
	85 and older	7	10	15	10	8	2	3
	Average	77 years	77 years	77 years	76 years	76 years	76 years	75 years
Male	64 and younger	0%	1%	4%	4%	4%	0%	4%
	65–74	33	35	25	37	32	46	39
	75–84	55	52	57	48	50	49	53
	85 and older	12	12	14	11	14	5	4
	Average	77 years	77 years	78 years	77 years	77 years	76 years	76 years

and entry fees. Since financial projections may involve a 20–30-year forecast of inflation, one should not be overly myopic with respect to recent inflation experience in making this estimate. While it is important to reflect recent inflation experience, it may be unwise to project the recent high experience over a long period of time. One approach is to select a graded inflation assumption, for example, starting at 10 percent in the first year and grading down to a long-run rate of 5 percent after 5 years.

In addition, the inflation rate used in financial forecasts need not, and probably should not, be an estimate of the CPI statistic. The CPI tends to overstate the true inflation rate in an environment of accelerating inflation and to understate it in an environment of decelerating inflation. The proper assumption to use is the community's internal rate of inflation, which may be substantially different from published indices such as the CPI. Moreover, in establishing the inflation assumption, it may be important to select different inflation rates—at least in the short run—for different categories of expenses and revenues. For example, health care expenditures have historically increased faster than other community expenditures, and this trend may continue. However, the authors caution against the use of a permanently greater rate of inflation on one component of expenses (or revenues) as compared to another component, since a difference in inflation for a period of 20 to 30 years can cause significant distortions.

There is no doubt that the inflation assumption is both difficult to select and important to the results of the financial forecast. It is therefore recommended that financial forecasts involve a sensitivity analysis which considers various optimistic and especially pessimistic scenarios. Generally speaking, if the inflation assumption enters into both revenues and expenses equally, the absolute value of the rate may be less crucial than one initially believes, a subject examined at a later point. There is without question, however, a major impact on the long-run financial forecasts of a community when the rate of inflation for revenues is different from the rate of inflation for various expense categories. If such scenarios make sense, then the authors recommend that extensive sensitivity analyses be performed.

Interest Rates

The second economic assumption is an estimate of future interest rates. This assumption is required for two reasons. The obvious reason is that, if the community has substantial cash balances (e.g., various reserves), it is important to take into account the expected interest returns on these funds. The second reason is that some of the financial analyses to be discussed later require the determination of today's value of money payable (or receivable) in future years. In order to assess properly the current worth of these future transactions, it is necessary to discount their value for the so-called time value of money. Consider a case where $1.10 is payable next year and the current rate of interest is 10 percent. The present value (or today's value) of this payment is $1. This is true because $1 invested at a 10 percent interest rate will indeed accumulate to $1.10 after one year. Similarly, $2.59 payable at the end of 10 years has a present value of $1, assuming a constant 10 percent interest assumption.

Interest rates are as difficult to select as inflation rates. The financial literature, however, indicates that over a period of years the real rate of interest on short-term securities, such as Treasury bills, is near zero. The real rate on intermediate and long-term fixed-income securities is between 2 and 3 percent. The expected rate of inflation is added to the real rate of interest to obtain the nominal rate of return, which is used in actuarial computations.

Thus, the selection of the inflation assumption should act as a guide in the selection of the interest rate. For example, if the inflation rate were selected as the graded example given above (i.e., 10 percent down to 5 percent over five years), then it might be reasonable to make an identical assumption for the short-term interest rate. On the other hand, short-term interest rates tend to follow the CPI, and if the community's inflation exposure is different from the CPI, there may be justification for having an interest rate different from the inflation rate. Again, as with the inflation assumption, it is wise to perform sensitivity analyses with regard to the interest assumption because of its potentially significant impact on the financial analyses of CCRCs.

Summary

This chapter discussed the types of actuarial assumptions needed for analyzing the long-term financial status of CCRCs. In this discussion, three categories of assumptions were described, and illustrative values were derived for several actual communities. There is a definite need for the development of a national, or regional, data base from which guidelines can be drawn in selecting the assumptions to be used for financial analyses of CCRCs. The development of CCRC morbidity rates is especially needed because, as this chapter points out, it is impossible to reflect the financial consequences of a continuing care contract with accuracy using only life expectancies and mortality rates. The actuarial assumptions to be used in making financial projections for the hypothetical community examined in the following chapters of this book are contained in Appendix B. ∎

Chapter Six

Population Projections for CCRCs

■ In order to make financial projections of a CCRC, it is necessary to forecast various characteristics of the community's population. For example, it is important to estimate the number of apartments that will be released each year, the temporary and permanent utilization of the health care facilities, the apartment density ratio (i.e., the ratio of apartment residents to total apartments, indicating the percentage of double occupancies), and other such population contingencies that will affect the community's revenues and expenses. Two characteristics that should be addressed by the methodology for projecting CCRC populations are the maturation process and the implications of random deviations due to the small population size.

CHARACTERISTICS OF IDEAL METHODOLOGY

Population Maturation

In the field of actuarial science, the concept of a mature population refers to a situation where the characteristics of a population (e.g., its age distribution, length of residency, distribution of double occupants, proportion of residents in the health care facility, and gender distribution) remain the same year after year. In practice, a perfectly mature population never occurs; however, the concept is important because eventually the population of most CCRCs will become reasonably stable from year to year after passing through a maturation period that may last anywhere from 10 to 15 or more years.

Generally, during the maturation period, apartment turnover rates increase, health care utilization increases, the apartment density ratio decreases, the percentage of females increases, average age and length of residency increase, and so forth. In addition to being in the immature or mature state, a CCRC's population can be overmature for a period of time. For example, if the ratio of health care center residents to apartment residents is 20 percent for a particular community in a mature state, this ratio could climb to 30 percent for a period of time due to a variety of factors. The population during this period would be considered overmature—at least with respect to the characteristic of health care.

Since the current and future maturity status of the community's population has an important impact on its revenues and expenses, it is essential that the population forecast methodology incorporate the maturing process. Moreover, since financial forecasts are designed to assess the long-term financial picture of the community under its current management policies *and* alternative policies, and since the adoption of alternative policies can affect the population's maturity status, the forecast methodology should be able to deal with this interaction as well.

Experience Deviations

CCRCs typically have fewer than 500 residents;[1] hence, there can be substantial deviations in the experience of CCRC populations relative to the expected experience suggested by a set of underlying mortality and morbidity rates. For example, if the apartment turnover rate for the upcoming year is expected to be 5 percent, it is important to be able to estimate the probability that the rate will be below 5 percent, because the financial implications of a lower rate are usually significant. Similarly, random deviations in health care utilization are crucial because of their financial importance, as are other experience deviations. Thus, the population forecast methodology should be able to estimate the likelihood of adverse experience of a population in order for management to conduct prudent financial planning.

With these two problem areas in mind, the analysis turns to two general types of forecast methodology: (1) approximation methods and (2) actuarial methods.

---

[1] Of the CCRCs responding to the question on community size, 89 percent indicated that they had fewer than 450 residents.

APPROXIMATION METHODS

Over the years, a number of general guidelines, or approximations, for forecasting future CCRC populations have been developed, including the following:

> *Apartment releases:* One percent of all apartments will be released during the first year of the community's operation, with this percentage increasing by one percentage point per year to an ultimate level of 8 percent.[2]

> *Health care utilization:* Approximately 17 percent of all community members will reside in the health care center on a permanent basis once the community has matured.[3]

> *Density ratio:* The ratio of total apartment residents to total apartments will be 1.25 during the life of the community.

> *Average age:* The average age of the community will increase by one half of an age for each two years of the community's operation, to an ultimate average of age 80.

> *Replacements:* The characteristics of new entrants to the community during the forecast period will be identical with the characteristics of those who vacate apartments due to death or permanent transfer to the health care center. Thus, the entry age distribution, gender distribution, double-occupancy distribution, and other population statistics are assumed to remain constant.

In addition to these rules of thumb, in some communities population forecasts are developed by assuming that the community's experience will follow precisely the experience of another community that has been in existence for 5 or 10 years. There are undoubtedly many other rules of thumb and/or approaches that logically fall under the approximation methodology, but the important point is that these do not capture the numerous variations in individual CCRCs that can invalidate such assumptions. This methodology makes assumptions about future population instead of making assumptions about the *determinants* of future populations (i.e., mortality rates, morbidity rates, entry age distributions, and so forth). Thus, it is risky, and possibly imprudent, to employ approximation methods as a basis for financial projections. Moreover, the approximation methodology does not address the prob-

---

[2] For an example of this rule, see "One Example of Accommodation Fee Funding," *Continuing Care: Issues for Nonprofit Providers,* Chapter VIII (Washington, D.C.: American Association of Homes for the Aging), page 37.

[3] The authors know of no rules of thumb for this statistic during the maturation period; however, there are undoubtedly some in current use, since 17 percent is a long-run statistic.

lem of year-to-year experience deviations which can have a significant effect on population forecasts and, hence, financial forecasts of CCRCs.

ACTUARIAL METHODS

There are two types of actuarial methods for forecasting CCRC populations: (1) the deterministic method and (2) the stochastic method. The second type represents an extension of the first type, as described below. The distinguishing characteristics of the actuarial methods are that they involve fundamental assumptions regarding mortality and morbidity rates which are then applied to the initial year's population in deriving the population of successive years'. Such statistics as apartment turnover, health care utilization, and dual occupancy are determined by this process as opposed to being predetermined.

Deterministic Forecast Method

Under this approach, the year-to-year population forecast follows the underlying assumptions precisely. For example, if there were 100 females at age 80 living in apartments and the applicable mortality rate were 5 percent, then the deterministic model would forecast 5 deaths and 95 survivors. The age of the survivors would be increased and the process repeated for each year throughout the forecast period.

The advantage of the deterministic population forecast method is that it deals automatically with the maturation process described earlier. The initial population will mature according to the underlying assumptions, the length of the maturity period depending on the assumptions used. In addition, the consequences of any management policies that might affect the future maturity status can also be analyzed under this method. For example, the effects on turnover (and other statistics) of accepting a larger proportion of couples into the community can be compared with the effects of a policy favoring single occupancies, whereas under approximation methods such analyses would be difficult or impossible.

The primary disadvantage of the deterministic method is that it does not take into account the implications of year-to-year experience deviations. The only way this method can be used to estimate such variability is to repeat the population forecast using alternative assumptions or to introduce a "shock" into the assumptions from one year to the next. For example, one could assume that mortality rates increase or decrease sharply during a specific year of the forecast and analyze the resulting impact on turnover and other statistics; however, it may be difficult to formulate a reasonable experimental design. It is this limitation that the stochastic method is designed to overcome.

Stochastic Forecast Method

This method represents an extension of the deterministic method. It, too, begins by applying underlying mortality and morbidity rates to the initial population; however, the application is somewhat different. Continuing with the above example involving 100 females at age 80, the stochastic model examines each individual separately and determines whether or not the individual survives the year. In each case, a random number from 1 to 100 would be generated and the individual would be assumed to die if the number was 5 or less (since the mortality rate was assumed to be 5 percent in the example) and assumed to live if the number exceeded 5. If this process were successively applied to all 100 individuals, the result would not be predetermined or ascertainable in advance. Although five are expected to die, the process might conclude with three deaths. The difference between the five expected deaths and the three actual deaths represents the random deviation for the year.

Moreover, if a new sequence of random numbers were generated and again applied to the 100 individuals, one might find that 7 died during the second iteration (or trial), and so forth for successive iterations. Therefore, the stochastic methodology involves multiple population forecasts, each one representing an "iteration" using a different set of random numbers.

Figure 6–1 illustrates the distribution of deaths that would occur if an infinite number of iterations were performed. This figure shows that

FIGURE 6–1
Distribution of Deaths among 100 Individuals *(death rate = 5 percent)*

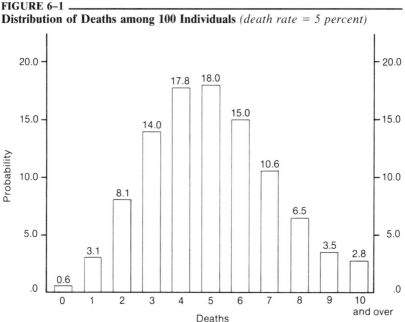

the expected number of deaths, five, has the highest probability of occurring. As the number of deaths increases or decreases, the probability of occurrence decreases somewhat symmetrically. In applying this approach, it is, of course, not feasible to generate an infinite number of iterations. Thus, a smaller number, such as 50, is generally used, and the resulting distribution, though not as smooth as the exact distribution, would tend to follow the pattern presented in Figure 6–1.

This example, of course, is an oversimplification of the stochastic process. However, it does serve to illustrate how this methodology incorporates random deviations into the population forecast, an element that should not be overlooked when dealing with small groups of individuals.

NUMERICAL ILLUSTRATIONS— HYPOTHETICAL COMMUNITY

The purpose of this section is twofold: (1) to illustrate the stochastic population forecast methodology and (2) to explore the population dynamics of CCRCs. A hypothetical community is used for illustrative purposes. The underlying actuarial assumptions and the physical configuration of the community for the baseline population forecast are given in Appendixes B and C, respectively.[4] Later in this section, changes in some of these parameters will be introduced to analyze the corresponding impact on the population forecasts.

Baseline Population Projection

Summary statistics for the baseline population forecast are given in Tables 6–1 through 6–4. Table 6–1 shows the number of residents in the apartment complex during each year throughout the 30-year forecast. Since the forecast methodology involves numerous iterations, the numbers shown in the table represent the *average* of the various iterations.[5] In addition to showing the number of residents by apartment type, the table also shows percentage of double occupancy.

A notable trend in Table 6–1 is that the total number of apartment residents decreases over the forecast period, beginning with 325 (a 1.44 density ratio) and scaling down by nearly 15 percent to 283 (a 1.26

---

[4] The actuarial assumptions were derived from the results of the case site experience studies and the authors' previous experience. It is not appropriate to apply these assumptions to existing or developing CCRCs.

[5] For illustrative purposes, the results in this section are based on 50 iterations of 30 years each. Additional iterations would be recommended in studying a specific community in order to develop somewhat tighter distributions than the ones underlying the data in these tables.

TABLE 6-1 ──
Baseline Apartment Population Forecast *(average values based on 50 iterations)*

Year	Studios (75) Number of residents	One bedroom (100) Number of residents	Density ratio	Two bedrooms (50) Number of residents	Density ratio	All apartments (225) Number of residents	Density ratio
1983	75	150	1.50	100	2.00	325	1.44
1984	75	149	1.49	99	1.98	323	1.43
1985	75	147	1.47	96	1.92	319	1.41
1986	75	145	1.45	93	1.86	312	1.38
1987	75	141	1.41	88	1.76	305	1.35
1988	75	138	1.38	85	1.70	298	1.32
1989	75	136	1.36	82	1.64	293	1.29
1990	75	134	1.34	80	1.60	288	1.28
1991	75	132	1.32	79	1.58	286	1.27
1992	75	131	1.31	78	1.56	284	1.26
1993	75	130	1.30	78	1.56	283	1.26
1994	75	131	1.31	78	1.56	283	1.26
1995	75	129	1.29	78	1.56	282	1.25
1996	75	129	1.29	78	1.56	282	1.25
1997	75	129	1.29	78	1.56	282	1.25
1998	75	130	1.30	79	1.58	284	1.26
1999	75	131	1.31	79	1.58	284	1.26
2000	75	130	1.30	79	1.58	284	1.26
2001	75	130	1.30	78	1.56	283	1.26
2002	75	131	1.31	78	1.56	284	1.26
2003	75	131	1.31	78	1.56	284	1.26
2004	75	131	1.31	78	1.56	284	1.26
2005	75	131	1.31	78	1.56	285	1.27
2006	75	132	1.32	79	1.58	286	1.27
2007	75	132	1.32	79	1.58	286	1.27
2008	75	132	1.32	79	1.58	286	1.27
2009	75	132	1.32	79	1.58	286	1.27
2010	75	132	1.32	79	1.58	286	1.27
2011	75	133	1.33	78	1.56	286	1.27
2012	75	133	1.33	78	1.56	286	1.27

density ratio) after 10 years and remaining at approximately that level thereafter. This trend is due to survivors maintaining their apartments after the death or permanent transfer of their spouse (or roommate). As indicated by the two-bedroom double-occupancy percentage, the ultimate proportion of double occupants is only about one half of the initial proportion. During the 10-year maturation period, revenues from monthly fees would also decrease—an important point to recognize in designing the pricing structure of a CCRC, and particularly the fees for double occupants. This trend would differ, of course, if the initial population had a greater or lesser number of couples, as dictated by the physical configuration of the community or by management policies. Thus, the authors reiterate an important principle: the community in question, with all of its nuances, must be simulated as opposed to using approximation methods that may or not be applicable.

Table 6–2 shows some additional statistics on the population of residents occupying apartments. The minimum, expected, and maximum turnovers experienced for the 50 iterations are shown. These data illustrate that the turnover rate will differ by apartment type and that there can be significant year-to-year variations in this statistic. Since turnover rates have an impact on the community's revenues, it would be risky to base a pricing structure on the aggregate expected apartment turnover rate alone. The financial impact of this problem and pricing methodologies designed to deal with the possibility of sustained adverse (i.e., low) turnover experience are examined in Chapters 6 and 7.

Table 6–3 provides statistics on health care utilization during the 30-year forecast period. It can be seen that the maturation period for the health care center is somewhat longer than that for the apartment complex, approximately 15 years in this case. At a mature state, about 18 percent of all residents are found to be living permanently in the health care center (i.e., there are 63 health care residents to 346 *total* residents). The variability in health care center residents is significant, ranging from about 50 to 80 residents in a mature state and having higher variability prior to this time. These data indicate that a 90-bed health care facility may be adequate, although when temporary transfers are considered, it may be somewhat small. Temporary transfers use approximately 3,200 bed-days per year in a mature state, or an *average* of about 9 bed-days per apartment resident per year.

Table 6–4 shows additional statistics on both apartment and health care center residents. A statistic of interest is the average years in the health care center for permanent residents, an average that eventually reaches four years. Based on an average daily cost of $50, this length of stay amounts to $73,000, excluding any inflationary increases in the cost of health care. It is therefore important that the morbidity rates as well as the mortality rates of health care center residents be developed carefully when making population and financial forecasts of CCRCs.

Effect of Aging Entry Age Distribution

Some communities experience an increase in the age of new entrants subsequent to the initial opening. This is undoubtedly caused by at least two factors. First, if the community develops a waiting list of prospective entrants, individuals on the waiting list become older as time passes. Second, as the initial population matures to an older average age, older individuals may be more attracted to enter the community and/or younger individuals may be less attracted. In any event, the aging of new entrants can affect the community's population and the

TABLE 6–2
Baseline Apartment Turnover Projection (*based on 50 iterations*)

Year	Studios (75)			One bedroom (100)			Two bedrooms (50)			All apartments (225)		
	Minimum	Expected	Maximum	Minimum	Expected	Maximum	Minimum	Expected	Maximum	Minimum	Expected	Maximum
1983	0	1	3	0	1	3	0	0	0	0	2	6
1984	0	2	4	0	2	4	0	0	2	1	3	7
1985	0	2	6	0	2	4	0	0	2	1	4	9
1986	1	4	10	0	3	7	0	1	2	2	8	16
1987	1	5	11	1	4	12	0	2	5	4	11	19
1988	0	5	10	1	5	12	0	2	6	7	12	23
1989	1	5	10	2	5	10	0	3	8	5	13	22
1990	2	6	10	2	6	11	0	3	8	7	15	20
1991	1	6	13	2	7	12	0	3	9	9	15	28
1992	0	5	9	1	7	13	0	3	7	7	15	25
1993	2	6	12	3	8	14	0	3	7	13	17	22
1994	2	6	10	2	7	12	0	3	9	8	15	23
1995	1	6	11	1	7	12	0	4	7	9	17	22
1996	2	6	12	2	8	15	0	3	7	11	17	22
1997	2	6	12	1	8	18	0	4	9	13	18	27
1998	2	6	12	2	8	13	1	4	7	9	18	26
1999	1	7	13	1	6	12	0	3	9	11	16	24
2000	2	6	12	2	8	18	0	3	6	11	17	25
2001	2	7	12	2	9	14	0	3	9	14	18	26
2002	1	7	13	4	8	18	0	3	9	10	17	29
2003	1	6	11	2	7	15	0	3	8	10	16	21
2004	2	6	11	3	8	12	1	4	8	11	17	27
2005	1	6	13	4	8	15	0	3	6	11	17	23
2006	2	6	13	4	8	15	0	3	8	7	17	28
2007	2	6	12	2	8	14	0	3	8	10	17	29
2008	1	5	12	2	8	14	0	3	7	10	17	21
2009	1	6	12	1	7	13	0	4	6	10	17	23
2010	1	7	12	3	8	16	0	3	9	9	17	24
2011	0	6	11	4	7	14	1	4	8	12	18	26
2012	0	7	12	2	7	11	0	4	8	11	18	23

TABLE 6–3
Baseline Health Care Center Population Forecast *(based on 50 iterations)*

Year	Number of residents			Annual transfers			Average number of temporary days
	Minimum	Expected	Maximum	Minimum	Expected	Maximum	
1983	0	0	0	0	3	7	766
1984	0	3	7	3	5	10	1,545
1985	3	7	12	1	7	14	2,306
1986	6	14	20	4	11	19	3,023
1987	12	22	34	7	14	21	3,666
1988	22	31	45	4	15	21	3,529
1989	28	39	55	8	15	23	3,413
1990	27	46	61	7	14	23	3,325
1991	36	51	71	8	15	22	3,263
1992	36	54	78	7	14	22	3,227
1993	45	57	72	8	15	23	3,199
1994	46	59	72	6	15	27	3,168
1995	48	60	73	6	15	22	3,160
1996	47	60	77	8	16	22	3,161
1997	51	62	81	11	16	21	3,146
1998	52	63	75	10	16	25	3,132
1999	49	63	78	6	14	23	3,127
2000	46	61	78	8	16	26	3,148
2001	43	62	78	10	16	23	3,154
2002	45	63	83	3	16	26	3,153
2003	50	63	82	9	15	23	3,144
2004	49	63	85	8	16	24	3,145
2005	46	63	83	5	16	24	3,155
2006	49	63	84	7	15	28	3,159
2007	45	63	84	6	15	27	3,164
2008	44	63	82	6	15	23	3,170
2009	44	63	80	8	15	27	3,186
2010	47	65	82	6	16	24	3,198
2011	52	66	89	10	16	23	3,187
2012	48	67	85	9	16	26	3,178

TABLE 6-4
Summary Statistics on Baseline Population Forecast (average values based on 50 iterations)

	Apartment center				Health care center			
Year	Number of residents	Average age	Years in community	Percentage female	Number of residents	Average age	Years in HCC	Percentage female
1983	325	75.7	.0	66.5%	0	.0	.0	.0%
1984	323	76.6	1.0	66.7	3	73.6	.0	45.7
1985	319	77.5	2.0	67.0	7	80.6	.3	56.7
1986	312	78.3	2.9	67.4	14	81.7	.6	63.3
1987	305	78.9	3.8	68.1	22	82.8	.8	62.4
1988	298	79.4	4.5	68.7	31	83.2	1.0	65.9
1989	293	79.8	5.2	69.1	39	83.7	1.3	68.9
1990	288	80.2	5.7	69.4	46	84.1	1.6	72.6
1991	286	80.4	6.2	69.7	51	84.6	1.9	74.8
1992	284	80.6	6.6	70.1	54	85.1	2.1	76.2
1993	283	80.8	6.9	70.2	57	85.5	2.4	78.1
1994	283	80.8	7.0	70.1	59	85.8	2.6	79.8
1995	282	80.9	7.2	70.4	60	86.2	2.7	80.2
1996	282	81.0	7.4	70.6	60	86.5	2.8	80.3
1997	282	81.0	7.4	70.6	62	86.9	2.9	80.1
1998	284	80.9	7.4	70.7	63	87.1	3.0	80.0
1999	284	80.9	7.4	70.5	63	87.2	3.0	80.6
2000	284	80.9	7.4	70.6	61	87.4	3.2	80.8
2001	283	80.9	7.5	71.1	62	87.5	3.2	80.1
2002	284	80.8	7.4	71.3	63	87.7	3.2	79.8
2003	284	80.8	7.4	71.3	63	87.7	3.3	80.2
2004	284	80.7	7.3	71.4	63	87.7	3.3	79.7
2005	285	80.7	7.3	71.4	63	87.8	3.4	79.2
2006	286	80.6	7.2	71.4	63	87.9	3.4	80.0
2007	286	80.6	7.2	71.5	63	87.9	3.5	79.6
2008	286	80.6	7.2	71.5	63	87.8	3.6	80.0
2009	286	80.7	7.2	71.4	63	87.8	3.6	80.7
2010	286	80.7	7.2	71.6	65	87.9	3.6	79.7
2011	286	80.7	7.2	71.4	66	87.9	3.7	79.6
2012	286	80.7	7.2	71.0	67	87.8	3.7	80.6

corresponding financial forecast. Thus, management should be aware of this phenomenon and adopt policies appropriate to the situation.

Table 6–5 shows the impact on the baseline population forecast of this phenomenon. For this experiment, it is assumed that the distribution of new entrants (which spans the ages from 65 to 85 and averages age 75 for the initial group of entrants) gradually increases for subsequent entrants by approximately one half of an age for each year after the community first opens, eventually stabilizing at age 80. The apartment density ratio is hardly affected by this change in assumption; however, the turnover statistics are increased, as would be expected. Although not shown in Table 6–5, the average age of apartment residents in a mature state increases from 81 in the base case to 83 in this experiment. Finally, the number of residents in the health care center increases for this forecast.

This experiment illustrates that a CCRC's population can change in response to a shift in entry ages and that making the population projection according to the actuarial methodology set forth previously can accommodate this possibility and others.

Effect of Alternative Policies Regarding Couples

The number of couples that enter the community is partially a function of management policy regarding new entrants. Some managements are indifferent to the dual-occupancy mix; others wish to discourage couples because they tend to lower turnover rates and corresponding entry fee revenues; and still others encourage couples to enter the community—sometimes for social reasons and sometimes for the short-run additional entry and/or monthly fee income.

Table 6–6 shows the results of a twofold management policy, namely, (1) increasing the number of coupled entrants (from 50 percent in one-bedroom apartments to 100 percent) and (2) requiring that the survivor of a couple move to a studio apartment after the death or permanent transfer of his or her spouse (or roommate), provided a studio apartment is available. The apartment density ratio increases significantly under this experiment, with the ultimate size climbing to nearly 1.51 (339 residents) as opposed to 1.27 (286 residents) under the baseline experiment, or a 20 percent increase in the ratio.

The other statistics of the community do not change significantly, there being only a modest increase in the number (and a decrease in the proportion) of health care center residents. Although most communities do not have strict policies requiring transfers, this may be an area that management should consider addressing, through either economic incentives or contract provisions, because of its potential for increasing revenues without a commensurate increase in costs. The financial

TABLE 6-5
Effect of an Increasing Entry Age Distribution

	Apartment center						Health care center					
	Density ratio		Turnover percentage				Health care ratio		Number of residents			
			Average value		Minimum value				Average value		Maximum value	
Year	Baseline	Experiment	Baseline	Experiment	Baseline	Experiment	Baseline	Experiment	Baseline	Experiment	Baseline	Experiment
1983	1.44	1.44	0.9%	0.9%	0.0%	0.0%	0.0%	0.0%	0	0	0	0
1984	1.43	1.43	1.3	1.3	0.0	0.0	0.8	0.8	3	3	7	7
1985	1.41	1.41	1.8	1.8	0.4	0.4	2.2	2.2	7	7	12	12
1986	1.38	1.38	3.6	3.6	0.9	0.9	4.1	4.1	14	14	20	20
1987	1.35	1.35	4.9	4.9	1.8	1.8	6.8	6.8	22	22	34	34
1988	1.32	1.32	5.3	5.3	2.7	2.7	9.5	9.5	31	31	45	45
1989	1.29	1.29	5.8	5.8	2.2	2.2	11.9	11.9	39	40	55	55
1990	1.28	1.28	6.7	6.7	3.1	3.1	13.6	13.7	46	46	61	61
1991	1.27	1.27	6.7	6.7	3.6	3.6	15.1	15.2	51	51	71	71
1992	1.26	1.26	6.7	7.6	3.1	4.4	16.1	16.3	54	55	78	79
1993	1.26	1.25	7.6	8.0	4.4	5.3	16.6	17.0	57	58	72	74
1994	1.26	1.25	6.7	8.0	3.6	4.0	17.3	17.8	59	61	72	75
1995	1.25	1.25	7.6	8.4	4.0	4.9	17.5	18.2	60	63	73	73
1996	1.25	1.25	7.6	8.9	4.9	5.3	17.6	18.3	60	63	77	82
1997	1.25	1.25	8.0	8.9	5.8	5.8	17.9	18.8	62	65	81	85
1998	1.26	1.25	8.0	8.9	3.6	5.3	18.1	18.9	63	66	75	77
1999	1.26	1.26	7.1	8.4	2.2	3.6	18.1	19.0	63	66	78	81
2000	1.26	1.25	7.6	9.3	4.4	4.0	17.7	18.8	61	65	78	84
2001	1.26	1.25	8.0	9.3	5.3	6.2	18.0	19.2	62	67	78	83
2002	1.26	1.25	7.6	9.3	4.4	4.0	18.2	19.2	63	67	83	81
2003	1.26	1.25	7.1	9.3	4.4	5.8	18.2	19.2	63	67	82	80
2004	1.26	1.26	7.6	9.3	4.9	5.8	18.2	19.3	63	67	85	93
2005	1.27	1.26	7.6	9.8	3.6	6.2	18.0	19.0	63	67	83	84
2006	1.27	1.27	7.6	9.3	3.1	5.8	18.1	19.0	63	67	84	87
2007	1.27	1.27	7.6	9.3	4.4	4.9	18.0	19.1	63	67	84	85
2008	1.27	1.26	7.6	8.9	3.6	4.9	18.0	19.2	63	68	82	89
2009	1.27	1.27	7.6	8.4	4.0	5.8	18.1	19.3	63	68	80	87
2010	1.27	1.26	7.6	9.3	4.0	5.3	18.5	19.7	65	70	82	86
2011	1.27	1.27	8.0	8.9	4.9	6.2	18.8	19.6	66	70	89	85
2012	1.27	1.27	8.0	9.8	4.9	5.3	18.9	19.6	67	70	85	88

TABLE 6-6
Effect of Survivor Transfer to Single Units

	Apartment center						Health care center					
	Density ratio		Turnover percentage				Health care ratio		Number of residents			
			Average value		Minimum value				Average value		Maximum value	
Year	Baseline	Experiment	Baseline	Experiment	Baseline	Experiment	Baseline	Experiment	Baseline	Experiment	Baseline	Experiment
1983	1.44	1.44	0.9%	0.9%	0.0%	0.0%	0.0%	0.0%	0	0	0	0
1984	1.43	1.43	1.3	1.3	0.0	0.0	0.8	0.8	3	3	7	7
1985	1.41	1.43	1.8	1.8	0.4	0.4	2.2	2.2	7	7	12	12
1986	1.38	1.41	3.6	3.1	0.9	0.9	4.1	4.1	14	14	20	20
1987	1.35	1.40	4.9	4.9	1.8	1.8	6.8	6.6	22	22	34	34
1988	1.32	1.39	5.3	5.3	2.7	2.7	9.5	9.2	31	32	45	45
1989	1.29	1.39	5.8	5.8	2.2	2.2	11.9	11.3	39	40	55	55
1990	1.28	1.40	6.7	6.2	3.1	2.7	13.6	12.8	46	46	61	63
1991	1.27	1.40	6.7	6.2	3.6	3.6	15.1	14.2	51	52	71	71
1992	1.26	1.41	6.7	6.7	3.1	3.6	16.1	15.0	54	56	78	80
1993	1.26	1.42	7.6	7.1	4.4	3.6	16.6	15.6	57	59	72	81
1994	1.26	1.44	6.7	6.7	3.6	2.7	17.3	16.2	59	63	72	78
1995	1.25	1.44	7.6	7.1	4.0	3.6	17.5	16.3	60	63	73	79
1996	1.25	1.45	7.6	7.1	4.9	4.0	17.6	16.4	60	64	77	82
1997	1.25	1.46	8.0	7.5	5.8	3.1	17.9	16.9	62	67	81	81
1998	1.26	1.47	8.0	7.5	3.6	4.0	18.1	17.3	63	69	75	86
1999	1.26	1.48	7.1	6.7	2.2	2.7	18.1	17.3	63	70	78	87
2000	1.26	1.48	7.6	6.7	4.4	3.6	17.7	16.9	61	68	78	87
2001	1.26	1.48	8.0	6.7	5.3	4.4	18.0	17.1	62	69	78	86
2002	1.26	1.48	7.6	7.1	4.4	4.0	18.2	17.3	63	70	83	88
2003	1.26	1.49	7.1	7.1	4.4	2.7	18.2	17.4	63	71	82	90
2004	1.26	1.49	7.6	7.1	4.9	4.0	18.2	17.6	63	72	85	87
2005	1.27	1.50	7.6	7.1	3.6	3.6	18.0	17.5	63	72	83	90
2006	1.27	1.50	7.6	7.1	3.1	4.0	18.1	17.7	63	73	84	100
2007	1.27	1.51	7.6	7.5	4.4	3.6	18.0	17.7	63	73	84	94
2008	1.27	1.51	7.6	6.7	3.6	3.6	18.0	17.8	63	74	82	102
2009	1.27	1.51	7.6	7.1	4.0	3.6	18.1	17.8	63	73	80	96
2010	1.27	1.51	7.6	6.7	4.0	2.7	18.5	18.1	65	75	82	106
2011	1.27	1.51	8.0	7.1	4.9	3.6	18.8	17.8	66	73	89	97
2012	1.27	1.51	8.0	7.1	4.9	4.9	18.9	18.0	67	74	85	93

impact of a change in policy could be analyzed by generating the cash flows associated with population projections for each policy.

Effect of Alternative Policies Regarding Permanent Transfers

In some instances, judgment is required as to whether an individual should be permanently transferred to the health care center. Some community administrators encourage such transfers in order to gain the entry fee revenue from apartment resales, a policy pursued even though having individuals live in the health care center is considerably more expensive. Other managers discourage such transfers until they are absolutely necessary.

Table 6–7 illustrates a management policy of encouraging transfers on a more rapid basis than the baseline case. Permanent transfer rates are assumed to increase by 25 percent; however, the overall life expectancy of residents remains unchanged.[6] This policy is seen to have little impact on the total number of apartment residents and the corresponding turnover statistics. However, the proportion of residents in the health care center increases dramatically. In a mature state, the number of such residents increases from the baseline value of approximately 63 to over 90.

NUMERICAL ILLUSTRATIONS— CASE STUDIES

The actuarial methodology for projecting future populations is applied to six existing communities in this section. The results of the mortality and morbidity experience studies given in the preceding chapter are used to estimate future apartment turnover and health care utilization, starting with the current resident census for each case study. Since the size and age of the community affect these projections, Table 6–8 describes each community by these criteria as well as by the community's location and health care guarantee.

The age characteristic refers to the year in which continuing care contracts were first offered. The community is considered *new* if it is 3 years or younger, *maturing* if it is 3 to 12 years old, and *mature* if it is over 12 years old. Size is categorized as *medium* for communities with 200 to 499 total residents and *large* for communities with 500 or more residents. The location description is based on the U.S. Census Bu-

---

[6] In order to simulate this policy, the mortality rates among apartment residents and health care residents were decreased in a way that maintained the same aggregate mortality for all residents combined.

TABLE 6–7
Effect of More Rapid Transfers to the Health Care Facility

	Apartment center						Health care center					
	Density ratio		Turnover percentage				Health care ratio		Number of residents			
			Average value		Minimum value				Average value		Maximum value	
Year	Baseline	Experiment	Baseline	Experiment	Baseline	Experiment	Baseline	Experiment	Baseline	Experiment	Baseline	Experiment
1983	1.44	1.44	0.9%	0.9%	0.0%	0.0%	0.0%	0.0%	0	0	0	0
1984	1.43	1.43	1.3	1.8	0.0	0.0	0.8	1.0	3	3	7	8
1985	1.41	1.41	1.8	2.2	0.4	0.4	2.2	2.8	7	9	12	14
1986	1.38	1.38	3.6	3.6	0.9	1.3	4.1	5.1	14	17	20	27
1987	1.35	1.35	4.9	5.8	1.8	2.7	6.8	8.6	22	28	34	38
1988	1.32	1.31	5.3	6.7	2.7	4.0	9.5	12.1	31	41	45	54
1989	1.29	1.29	5.8	6.2	2.2	2.2	11.9	15.2	39	52	55	74
1990	1.28	1.28	6.7	7.1	3.1	3.1	13.6	17.6	46	61	61	76
1991	1.27	1.27	6.7	7.1	3.6	3.6	15.1	19.4	51	68	71	86
1992	1.26	1.26	6.7	7.5	3.1	3.6	16.1	20.7	54	74	78	95
1993	1.26	1.25	7.6	8.4	4.4	5.3	16.6	21.6	57	78	72	94
1994	1.26	1.26	6.7	8.0	3.6	4.4	17.3	22.5	59	82	72	97
1995	1.25	1.25	7.6	8.0	4.0	4.4	17.5	23.0	60	84	73	99
1996	1.25	1.25	7.6	8.4	4.9	5.3	17.6	23.1	60	85	77	100
1997	1.25	1.26	8.0	8.9	5.8	4.4	17.9	23.4	62	87	81	100
1998	1.26	1.26	8.0	8.4	3.6	4.4	18.1	23.8	63	89	75	102
1999	1.26	1.27	7.1	7.1	2.2	3.6	18.1	23.9	63	89	78	110
2000	1.26	1.26	7.6	8.0	4.4	4.4	17.7	23.6	61	88	78	103
2001	1.26	1.26	8.0	8.9	5.3	5.3	18.0	23.9	62	89	78	104
2002	1.26	1.26	7.6	8.4	4.4	4.4	18.2	23.9	63	89	83	107
2003	1.26	1.26	7.1	8.4	4.4	4.4	18.2	24.1	63	90	82	106
2004	1.26	1.26	7.6	8.0	4.9	4.4	18.2	24.5	63	92	85	108
2005	1.27	1.26	7.6	8.4	3.6	4.4	18.0	24.3	63	91	83	105
2006	1.27	1.27	7.6	8.0	3.1	4.4	18.1	24.3	63	92	84	115
2007	1.27	1.27	7.6	8.0	4.4	4.0	18.0	24.2	63	91	84	111
2008	1.27	1.27	7.6	8.0	3.6	4.0	18.0	24.3	63	92	82	115
2009	1.27	1.27	7.6	8.4	4.0	5.3	18.1	24.4	63	92	80	114
2010	1.27	1.27	7.6	8.0	4.0	4.4	18.5	24.8	65	94	82	113
2011	1.27	1.27	8.0	8.0	4.9	4.9	18.8	25.1	66	96	89	115
2012	1.27	1.27	8.0	8.4	4.9	4.9	18.9	25.2	67	96	85	112

TABLE 6–8
General Characteristics of Case Study CCRCs

Characteristics	Case 1	Case 2	Case 3	Case 4	Case 5	Case 6
Age	Maturing	Maturing	Mature	New	Maturing	Mature
Size	Medium	Large	Large	Large	Medium	Large
Location	Northeast	South	North Central	South	North Central	West
Health care guarantee	Extensive	Extensive	Both	Extensive	Extensive	Extensive

reau's categories for Northeast, South, North Central, and West. All the CCRCs offer extensive health care guarantees (one offers both extensive and limited guarantees), meaning that the resident pays the same monthly fee in the health care center which he or she paid prior to permanent transfer.[7]

Apartment Turnover Percentage

The expected rate of apartment turnover typically increases as the community ages and eventually stabilizes as the community reaches maturity. As noted previously, this statistic is needed for estimating future entry fee revenues. Table 6–9 contains the average apartment

TABLE 6–9
Apartment Turnover % and Cause of Apartment Turnover for Case Study CCRCs

Statistic	Fiscal years	Case 1	Case 2	Case 3	Case 4	Case 5	Case 6
Average expected apartment turnover	1982 through 1986	8.5%	8.1%	15.9%	6.2%	6.1%	7.3%
	1987 through 1991	9.0	9.0	15.5	8.1	7.0	7.9
Apartment turnover caused by death	1982 through 1986	44%	42%	5%	50%	69%	52%
	1987 through 1991	43	43	7	51	71	50

turnover percentages for five-year intervals, from 1982 through 1986 and from 1987 through 1991. This table shows a slight increase in the second five-year interval for all cases except Case 3. The range in expected turnover percentages is 6 percent to 9 percent, excluding Case 3, which is an outlier showing 15 percent.[8]

---

[7] The exact definition for health care guarantee used in this study is given in Chapter 2.

[8] This community appears to have an aggressive permanent transfer policy of moving residents to its personal and nursing care facilities.

The bottom portion of Table 6–9 shows the percentage of apartment turnovers caused by the death of a resident. This percentage is consistently over 40 percent for all cases except Case 3, where it is less than 10 percent. The variation in these percentages is explained somewhat by differences in the morbidity assumptions which are affected by management policies on permanent transfers.

FIGURE 6–2A
Apartment Turnover Projection for Case 1

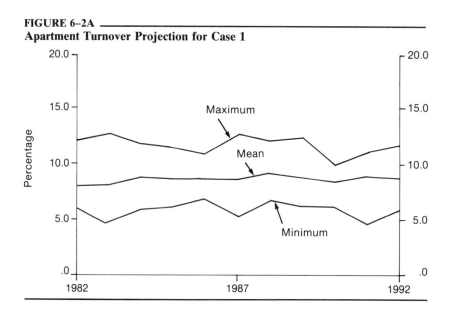

FIGURE 6–2B
Apartment Turnover Projection for Case 2

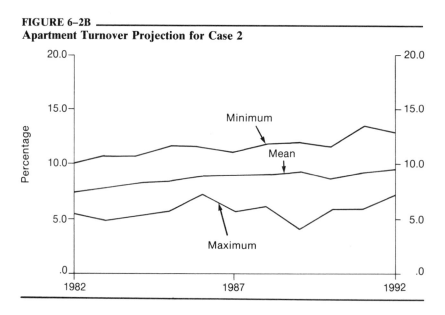

As noted earlier, the stochastic methodology allows one to analyze the risks associated with random deviations that might take place in the population forecast. An example is presented in Figures 6–2A through 6–2F, where the mean, minimum, and maximum apartment turnover percentages for the 6 case studies are shown. The minimum and maxi-

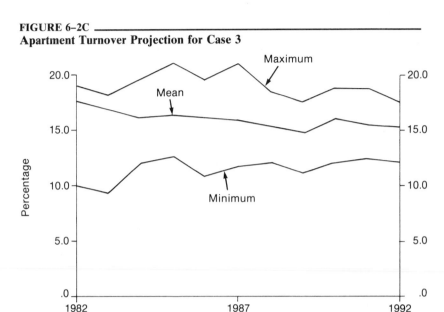

FIGURE 6–2C
Apartment Turnover Projection for Case 3

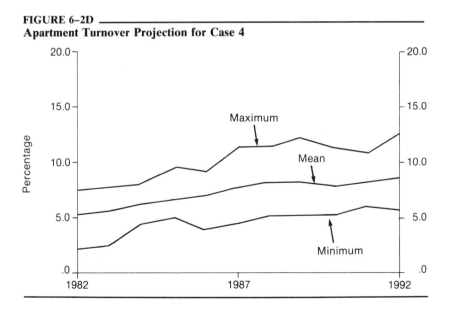

FIGURE 6–2D
Apartment Turnover Projection for Case 4

FIGURE 6–2E ——————————————————————————————
Apartment Turnover Projection for Case 5

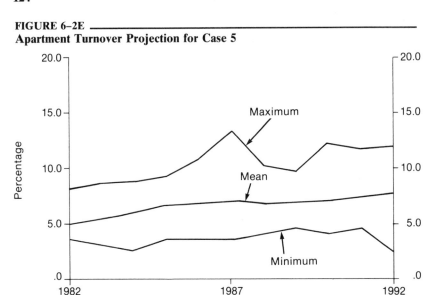

FIGURE 6–2F ——————————————————————————————
Apartment Turnover Projection for Case 6

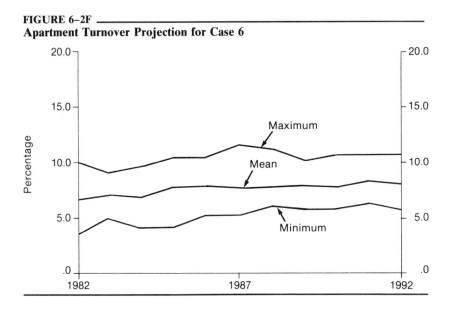

mum variation in these examples ranges from positive 5 to negative 5 percentage points from the expected (mean) values.

Health Care Utilization

Health care utilization is another key statistic generated by a population projection. This statistic is used both for financial projections and

TABLE 6–10 ————————————————————————————————————
Projected Health Care Ratios for Case Study CCRCs

Fiscal year	Case 1	Case 2	Case 3	Case 4	Case 5	Case 6
1982	11.1%	13.5%	25.5%	2.5%	4.0%	12.7%
1983	12.0	14.6	28.1	4.7	4.6	11.2
1984	12.5	15.4	26.8	6.7	5.1	10.9
1985	13.4	16.0	28.8	8.2	5.1	10.5
1986	13.8	16.6	30.0	9.6	6.0	10.4
1987	14.0	17.2	30.9	10.2	6.7	10.5
1988	14.1	17.6	31.8	11.0	6.7	10.5
1989	14.4	17.8	32.4	11.7	6.6	10.5
1990	14.6	18.2	32.8	12.2	6.5	10.5
1991	14.8	18.5	33.3	12.6	6.9	10.9

for estimating the ultimate size of the health care center. Table 6–10 contains a statistic summarizing the permanent health care usage by continuing care contractholders. This statistic is the health care ratio, which equals the number of permanent health care residents divided by the total number of continuing care contractholders. The results of our survey showed that the average ratio was 13.1 percent for CCRCs that had nursing care only and offered contracts with *extensive* health care guarantees; the average for CCRCs that had personal care and nursing care was 15.6 percent. The average health care ratio during the 10th year of the projection for the six CCRCs studied here is 16 percent, ranging from a low of 6.9 percent to a high of 33.3 percent. This variation is caused by differences in the communities' initial population maturity and the underlying assumptions. Variation of this magnitude

FIGURE 6–3A ————————————————————————————————————
Projection of Total Health Care Requirements for Case 1

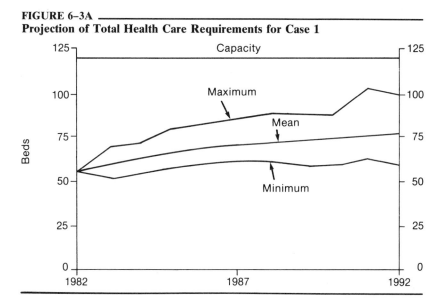

also point to the weakness of using rules of thumb for estimating health care utilization.

In order to estimate whether the current health care capacity of each community was adequate, the stochastic model was used to estimate the distribution of total health care utilization, including the health care beds required by permanent residents and apartment residents using

FIGURE 6–3B
Projection of Total Health Care Requirements for Case 2

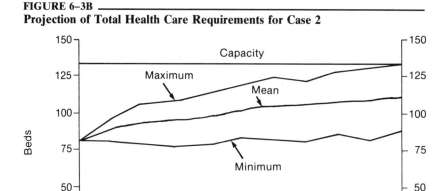

FIGURE 6–3C
Projection of Total Health Care Requirements for Case 3

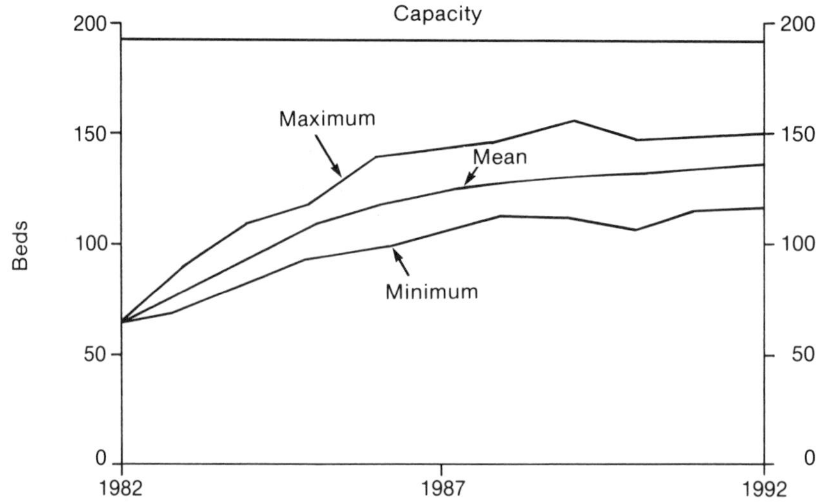

FIGURE 6–3D
Projection of Total Health Care Requirements for Case 4

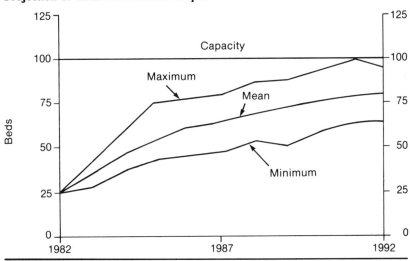

FIGURE 6–3E
Projection of Total Health Care Requirements for Case 5

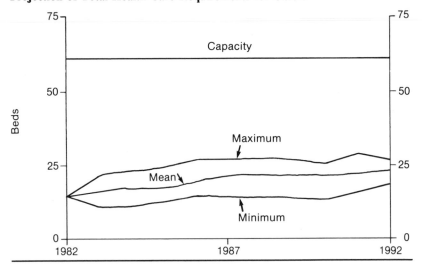

the health care facility on a temporary basis.[9] Figures 6–3A through 6–3F show each community's current capacity and the minimum and maximum requirements based on 25 iterations. The maximum expected

---

[9] The health care utilization estimates do not reflect needs during an epidemic or due to seasonal variations. Hence, it is possible that requirements may exceed the maximum number indicated.

128

FIGURE 6–3F ───────────────────────

Projection of Total Health Care Requirements for Case 6

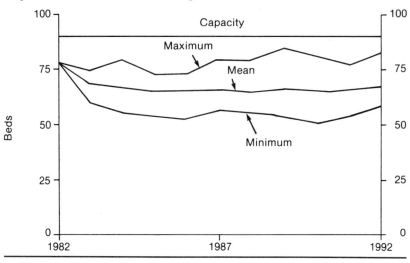

requirements for Cases 2 and 4 approach their capacity. Combining this observation with the fact that the projections do not reflect seasonal variations, these communities may need to start planning for the future expansion of their facilities. Case 5 has projected requirements that are far below its capacity (its health care ratio was also the lowest of all cases). However, this community is relatively new and its actuarial data base is sparse. The cash flow projections associated with this population projection should be reviewed carefully, and perhaps alternative projections should be generated to reflect more typical health care usage.

Summary

The projection of future population flows is an important component in performing financial analyses of CCRCs. Current practice is to use rules of thumb, or approximation methods, to estimate statistics required for cash flow projections such as apartment turnover and health care utilization. However, this approach has several deficiencies. First, rules of thumb are based on the assumption that all communities have approximately the same mortality and morbidity rates, management policies, and demographic profiles. Second, this approach does not allow management to determine the impact of random deviations from the assumptions due to the small size of the population. Moreover, approximation methods do not allow management to explain the effects of different management policies.

Two actuarial methods, deterministic and stochastic, for projecting future population flows were described, and a numerical example was developed using the stochastic method to illustrate the impact of changes in assumptions regarding entry age distribution and changes in policies toward admission of couples. The actuarial projection model was applied to the six case studies in generating population projections using mortality and morbidity assumptions derived from their experience studies. These projections showed that the population flows for the communities will vary due to differences in underlying assumptions and the current resident profile. ■

Chapter Seven _____
New Entrant
Pricing Theory

■ Continuing care retirement communities offer contracts that last for more than one year and promise shelter and health care to their residents. In exchange for this promise, residents pay a one-time entry fee and monthly service fees thereafter, subject to periodic increases for inflation. The purpose of this chapter is to describe the application of actuarial principles for (1) estimating the total liabilities (or costs) associated with a new entrant to a CCRC and (2) funding these liabilities (i.e., determining actuarially adequate fees). The actuarial methodology described in this chapter is the first component of a three-component management tool for assessing the long-term financial implications of CCRC contracts, the other two components being discussed in Chapters 8 and 9.

ACTUARIAL LIABILITIES

The actuarial liability for a continuing care contract represents the present value of expected future costs associated with an individual during his or her residence in a CCRC. The value of this liability is dependent on several factors for any given individual: (1) demographic factors such as age, sex, health status, and the number of residents per apartment (all of which, in turn, determine the appropriate mortality and morbidity rates to be used in calculating the liability); (2) contractual factors relating to refund provisions and health care guarantees; (3) accounting factors such as expense allocations; and (4) economic factors such as inflation rates and interest rates. For a given set of facts (such as entry age and sex) and a given set of actuarial assumptions, the resulting actuarial liability is unique and predetermined for each individual resident. Management cannot change the expected value of this liability without altering the provisions of the CCRC contract. The funding of the liability (or the setting of fees), on the other hand, can be affected by management, provided that the fees selected, on either an individual or group basis, fully meet the liability of the individual or group. Therefore, the first step in formulating a pricing policy is to accurately determine a CCRC's actuarial liabilities.

Actuarial Liability Calculation

Calculating the actuarial liability for a cohort group of residents requires the use of a closed-group (assuming no new entrants) population projection that estimates the probability of survival, by living status, to each future year.[1] The population projection is then combined with assumptions about future expenses, with expenses being proportionately allocated to surviving residents so that they pay their fair share of the cost of future services. The present value, or today's value, of this expense stream is referred to as the present value of future expenses (PVFE) and is, in fact, the actuarial liability for the group. The details of this calculation are presented in Appendix D, while a simplified example is given in Table 7-1.

The values in Table 7-1 are based on mortality and morbidity rates applicable to a female entrant at age 75.[2] Expenses while residing in an apartment unit are initially assumed to be $700 per month ($8,400 annually), while health care center expenses are assumed to be $46 per day ($16,800 annually). Both apartment and health care expenses are assumed to increase 10 percent annually, and their present values are determined using a 12 percent interest discount rate.

Columns 3 through 7 contain the values required to determine the present value of future expenses. Column 3 contains the present value of $1 payable in future years (i.e., the interest discount factor). For example, the present value of $1 payable at the end of four years is 64 cents. Another way of viewing this is that 64 cents invested today at a 12 percent rate of interest will accumulate to $1 at the end of four years.

The probability of survival over the next 20 years in either an apartment or the health care center is given in columns 4 and 5, respectively. At the end of 10 years, for example, 70.3 percent of the original group

---

[1] The actuarial mathematics used to develop this model are referred to as the "multiple decrement model." For an explanation of the underlying theory, see C. Wallace Jordan, *Life Contingencies* (Chicago: Society of Actuaries, 1975), chaps. 14–16.

[2] These rates are the same as the illustrative mortality and morbidity rates given in Appendix B.

TABLE 7-1
Illustration of Actuarial Liability Calculation

Beginning of year (t)	Age	Present value of $1 promised in year t	Illustrative Probability of survival Apartment center	Health care center	Projected apartment center expenses	Projected health care center expenses	Present value of apartment expenses	Present value of health care expenses
0	75	1.00000	100.0%	0.0%	$ 8,400	$ 16,800	$ 8,400	$ 0
1	76	.89286	96.3	2.4	9,240	18,480	7,942	402
2	77	.79719	92.2	4.9	10,164	20,328	7,472	799
3	78	.71178	87.8	7.5	11,180	22,361	6,991	1,187
4	79	.63552	83.2	9.9	12,298	24,596	6,500	1,558
5	80	.56743	78.2	12.4	13,528	27,057	5,999	1,905
6	81	.50663	72.8	14.7	14,881	29,762	5,492	2,218
7	82	.45235	67.3	16.8	16,369	32,738	4,980	2,487
8	83	.40388	61.5	18.6	18,006	36,012	4,469	2,702
9	84	.36061	55.5	19.9	19,807	39,613	3,962	2,854
10	85	.32197	49.4	20.9	21,787	43,575	3,466	2,934
11	86	.28748	43.3	21.3	23,966	47,932	2,985	2,937
12	87	.25668	37.3	21.1	26,363	52,726	2,526	2,860
13	88	.22917	31.5	20.3	28,999	57,998	2,096	2,705
14	89	.20462	26.1	18.9	31,899	63,798	1,701	2,479
15	90	.18270	21.0	17.2	35,089	70,178	1,349	2,198
16	91	.16312	16.6	14.9	38,598	77,196	1,043	1,883
17	92	.14564	12.7	12.6	42,458	84,915	787	1,557
18	93	.13004	9.6	10.2	46,703	93,407	580	1,243
19	94	.11611	7.0	8.0	51,374	102,747	417	960

Sum* $80,034 $40,170

Actuarial Liability $120,204

* Column totals reflect projected revenues and expenses to age 110.

of entrants are expected to be alive, of whom 49.4 percent are living in their apartments and 20.9 percent are living in the health care center. The relative change in the living status of surviving residents is illustrated in Figure 7–1. The life expectancy for this group of entrants, not

FIGURE 7–1 _____
Probability of Survival by Living Status

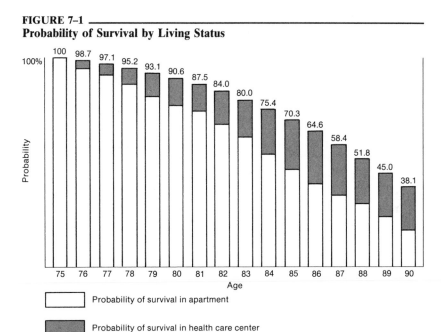

Probability of survival in apartment

Probability of survival in health care center

shown in Table 7–1, is 13.6 years (10.6 years of expected apartment residence and 3.0 years of expected health care center residence).

Projected expenses are given in columns 6 and 7. The present value of apartment expenses, which is the product of (1) the interest discount factor (column 3), (2) the probability of survival in the apartment center (column 4), and (3) projected apartment center expenses (column 6), is given in column 8 and sums to $80,034. The present value of health care expenses, equal to the product of columns 3, 5, and 7, is given in column 9. Its sum is $40,170. Hence, in this example, the total PVFE, or actuarial liability, for an age-75 female entrant is $120,204.

The preceding example is a simplified illustration of the actuarial liability calculation. For an actual case, the liability would include the costs of both temporary and permanent health care utilization and would recognize that some expenses (e.g., capital assets) may necessarily be part of the projected expense stream for a limited time period or may increase more slowly than the assumed inflation rate. The subsequent tables presented in this chapter are based on a more realistic calculation using assumptions presented in Appendixes B and C. The derived actuarial liability for an age-75 female entrant is $151,951.

Demographic Factors

Since demographic factors (age, sex, health care, and couple status) affect the mortality and morbidity assumptions used to develop the probabilities of survival, the PVFE varies according to these factors. For example, since younger entrants are expected to live longer, their PVFE at entry is larger than the PVFE for older entrants. Females are expected to live longer than males, as well as require more health care, and therefore their PVFE is higher than males at the same age. The PVFE for a couple, even though less than the sum of two single-entrant PVFEs, is larger than that for a single entrant, since a couple is expected to occupy an apartment longer and to experience twice the health care costs of a single resident. The impact of variations in health status is not as straightforward. While less healthy entrants will require more health care and thus incur higher costs, their shorter life expectancy might offset this increase.

The relative impact of age, sex, and couples on the PVFE, or actuarial liability, at entry is shown in Table 7–2. With regard to the age

TABLE 7–2
Illustration of Age, Sex, and Couples on Actuarial Liabilities
(age-75 female actuarial liability = 100 percent)

Entry age	Female	Male	Couple
70	118%	97%	178%
75	100	82	153
80	81	67	126

dimension, the PVFE changes by 15–18 percent for each five-year age interval, or an average of about 3 percent per year. The change is the same for couples (where both entrants are assumed to be the same age) as for single entrants, or 16 percent [(178 ÷ 153) − 1] per five years. Along the sex and couple dimension, the PVFE for age-75 females is approximately 22 percent [(100 ÷ 82) − 1] more than the PVFE for males, while a single female entrant has a PVFE approximately 35 percent [1 − (100 ÷ 153] less than that for a couple. It should be noted that even though there may be a specific relationship among PVFE's with regard to demographic factors, as well as other cost determinants, it does not necessarily follow that fees must exhibit these differentials. Fees, as illustrated later, can be developed to match a wide range of management objectives. The only restriction must be that the aggregate fees for all residents must equal their aggregate PVFE.

Contractual Factors

One way that management can alter the actuarial liability associated with a new entrant is by changing the contractual provisions. Two commonly modified areas are the health care guarantee and the refund provision. While it is true that the total actuarial liability faced by an individual resident is the same regardless of the type of health care guarantee offered, the portion faced by the individual himself versus the amount faced by the community is affected by the CCRC's health care guarantee. An example of this effect is given in Table 7–3.

TABLE 7–3 ————————
**Illustration of Alternative
Health Care Guarantees on
Actuarial Liabilities**
(*extensive guarantee for
each age = 100 percent*)

Entry age	Co-pay provision		
	0%	25%	50%
70	100%	90%	82%
75	100	90	81
80	100	90	79

The relative change in the liability faced by the community for a 0 percent, 25 percent, and 50 percent co-pay contract is given in Table 7–3 for female entrants ages 70, 75, and 80. Under a co-pay provision, the resident pays a percentage of the per diem health care charge in addition to his or her monthly fee while utilizing the health care center. For example, if the per diem charges are $46, the resident would pay $11.50 per diem under a 25 percent co-pay contract and $23 per diem under a 50 percent co-pay contract.[3]

This table shows that, as a percentage of the 0 percent co-pay provision (or extensive guarantee), a 25 percent co-pay contract reduces the total actuarial liability (apartment and health care combined) by 10 percent. A 50 percent co-pay contract reduces the total liability by 20 percent. The trade-off in offering a limited health care guarantee is that the community may experience an increase in its financial aid liability if

---

[3] A comprehensive discussion of the relative costs of health care guarantees is presented in Howard E. Winklevoss and Alwyn V. Powell, "Retirement Communities: Assessing the Liability of Alternative Health Care Guarantees," *Journal of Long-Term Care Administration 9*, no. 4 (Winter 1981) pages 8–33.

the financial requirements at admission are not strengthened, and such strengthening may, in turn, restrict the market of potential CCRC residents. The financial aid liability is not easily quantified; however, it is an important consideration in analyzing the risks of a specific guarantee since communities rarely terminate a contract due to the resident's inability to pay fees.[4]

Entry fee refund provisions at death or withdrawal are often used as a marketing tool to promote an "open door" effect for residents. However, liberal refund provisions increase the actuarial liability.[5] The expected increase in net entry fees (i.e., entry fees associated with no refunds) for several refund provisions is given in Table 7–4. Column 2 contains the increase for 100 percent death refunds for 1 to 25 years, while column 3 shows the effect for a prorated refund. For example, the cost of a 100 percent entry fee refund for five years is 11.3 percent of the initial entry fee, while the cost of a prorated refund is 5.5 percent. Columns 4 and 5 show the entry fee increase associated with withdrawal refunds. These costs are substantially less than death refunds only because the probabilities of withdrawal are assumed to be less than death rates. Alternative withdrawal assumptions may affect these ratios dramatically.

Accounting Factors

Accounting factors refer to management decisions regarding the allocation of future expense values used in the PVFE calculation. These decisions include the methodology used for *expensing* fixed assets (actuarial versus accounting methodology), the *allocation* of aggregate expenses to individual residents, and the *timing* of when expenses are assumed to occur for the replacement of equipment and furnishings, the generation of reserves for future building refurbishments, and the eventual replacement of the current facility. Management decisions on each of the accounting factors must be somewhat subjective, there being no specific guidelines for such decisions.

Actuarial versus Accounting Methodologies. The basic issue here is whether the method used for financing a fixed asset should be a factor in determining the expense stream associated with that asset. Actuarial expenses for a fixed asset are determined such that the present value of those expenses equals its cost. For example, if an asset cost $15 million and is assumed to have a useful lifetime of 40 years, the annual actuar-

---

[4] Results of the survey conducted for this study indicate that none of the surveyed communities had ever terminated a contract so long as the resident did not willfully dissipate his or her financial resources.

[5] Actuarially, the refund can be any value even though traditionally it is based on the original entry fees.

TABLE 7–4
Illustrative Relative Increase in Entry Fees for Alternative Entry Fee Refund Provisions
(age-75 female entrant)*

Refund period (years)	Increase in entry fee for death refunds		Increase in entry fee for withdrawal refunds†	
	100 percent refund	Prorated refund‡	100 percent refund	Prorated refund‡
1	2.2%	1.1%	0.9%	0.5%
2	4.4	2.2	1.7	0.9
3	6.7	3.3	2.4	1.3
4	9.0	4.4	3.0	1.6
5	11.3	5.5	3.9	2.3
6	13.8	6.6	3.9	2.3
7	16.3	7.7	4.3	2.5
8	18.9	8.9	4.6	2.8
9	21.6	10.0	4.8	3.0
10	24.3	11.2	5.0	3.1
11	27.0	12.3	5.1	3.3
12	29.7	13.5	5.2	3.5
13	32.3	14.7	5.3	3.6
14	34.8	15.9	5.4	3.7
15	37.0	17.0	5.4	3.8
16	39.0	18.1	5.4	4.0
17	40.7	19.2	5.4	4.0
18	42.1	20.3	5.5	4.1
19	43.1	21.3	5.5	4.2
20	43.9	22.2	5.5	4.3
21	44.4	23.1	5.5	4.3
22	44.8	24.0	5.5	4.3
23	45.1	24.7	5.5	4.4
24	45.2	25.5	5.5	4.4
25	45.3	26.2	5.5	4.5

* The values given represent the amount by which entry fees would have to be increased to cover the cost of expected refunds, based on an age-75 female entrant.

† Withdrawal rates are assumed to be 1 percent per year regardless of age, sex, and length of stay in the community.

‡ This provision means that the amount refunded is prorated over the time period given; thus, a prorated refund over five years implies that 20 percent is deducted annually.

ial expense would be $1,625,000 ($15,000,000 ÷ 9.23303, where 9.23303 is the present value of $1 payable at the beginning of each year for 40 years). The actuarial expense methodology generates the same expenses for a fixed asset irrespective of its financing. The rationale for this is that the asset provides the same services to the community and, therefore, is consumed in the same fashion by residents irrespective of the method by which it is financed. The accounting expense methodology, on the other hand, generates expenses that vary according to the financing method (the depreciation expense is fixed, but the interest expense varies). This implies that the PVFE derived from accounting methodology differs, depending on the financing method, a concept at odds with the true economic expense of the asset. The actuarial expensing methodology is used to develop the numerical illustrations presented in this book.

Expense Allocations. Two sets of allocation factors are required in developing actuarial liabilities. The first set is used to distribute aggregate expenses between the apartment cost center and the health care cost center (if the community offers both personal care and nursing care, a further allocation is required). The second set is used to indicate the portion of each cost center's expenses that vary on a per capita basis versus a per unit basis (square footage). These allocation percentages may be difficult to derive precisely, requiring some judgment by management.

Table 7–5 contains the relative cost differentials for a single entrant to a studio unit, a one-bedroom unit, and a two-bedroom unit. This

TABLE 7–5
Illustrative Comparison of Actuarial Differentials for Three Apartment Types *(age-75 female entrant)*

Apartment type	Ratio of present value of future expenses for one- and two-bedroom units to studio units		
	Capital costs	Operating costs	Total costs
Studio	1.00	1.00	1.00
One bedroom	1.28	1.09	1.18
Two bedrooms	1.55	1.18	1.33

table contains differentials for the PVFE associated with capital expenses, operating expenses, and total expenses (capital and operating combined). For example, if a community adopted a pricing policy in which entry fees covered only capital expenses, then the one-bedroom entry fee should be 1.28 times the studio entry fee and the two-bedroom entry fee should be 1.55 times the studio fee. One-bedroom and two-bedroom monthly fees, which in this illustration are designed to cover operating expenses, should be 1.09 and 1.18 times the studio monthly fee, respectively. On the other hand, if the community employed a pricing philosophy that allocated a portion of the total PVFE to entry fees and the residual to monthly fees, then both entry fees and monthly fees for the one-bedroom unit should be 1.18 times the studio fees (column 3), while the two-bedroom fees should be 1.33 times the studio fees.

Timing of Capital Expenses. The inclusion of expenses for the replacement of capital assets poses interesting equity questions for the management of a CCRC. On the one hand, since it is not possible to predict exactly the incidence of future replacement expenditures, one might factor into the PVFE calculation a "smooth" stream of replacement expenses that anticipates future expenditures. It could be argued that this approach is not equitable to current residents, who are not likely to receive any benefit from future expenditures. The counterargument is that since current residents are using (consuming) the community's capital assets, they should replace those assets to maintain the community's attractiveness to future residents. The rationale for this argument is that residents do not have ownership rights in the community and therefore can be assessed charges to minimize its physical deterioration. Alternatively, the expenses for capital assets could be incorporated into the PVFE when these assets are actually replaced. The advantage of this approach may be its equity, since the residents who receive the benefit of the new asset fund its purchase. The disadvantage is that the resulting expense stream is not likely to follow inflation, creating an undesirable pattern of fee increases.

The numerical examples presented in this chapter are based on a smooth expense pattern in connection with replacing equipment and furnishings and with refurbishing and/or modernizing the current facility. Building replacement expenses are factored into the PVFE based on the resident's expected lifetime in the new facility. Thus, early generations will have a small value for this expense, while later generations will have an ever-increasing value. An alternative approach for building replacement (not illustrated in this chapter) is to advance-fund a predetermined portion of the estimated replacement cost. This approach will generate larger liabilities than the first method during the early years of a community and smaller liabilities when replacement is needed.

Economic Factors

The actuarial liability is significantly affected by the two economic factors of inflation and interest rates. Since inflation is used to project the cost of future services, the higher the rate of inflation, the higher will be the actuarial liability. The interest rate, on the other hand, is used to find the present value of such future costs. Thus, the higher the interest rate, the lower will be the actuarial liability. If the interest rate and the inflation rate are both increased (or decreased) by the same amount, they will have little impact on the actuarial liability because their individual effects will be offset. Therefore, the crucial economic factor is the *difference* between the two rates. Generally, the long-run equilibrium relationship is one where the interest rate is one or two percentage points above the inflation rate; however, there have been many short-term periods during which this relationship has not held.

TABLE 7-6 _____

Illustrative Effect of Economic Factors on
Actuarial Liability *(age-75 female entrant with*
10 percent inflation and 12 percent interest =
100 percent)

Inflation rate	Interest rate			
	8%	10%	12%	14%
6%	96.0%	88.9%	83.3%	78.8%
8	107.4	98.1	90.9	85.1
10	121.5	109.4	100.0	92.6
12	139.0	123.2	111.1	101.6

Table 7-6 shows the relative impact of alternative inflation and interest rates on the actuarial liability for an age-75 female entrant. As can be seen, as long as the differential between the rates is constant, the actuarial liability is minimally affected; however, when this relationship is altered, the economic factors are seen to have a significant impact.

SETTING FEES TO FUND ACTUARIAL LIABILITIES[6]

As noted in the preceding section, the actuarial liability for an individual resident, or a group of residents, is fixed for a given set of facts and assumptions. However, the fees selected to fund that liability can be structured to match a wide range of criteria set forth by management. By using the actuarial liabilities previously calculated, management can apply actuarial theory in developing fees that are both adequate and equitable on an individual, or micro, basis. This means that fees would vary according to the resident's age, sex, health status at entry, apartment type, year of entry, and so forth. Alternatively, management may desire to offer a less complicated fee structure, choosing to socialize, or share, costs among all residents. For example, fees may vary

---

[6] The funding discussion is based on the assumption that fees are set to cover *expected* liabilities (i.e., those liabilities that will accrue if experience exactly follows the actuarial assumptions). In practice, the so-derived fees, or "pure premiums," would be increased either implicitly or explicitly to recognize the potential for larger liabilities due to the uncertainty of the underlying assumptions. Implicit or explicit adjustments are referred to as contingency factors. An implicit contingency factor means that more conservative assumptions (as compared to one's best estimate) are used to generate actuarial liabilities, thus producing higher fees. An explicit contingency factor means that the pure premiums are increased by an explicit amount based on a statistical estimate of the potential variation in the expected liability. An example of an explicit contingency factor calculation for a group of residents is given in Chapter 8 in the discussion of the buffer fund method used to deal with financial gains and losses.

according to the resident's apartment type and number of occupants only. In this case, management need only be concerned that fees in the aggregate, or on a macro basis, for a group of residents be adequate.

Fee Structure Objectives

Actuarial theory gives management considerable flexibility in designing the pricing structure of a CCRC. However, this flexibility may be disadvantageous in the sense that there are no prescribed guidelines or objectives for developing fees. Without guidelines and objectives, management may not be able to explain (or defend) changes in fees to residents. Two logical and desirable goals for setting fees that will both provide guidance to management in adjusting fees and allow it to defend such adjustments to residents are discussed below.

Group Equity. On a macro level, this goal requires that the pricing structure for a cohort group of new entrants be self-supporting. In other words, the total revenues anticipated from a group of entrants should cover the total expenses anticipated for the services provided to them by a CCRC. A pricing structure meeting this objective ensures that the fees associated with future groups will not be needed to pay for the services used by prior groups (assuming that the community's future experience matches the underlying assumptions). On a micro level, this objective implies that different fees would have to be charged to individual residents with different characteristics as to age, sex, health status, apartment type, and so forth. The micro interpretation of group equity, however, need not be fully implemented. Fees could vary by some factors (such as apartment type) and not others (such as age, sex, and health status). Thus, the group equity objective can be met on a macro level. Pricing structures based on the group equity concept are, by definition, actuarially adequate.

The group equity concept also has implications for the types of expenses that should be allocated to the current group. For example, one issue is whether it is equitable to include amounts for future refurbishments in the fees for current residents, since many will have died by the time such expenditures are made. Another issue is the expensing of the physical facility in such a manner that each generation pays its fair share of its costs.

The group equity concept, on either a micro or macro level, is the keystone of any actuarially sound pricing methodology. Its acceptance has manifold ramifications for establishing fees.

Inflation-Constrained Increases in Monthly Fees. The second desirable goal is to limit the annual increase in monthly fees to the rate of increase in the community's expenses (i.e., the community's internal inflation rate). Inflation-constrained fee increases are intended to insulate residents from the higher costs associated with increased health care utilization during the community's maturation period.

The desirability of inflation-constrained fee increases is based on the assumption that residents move to a community, in part, to avail themselves of a continuing care program that has a reasonably predictable future cost. Under this assumption, the overseers of the community have a moral and implied commitment to develop a long-term pricing strategy that is not anticipated to require monthly fees to increase faster than the community's internal inflation rate.

One important implication of inflation-constrained increases in monthly fees is that the community's fee structure will automatically build up funds to cover the future shortfall between expenses and monthly fees as the community matures and health care utilization increases. These funds represent the prefunding of future health care costs and other deferred liabilities.

Illustrative Actuarially Based Fee Structures

Actuarially adequate fees structures that meet both of the above pricing objectives can be determined by equating the present value of future revenues with the present value of future expenses for an individual entrant or a cohort group of entrants. The present value of future revenues consists of the entry fee plus the present value of future monthly fees. The general relationship between revenues and expenses can be represented as follows:

$$PVFR = PVFE[7]$$
$$EF + PVMF = PVFE$$

where

$PVFR$ = Present value of future revenues
$PVFE$ = Present value of future expenses (or actuarial liability)
EF = Entry fee.
$PVMF$ = Present value of monthly fees (inflation-constrained)

This formula can be used to determine actuarially adequate entry fees for a given monthly fee, and vice versa, once the PVFE (or actuarial liability) is calculated.

Table 7–7 contains several actuarially adequate fee combinations where the PVFE is assumed to equal $151,951. This table shows that if the community were to charge no monthly fee, then the actuarially adequate entry fee would be $151,951. Alternatively, if no entry fee were charged, the actuarially adequate monthly fee would be $1,062 (an amount that would also have to be paid after permanent transfer to

---

[7] The underlying mathematics of this formula is explained in detail in Appendix D.

TABLE 7–7
Illustration of Actuarially Equivalent Pricing Structures *(age-75 female entrant)*

Actuarial liability	Entry fees	Monthly fees	Present value of monthly fees
$151,951	$151,951	$ 0	$ 0
151,951	125,000	188	26,951
151,951	100,000	363	51,951
151,951	75,000	568	76,951
151,951	50,000	713	101,951
151,951	25,000	898	126,951
151,951	0	1,062	151,951

the health care facility). If the entry fee were set at $50,000, then the present value of monthly fees would be $90,000 and the derived monthly fee would be $713.[8] As Figure 7–2 illustrates, an infinite number of actuarially adequate entry fee/monthly fee combinations can be

FIGURE 7–2
Entry Fee/Monthly Fee Trade-off

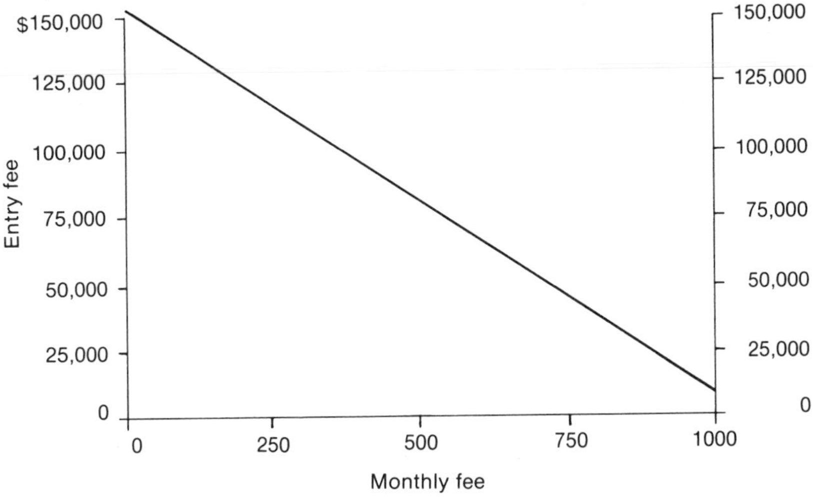

derived using the actuarial pricing equation. Any point along the line in Figure 7–2 represents an acceptable entry fee and monthly fee combination. In this example, the trade-off between monthly fees and entry fees is such that for every $1 increase in monthly fees, entry fees can be reduced by $143. The final selection of an entry fee/monthly fee combi-

---

[8] This value is determined by dividing the PVMF by the product of 12 times the present value of $1 increasing annually for inflation, or 12 × 11.92 in this example.

nation depends on marketing considerations and management's philosophy regarding the expenses to be covered by entry fees and those to be covered by monthly fees. However, the authors strongly discourage the policy of charging only an entry fee because the risks associated with misestimation of assumptions are extremely large, and if only an entry fee is charged, the community has no way to adjust fees to compensate for misestimation or variations due to random fluctuations in experience.

Entry Fee/Monthly Fee Trade-off

The issue regarding those expenses that should be covered by entry fees versus those that should be covered by monthly fees can also be viewed simply as what portion of the PVFE should be allocated to entry fees and what portion should be allocated to monthly fees. Clearly, the larger the portion of the PVFE allocated to entry fees, the more the community is exposed to risks of underpricing due to misestimation of assumptions such as inflation, mortality, and morbidity. On the other hand, one advantage of collecting as much as possible in entry fees is that residents will not be able to divest themselves of those funds, thus minimizing the community's financial aid risk.

Alternatively, the community could collect most of its revenues through monthly fees and minimize its inflation risk. The extreme example of this alternative is the case where monthly fees are the only charges. The advantage of covering a larger portion of the PVFE by monthly fees is that such fees can be adjusted to cover unfavorable deviations in the underlying assumptions. One disadvantage, again, is that the financial aid risk is increased, since monthly fees are more likely to exceed the monthly income of some residents and eventually exhaust all of their financial resources.

One approach to the entry fee/monthly fee trade-off is to combine the real estate concept of pricing with the actuarial concept. Under this approach, entry fees are set to cover capital expenses, which initially increase less than inflation. Monthly fees are set to cover the residual operating expenses. The advantage of this approach is that since entry fees are set to cover relatively fixed expenses, the required increase in entry fees is substantially less than the overall inflation rate, thereby minimizing the community's exposure to inflation misestimation. The disadvantage is that the level of entry fees is somewhat predetermined by capital expenses and may not give management sufficient flexibility in selecting fees.

Another approach to minimizing the community's inflation exposure, as well as the risk associated with unfavorable mortality and morbidity experience, is to limit the portion of the PVFE allocated to entry fees. No objective guidelines can be given for the correct proportion that should be allocated to entry fees, but the authors believe that this percentage probably should not be less than 20 percent or more than 50 percent to minimize the inflation risk without unduly increasing the financial aid risk. A possible disadvantage is that there is no clear identification regarding the expenses to be covered by each revenue component, although this does not affect actuarial adequacy.

An example of fees under two approaches for an age-75 female entrant is given in Table 7–8. In both cases, it is assumed that the

TABLE 7–8

Illustrative Comparison of Actuarially Adequate Fee Structures under Real Estate/Actuarial and Percentage of PVFE Pricing Approaches *(age-75 female entrant)*

	Entry fees		Monthly fees	
Apartment type	Real estate/ actuarial approach	30 percent of PVFE approach	Real estate/ actuarial approach	30 percent of PVFE approach
Studio	$42,180	$39,619	$628	$646
One bedroom	53,846	45,585	686	744
Two bedrooms	65,511	51,551	743	841

resident pays the same monthly fee after permanent transfer to the health care center, although this assumption is not necessary. The entry fee under the percentage approach is set to cover 30 percent of the total PVFE.

In this example, the entry fees under the real estate/actuarial approach are consistently more than those under the 30 percent of PVFE approach, while the reverse is true for monthly fees. The point of this illustration is that actuarial theory provides a multitude of ways for management to set fees that are actuarially adequate, while selecting an entry fee/monthly fee combination that meets other criteria in addition to actuarial adequacy.

ACTUARIALLY EQUITABLE FEE DIFFERENTIALS

The concept of fee equity is not well defined, depending primarily on management philosophy. Actuarial theory can provide actuarially equitable fee differentials for a given set of demographic, contractual, accounting, and economic factors, as well as a specific pricing philosophy. However, management may choose to ignore the actuarial differentials and simply use actuarial theory to establish a fee structure that is, overall, actuarially adequate (i.e., each group of residents is anticipated to pay its own way) while meeting other specific objectives. Many communities choose to establish fee differences along the lines of apartment type and number of occupants, ignoring sex and age differences.[9] These two dimensions are discussed in the following paragraphs.

It will be noted that the fee differentials shown in Table 7–8 for different apartment types vary according to the pricing philosophy assumed. The real estate/actuarial approach has entry fee differentials (or ratios) for studio, one-bedroom, and two-bedroom units of 1.00, 1.28, and 1.55[10] compared to the square footage differentials among the units, which equal 1.00, 1.50, and 2.00. The reason the fee differentials do not equal the square footage differentials is that some of the capital expenses allocated to entry fees are shared equally among all residents and are therefore allocated on a per capita basis. The monthly fee differentials under the real estate/actuarial approach are 1.00, 1.09, and 1.18. These differentials are less than the entry fee differentials since more of the operating expenses are allocated on a per capita basis than was the case for capital expenses. Entry fee and monthly fee differentials are identical under the percentage of PVFE approach, equal to 1.00, 1.18, and 1.33 for studio, one-bedroom, and two-bedroom units, respectively.

Even though the two pricing approaches generate different fee differentials, both are correct for the approach assumed. Moreover, other pricing philosophies will generate a different set of differentials. It should also be noted that even though a community's pricing structure may not be in actuarial balance (i.e., the PVFR is not equal to the PVFE), these actuarial differentials can still be applied to that structure. Finally, the actuarial differentials may change as the community's expense pattern matures or if some of the underlying assumptions are changed; hence, they should be reassessed periodically.

Couples pose a special problem for CCRCs. Not only is the last survivor of a couple expected to occupy an apartment longer than a single resident, but the community is also exposed to approximately twice the health care utilization, affecting two critical financial factors of the community. Currently, most communities differentiate monthly fees by the number of occupants, while few differentiate entry fees. Charging the same entry fee regardless of the number of entrants is reasonable, provided that the differential in monthly fees is adequate or that the shortfall is made up elsewhere in the community's pricing structure.

---

[9] Less than 10 percent of the CCRCs responding to the Wharton School survey said that they varied fees by age or sex.

[10] These differentials are determined by dividing fees for all units by the studio fee.

TABLE 7–9
**Illustrative Comparison of Actuarially Based
Second-Person Fee Differentials***

Variation	Entry fee differential	Monthly fee differential
Equal entry fee and monthly fee differentials	51%	51%
Zero entry fee differential	0	91
Zero monthly fee differential	118	0

* Based on age-75 entrants to one-bedroom units.

Table 7–9 contains the appropriate fee differentials for three varia-tions.[11] The first variation is based on the assumption that the differen-tial between one- and two-person entry fees is the same as the monthly fee differential. This example shows that two-person monthly and en-try fees should be 51 percent more than one-person fees. The second variation is based on the assumption that entry fees are the same for one or two entrants (i.e., 0 percent entry fee differential). The required monthly fee differential in this case is 91 percent. The third variation is based on the assumption that monthly fees do not change with the number of entrants. This case requires that the entry fee differential be 118 percent.

Actuarial theory can be used to determine an infinite set of actuari-ally fair fee differentials.

Summary

This chapter described the theory and implications of the actuarial liability associated with a continuing care contract and methods for setting fees to actuarially fund that liability. The actuarial liability (PVFE) is dependent on demographic, contractual, accounting, and economic factors. For a given set of factors, the liability is fixed and cannot be altered by management. However, the fee structure used to fund the liability can be adjusted by management to match its objec-tives regarding equity, marketability, and so forth.

In summary, the methodology for funding the actuarial liability does not require that specific characteristics (e.g., sex, age, and apartment

---

[11] These differentials are independent of the pricing philosophy used.

type) be incorporated in designing a CCRC fee structure. The guidelines set forth in this chapter require that, for a group of new entrants, fees in aggregate be actuarially adequate. Actuarial theory can be used by management to develop a fee structure that reflects its philosophy without jeopardizing the community's long-term financial soundness. ■

Chapter Eight

Actuarial Valuations: Methodology for Determining Fee Adjustments

■ In the preceding chapter, actuarially adequate fees were derived from a set of underlying assumptions, including future mortality, morbidity, inflation, and interest. If the community's experience were to follow these assumptions exactly and if fees were increased according to the inflation assumption, then the community would maintain its actuarially adequate position. Since this is an unlikely scenario, management needs a tool to assess the financial consequences of annual experience "deviations" so that fees can be adjusted accordingly. The actuarial valuation methodology, which is traditionally applied to pension plans for setting annual contributions to keep the plans actuarially sound, is the approach the authors recommend for generating the needed information for making CCRC fee adjustments.

The authors believe that the age of a community can have an impact on the frequency with which actuarial valuations should be undertaken and the manner in which the results are used. For a *maturing* CCRC, where expenses for continuing care contractholders are increasing faster than their corresponding revenues because of the adoption of inflation-constrained monthly fees, management will need to examine the relationship between its long-term assets and liabilities annually. In this case, the community's demographic profile is changing rapidly, generating significant and frequent shifts in the asset/liability relationship. By closely monitoring this relationship, management may be able to make relatively minor annual fee adjustments for eliminating any imbalance, whereas, if such adjustments are not made, more severe changes might be required in the future.

149

For a *mature* CCRC, where the rate of increase in expenses and revenues has stabilized and is approximately equal to the rate of increase in revenues, there is less of a need for annual valuations since the asset/liability relationship is less likely to change as quickly or as much as is the case for a maturing CCRC. Moreover, if an actuarial imbalance exists between assets and liabilities, the long-term financial position for a mature community may not be seriously threatened, provided the community's cash flow is projected to be adequate and management intends to offer continuing care contracts throughout the indefinite future. Therefore, in the authors' judgment, it is reasonable to make a different use of the valuation results for each CCRC, depending on its age and other financial characteristics, and possibly even to apply a different type of valuation philosophy regarding the definition of future liabilities to communities that differ in age.

One by-product of an actuarial valuation is the determination of the actuarial reserves that should be held by a CCRC. Conceptually, actuarial reserves are the amount a community should hold to offset the difference between its future expenses and its future revenues. The assets backing up an actuarial reserve may be both liquid, such as cash, and nonliquid, such as land and physical plant. One financial issue not addressed by actuarial valuations is the desired level of liquid assets. The liquid asset issue is often raised by legislators who wish to establish funding requirements for actuarial reserves. The "correct" amount of liquid assets, which depends on the community's debt load and the proportion of revenues generated from monthly fees versus entry fees, can be determined through accounting and/or cash management techniques. Nevertheless, it is generally true that an actuarially priced CCRC will generate liquid assets far in excess of those deemed necessary from an accounting viewpoint. Thus, there will be little concern over liquid asset requirements for a CCRC in actuarial balance under the closed-group approach.

THEORY OF ACTUARIAL VALUATIONS

Actuarial valuations compare a CCRC's aggregate assets with its aggregate liabilities. Aggregate assets are the community's tangible assets (liquid assets and physical plant) plus the present value of future monthly revenues, which can be considered an intangible or prospective asset. Aggregate liabilities, on the other hand, are the community's current and long-term liabilities plus the present value of future expenses associated with the services promised to continuing care contractholders. If aggregate assets equal aggregate liabilities, the community's pricing structure is in actuarial balance and monthly fees need be increased only by the community's inflation rate (i.e., the community's internal inflation rate) in order to maintain this balance. If aggregate assets are less than aggregate liabilities, then monthly fees would have to be increased by more than the assumed inflation rate to bring the community into actuarial balance, and vice versa.

It was pointed out previously that there is more than one way to define a community's future liabilities, resulting in two types of valuations: (1) closed-group and (2) open-group. The liability calculation under the closed-group method takes into account *current* residents only. This means that the present value of future expenses is derived from an expense projection that may extend for 30 years or more to reflect the probability that some residents may live for that length of time. The liabilities and corresponding assets associated with new entrants are ignored. Valuations using the closed-group approach test whether the community's tangible and prospective assets on behalf of *current* residents equal their existing and future liabilities. This method is consistent with a management policy to minimize intergenerational subsidies, implying a self-supporting fee structure. Moreover, a pricing policy meeting this test will generate sufficient resources for management to liquidate the continuing care obligations for existing residents without having to increase future fees by more than inflation.

The open-group method differs from the closed-group method in two respects. First, the financial impact of new entrants is taken into consideration. Under the closed-group method, new entrants are assumed to be priced on a break-even basis and, thus, are assumed to have no financial consequence.[1] New entrants can generate either a positive or negative financial impact under the open-group method. Second, the CCRC's liability is based on both current and future residents *over a fixed time period*. The authors recommend that this time period be at least 15 years to ensure that decisions are based on a stabilized pattern of revenues and expenses. An actuarially balanced position using this method could be achieved with lower fees than those required under the closed-group method because the highest expenses for a group of residents (toward the end of their life span when they are likely to require health care) are deferred to future generations. Therefore, this method is consistent with the management philosophy of accepting intergenerational transfers of funds and the assumption that management will always offer continuing care contracts.

The appropriateness of either method depends on management's goals and the community's age. Achieving actuarial adequacy under the closed-group method for a mature community might be difficult if

---

[1] If the combination of entry fees and monthly fees is not adequate, the new entrant pricing methodology (see Chapter 7) would be applied to derive adequate entry fees.

previous fees were not set with this goal in mind. For such cases, an open-group valuation may be appropriate, provided that projected cash flows are adequate. Also, the open-group method may be appropriate for a maturing CCRC provided that management agrees with the above-mentioned constraints. The closed-group methodology is described in this book because it represents the highest standard for the financial evaluation of a CCRC.

Actuarial Valuation Statement

The primary question that an actuarial valuation answers is whether the community's assets are equal to its liabilities, as summarized below:

Actuarial Valuation Statement

Aggregate assets		Aggregate liabilities
1. Short-term assets		1. Short-term liabilities
+		+
2. Actuarial value of fixed assets	$\overset{?}{=}$	2. Long-term liabilities
+		+
3. Prospective assets		3. Prospective liabilities

If these two components of a CCRC are not equal, the balancing item is termed the unfunded liability (a negative unfunded liability represents a surplus).

If the relationship does not hold for a given CCRC, the results of an actuarial valuation provide guidelines on how to adjust fees to eliminate the imbalance. If an imbalance exists (particularly if aggregate assets fall short of aggregate liabilities) and management does not change its fees to eliminate that imbalance, the actuarial deficit may grow over a period of years to the point where a severe adjustment in fees would be necessary in order to prevent a financial crisis.

In this sense, an actuarial valuation serves as an early warning device, allowing management to uncover deficiencies in its pricing policies far in advance of a financial crisis. Using this tool may allow management to make relatively modest fee adjustments currently to avoid future financial problems that would require more dramatic changes. The information generated by an actuarial valuation is extremely important during the maturation period of a CCRC when a robust cash flow position, which will deteriorate in a few years, could lead management to mistakenly believe that the community is financially sound (e.g., see the cash flows associated with Case 2 in Chapter 4).

For an initial move-in population, an actuarial valuation would show that the community is in actuarial balance (i.e., the unfunded liability would be zero) if fees were based on the actuarial pricing methodology described in the preceding chapter. Moreover, if experience matches the underlying assumptions and the fees for new entrants are also actuarially determined, then future valuations would show a zero unfunded liability. To demonstrate this point, a simplified example of projected valuations on a closed group of residents follows.

Projected Closed-Group Valuation

In this example, it is assumed that the community has 100 females at age 75 entering its one-bedroom apartment units and that fees are actuarially balanced at entry. The fees for these residents involve an entry fee of $53,846 and a monthly fee of $686 (values that were derived in Chapter 7). Monthly fees are assumed to increase 10 percent annually. The actuarial liability, or PVFE, associated with these residents is $15,195,100. Table 8–1 contains projected actuarial valuations and cash flows associated with the surviving members from the original 100 residents over their potential lifetimes (to age 110) in the community.

The first three columns of Table 8–1 contain the year of operation, the age of surviving residents, and the number of surviving residents. The next three columns contain items from the cash flow projection based on the surviving residents: total revenues, total expenses, and net cash flow. The last four columns contain items included in an actuarial valuation statement: aggregate assets, which consist of liquid assets and the present value of future revenues (PVFR); aggregate liabilities which in this example include only the present value of future expenses (PVFE); and the unfunded liability.

The flow through this table is explained as follows. Liquid assets are initially $5,385,000, a value equal to the sum of all entry fees paid by the 100 entrants. Liquid asset values in future years are calculated by adding the net cash flow, equal to the difference between revenues and expenses, to the prior year's liquid asset balance. The present value of future revenues (PVFR) is the discounted value (discounted for both interest and mortality) of future monthly fees to be collected from current residents. The present value of future expenses is the discounted value of the costs of providing shelter and health care to surviving residents. During the first year, this value equals the sum of liquid assets and PVFR, or $15,195,000, since the fee structure was established to be in actuarial balance. The unfunded liability for each year is determined by subtracting aggregate assets from aggregate liabilities.

Several observations can be made from this table. First, a long-term projection is mandatory for financial analysis of continuing care con-

154

TABLE 8–1
Projected Cash Flow and Actuarial Valuation Statements
for 100 Age-75 Female Entrants *($000)*

			Cash flow		
Year (t)	Age (x)	Number of survivors	Total revenues	Total expenses	Net income
0	75	100.0	—	—	—
1	76	98.7	$1,413	$1,290	$ 123
2	77	97.1	1,497	1,376	121
3	78	95.3	1,582	1,471	111
4	79	93.1	1,669	1,574	95
5	80	90.6	1,755	1,686	69
6	81	87.6	1,837	1,803	34
7	82	84.1	1,911	1,924	(13)
8	83	80.0	1,975	2,045	(70)
9	84	75.5	2,025	2,162	(137)
10	85	70.3	2,055	2,267	(212)
11	86	64.6	2,066	2,299	(233)
12	87	58.5	2,050	2,356	(306)
13	88	51.9	2,003	2,376	(373)
14	89	45.1	1,920	2,353	(433)
15	90	38.2	1,803	2,278	(475)
16	91	31.5	1,655	2,152	(497)
17	92	25.3	1,480	1,978	(498)
18	93	19.8	1,291	1,767	(476)
19	94	15.0	1,096	1,533	(437)
20	95	11.1	906	1,292	(386)
21	96	8.1	731	1,059	(328)
22	97	5.7	443	846	(270)
23	98	3.9	443	659	(216)
24	99	2.6	332	501	(169)
25	100	1.7	244	372	(128)
26	101	1.1	174	268	(94)
27	102	0.7	121	188	(67)
28	103	0.4	80	127	(47)
29	104	0.2	53	83	(30)
30	105	0.1	31	51	(20)
31	106	0.1	19	30	(11)
32	107	0.0*	11	17	(6)
33	108	0.0*	5	9	(4)
34	109	0.0*	3	4	(1)
35	110	0.0*	0.8	1.7	(0.9)

* Less than 0.1, but greater than 0.

tracts since a significant portion of residents will survive 10 years or more. In this example, more than 10 percent of the original group survives for at least 20 years. Second, the actuarial liability for a group of residents increases for the first few years after entry even though not all the residents survive. Third, and perhaps most important, the un-

Aggregate assets

Liquid assets	PVFR	Aggregate liabilities PVFE	Unfunded liability
$5,385	$ 9,810	$15,195	$0
5,508	10,066	15,574	0
5,629	10,273	15,902	0
5,740	10,422	16,162	0
5,835	10,503	16,338	0
5,904	10,507	16,411	0
5,938	10,423	16,361	0
5,925	10,244	16,169	0
5,855	9,963	15,818	0
5,718	9,577	15,295	0
5,506	9,086	14,592	0
5,273	8,495	13,768	0
4,967	7,815	12,782	0
4,594	7,060	11,654	0
4,161	6,257	10,418	0
3,686	5,430	9,116	0
3,189	4,611	7,800	0
2,691	3,829	6,520	0
2,215	3,109	5,324	0
1,778	2,468	4,246	0
1,392	1,916	3,308	0
1,064	1,455	2,519	0
794	1,080	1,874	0
578	782	1,360	0
409	553	962	0
281	380	661	0
187	253	440	0
120	162	282	0
73	100	173	0
43	58	101	0
23	33	56	0
12	17	29	0
6	8	14	0
2	4	6	0
1	1	2	0
0.1	0.3	0.4	0

funded liability is zero for every year during the projection. In other words, an actuarial valuation of current residents who enter at different years is expected to have a zero unfunded liability, provided fees are in actuarial balance and experience follows the underlying assumptions.

ACTUARIAL VALUATION: NUMERICAL EXAMPLE

The preceding example was based on the simplistic assumption that all residents were of the same sex and age at entry and that all assets and expenses were expressed in terms of cash. In reality, a community will consist of both males and females whose ages may range from 65 to 100. Also, some of the community's assets will be held in nonliquid items such as buildings and equipment. Values for these assets must be expressed in terms of their actuarial equivalents.[2] Table 8–2 contains a more realistic actuarial valuation based on a hypothetical community serving 350 residents.

Assets are given on the left-hand side and liabilities on the right-hand side of the valuation statement. In this example, aggregate assets and liabilities are separated into three components, as described below.[3] The unfunded liability, equal to the difference between aggregate liabilities and assets, is recorded on the liability side of the valuation statement.

Aggregate Assets

Short-Term Assets. Short-term assets typically include cash, marketable securities, inventory, and accounts receivable. These items are recorded at their market value to reflect their current economic worth to the community. This example has two short-term assets, cash (component 1*a*) and trusteed funds (component 1*b*). Cash, which equals the portion of entry fees not used for plant financing plus working capital and contingency funds, is slightly less than $5 million. The trusteed funds are approximately $6 million and are equal to the debt service reserve required by the financing agreement. Total short-term assets equal $10,629,917, or 17.2 percent of aggregate assets.

Actuarial Value of Fixed Assets. The actuarial value of fixed assets (AVFA) represents the present value of services provided by fixed assets for investments in land, buildings, equipment, and furnishings and amortization of start-up costs. In future years, the actuarial values for additions or improvements to fixed assets are added to this component and deductions are made according to an actuarial amortization schedule. Initially, the building value (component 2*b*), which includes construction plus start-up costs, is the largest portion of the AVFA. The building value in this example is almost $19 million, or 91.7 percent

---

[2] The actuarial equivalent value for a fixed asset is based on the method used to expense that asset. The actuarial value for a fixed asset is defined to be the present value of expenses associated with that asset over its remaining useful lifetime.

[3] In some cases, an additional liability is recorded for fund balances. This component would include liabilities for future asset replacement and for contingencies.

TABLE 8–2

Actuarial Valuation Statement
XYZ RETIREMENT COMMUNITY
As of December 31, 1982

Assets

1. Short-term assets:
   a. Cash.................................. $ 4,679,917 — 7.6%
   b. Reserved funds .... 5,950,000 — 9.6
      Total liquid assets.................. 10,629,917 — 17.2

2. Actuarial value of fixed assets:
   a. Land .... 500,000 — 0.8
   b. Buildings............................ 18,750,000 — 30.4
   c. Equipment and furnishings .... 1,200,000 — 2.0
      Total fixed assets .... 20,450,000 — 33.2

3. Prospective assets:
   a. Present value of
      future revenues (PVFR)............... 30,571,322 — 49.6
   b. Present value of supplemental fees ... 0 — 0.0
      Total prospective assets .... 30,571,322 — 49.6

   Aggregate assets........................ $61,651,239 — 100.0%

Liabilities

1. Short-term liabilities:
   a. Current portion of debt .... $ 62,155 — 0.1%
      Total short-term liabilities......... 62,155 — 0.1

2. Long-term liabilities:
   a. Debt................................. 14,937,845 — 24.2
      Total long-term liabilities.......... 14,937,845 — 24.2

3. Prospective liabilities:
   a. Present value of
      future expenses (PVFE)............... 46,651,239 — 75.7
   b. Unamortized actuarial losses (gains).. 0 — 0.0
      Total prospective liabilities .... 46,651,239 — 75.7

   Aggregate liabilities.................. $61,651,239 — 100.0%
   Unfunded liabilities................... 0 — 0

of the combined fixed asset values. The total AVFA is $20,450,000, or 33.2 percent of aggregate assets.

Prospective Assets. Prospective assets represent the actuarial value of future revenues to be received from current residents. This component includes the present value of future monthly fees or revenues (PVFR) and the present value of supplemental monthly fees, if any, that are required to fund experience deviations (see later discussion).[4] The PVFR is equal to $30.6 million in this example, while the value for supplemental fees is zero since the initial pricing structure was designed to be in actuarial balance. Total prospective assets are 49.6% of the aggregate assets.

Aggregate Liabilities

Short-Term Liabilities. Short-term liabilities represent those amounts that will become due in the current year. Examples are the current portion of debt, accounts payable, and accrued wages. The value recorded for the current portion of debt (component 1*a*) is $62,155. The value of other short-term liabilities is assumed to be zero and is not recorded on this statement. Typically, short-term liabilities in this example will be an insignificant portion of aggregate liabilities, and in this case amount to less than 0.1 percent.

Long-Term Liabilities. Long-term liabilities are liabilities payable over a period of years but are not contingent on the survival of current residents (the value for the latter liability is recorded under prospective liabilities). The primary component of long-term liabilities is debt (component 2*a*). Debt, which is about $15 million, is the only long-term liability in this illustrative example, representing 24.2 percent of aggregate liabilities.

Prospective Liabilities. Prospective liabilities consist of the present value of future expenses (PVFE, component 3*a*) and, if any, unamortized actuarial gains or losses (component 3*b*). The PVFE, which totals $46.7 million, is the major element of prospective liabilities. Table 8–3 shows a breakdown of the PVFE by cost center and type of expense. Future health care expenses in this example represent 37.5 percent of the total expenses, while future apartment expenses represent 62.5 percent. Note that the total present value of future *operating* expenses in Table 8–3 ($13,930,463 + $16,640,869 = $30,571,322) is equal to the present value of future revenues (i.e., monthly fees) in Table 8–2, by definition of the pricing philosophy.

---

[4] Other revenue sources that might be included with this component include the present value of future reimbursement from outside agencies and the present value of any voluntary contributions from residents.

TABLE 8-3 ───────────────────────────────
Present Value of Future Expenses by Cost Center and Type

Type of expense	Amount	Percentage of total PVFE
Health care cost center:*		
Operating	$13,930,463	29.9%
Building	1,988,920	4.3
Building replacement	4	0.0
Land	52,468	0.0
Original equipment and furnishings	296,273	0.6
Equipment replacement	595,095	1.3
Refurbishment/modernization	646,659	1.4
Subtotal	17,509,882	37.5%
Apartment cost center:		
Operating	16,640,859	35.7
Building	10,415,211	22.3
Building replacement	3	0.0
Land	274,754	0.6
Original equipment and furnishings	651,584	1.4
Equipment replacement	572,670	1.2
Refurbishment/modernization	586,276	1.3
Subtotal	29,141,357	62.5%
Total PVFE	$46,651,239	100.0%

* These costs include all liabilities under the contract offered by the community. This liability includes only future nursing care in some communities, while in others it may include some acute or physician's care. This example is based on the assumption that the contract covers nursing care only.

No actuarial gains or losses are shown on the illustrative actuarial valuation statement in Table 8–2. Values for this component will be determined in future years by comparing the following year's *expected* actuarial position with the *realized* actuarial position. The total prospective liabilities are 75.7 percent of the aggregate liabilities.

Actuarial Reserves and Unfunded Liabilities

Actuarial reserves are equal to the difference between prospective assets and prospective liabilities.[5] Actuarial reserves represent the present value of future obligations to current contractholders that are not covered by their anticipated monthly fees. In this example, where monthly fees are assumed to be inflation-constrained, the actuarial reserve is $16,079,917 ($46,651,239 − $30,571,322).

The net assets of a community are equal to the difference between (1) short-term assets plus the actuarial value of fixed assets

───────────
[5] If the community explicitly calculates a liability for contingencies, this value would also be added to actuarial reserves.

($10,629,917 + $20,450,000) and (2) short- and long-term liabilities ($62,155 + $14,937,845). In this case, the community's net assets are equal to its reserves (i.e., $16,079,917). If net assets are equal to actuarial reserves, the community is in "actuarial balance" and has a zero unfunded liability. An actuarial imbalance exists if net assets are not equal to actuarial reserves, and the community will then have a positive or negative unfunded liability. An equivalent and easier way to determine the unfunded liability is simply to subtract aggregate assets from aggregate liabilities.

The size of a community's unfunded liability provides a barometer for assessing its long-term financial position. A small unfunded liability (less than 10 percent of aggregate assets) does not usually imply a near-term cash flow problem. However, if the liability is not funded, it will grow with the interest rate assumed in the valuation and may result in a cash flow problem in later years.

TABLE 8–4
Experimental Design for Valuation
Sensitivity Analysis

Experiment	Assumption changes
1	Baseline; no changes
2	1% increase in inflation (from 10% to 11%)
3	2% increase in inflation (from 10% to 12%)
4	1% decrease in inflation (from 10% to 9%)
5	2% decrease in inflation (from 10% to 8%)
6	1% increase in interest (from 12% to 13%)
7	2% increase in interest (from 12% to 14%)
8	1% decrease in interest (from 12% to 11%)
9	2% decrease in interest (from 12% to 10%)
10	25% increase in mortality rates
11	25% decrease in mortality rates
12	25% increase in morbidity rates
13	25% decrease in morbidity rates
14	25% increase in mortality rates and 25% decrease in morbidity rates
15	25% decrease in mortality rates and 25% increase in morbidity rates
16	2% decrease in inflation (from 10% to 8%), 25% increase in mortality rates, and 25% decrease in morbidity rates
17	2% increase in inflation (from 10% to 12%), 25% decrease in mortality rates, and 25% increase in morbidity rates
18	2% increase in interest (from 12% to 14%), 25% increase in mortality rates, and 25% decrease in morbidity rates
19	2% decrease in interest (from 12% to 10%), 25% decrease in mortality rates, and 25% increase in morbidity rates

Even though a community may have a modest unfunded liability under a given set of assumptions, management may be concerned with the relative importance of specific assumptions on the unfunded liability. In performing an actuarial valuation for CCRCs, it is a reasonable and sensible practice to generate alternative valuations under different sets of assumptions because the data base used to develop these assumptions is often not as credible as one would like to have them. This practice is referred to as a sensitivity analysis. Table 8–4 contains an experimental design for performing a sensitivity analysis that includes favorable and unfavorable changes in mortality, morbidity, inflation, and interest assumptions.

Table 8–5, which contains the results of the sensitivity analysis, shows the actuarial reserve, the unfunded liability, and the ratio of the unfunded liability to the aggregate assets. The actuarial reserve

TABLE 8–5
Sensitivity Analysis *($000)*

Experiment	Actuarial reserves*	Unfunded liability	Ratio of unfunded liability to aggregate assets
1 Baseline	$16,080	$ 0	0.0%
2 +1% inflation	16,904	834	1.3
3 +2% inflation	17,930	1,850	2.8
4 −1% inflation	15,393	(687)	(2.0)
5 −2% inflation	14,824	(1,256)	(3.6)
6 +1% interest	15,952	(1,046)	(1.7)
7 +2% interest	15,855	(1,952)	(3.4)
8 −1% interest	16,249	1,213	1.9
9 −2% interest	16,469	2,630	4.0
10 +25% mortality	14,070	(2,010)	(3.4)
11 −25% mortality	19,099	3,019	4.0
12 +25% morbidity	17,001	921	1.5
13 −25% morbidity	15,009	(1,071)	(1.7)
14 +25% mortality −25% morbidity	13,165	(2,915)	(4.8)
15 −25% mortality +25% morbidity	20,195	4,115	6.5
16 −2% inflation +25% mortality −25% morbidity	12,417	(3,663)	(6.3)
17 +2% inflation −25% mortality +25% morbidity	23,115	7,035	10.5
18 +2% interest +25% mortality −25% morbidity	13,403	(4,404)	(7.7)
19 −2% interest −25% mortality +25% morbidity	21,525	7,686	11.3

* Actuarial reserves = PVFE − PVFR.

(column 2) is the difference between the PVFE and the PVFR, representing the amount of unencumbered assets that the community should hold to be in actuarial balance. The reserve under the baseline assumptions is $16 million and ranges from $13 to $23 million under alternative assumptions. Experiments 5 through 9 show that the prospective assets and liabilities are approximately equal for the interest sensitivities since the actuarial reserve is relatively constant for these experiments.

Like the variance in actuarial reserves, the absolute value of the unfunded liability associated with unfavorable assumptions is greater than the value associated with favorable assumptions. The unfunded liability as a percentage of aggregate assets ranges from a positive 11 percent (implying an actuarial deficit) to a negative 8 percent (implying an actuarial surplus). This relatively modest range for rather significant assumption changes suggests that the continuing care concept is financially viable for small groups.

Methods for Funding Unfunded Liabilities

If a community is not in actuarial balance (i.e., there is an actuarial deficit or surplus), management can select several funding methods to eliminate the imbalance. The discussion of funding methods is based on the assumption that the community has a deficit; hence, the methods are described in terms of fee increases. If a surplus exists, similar decreases in fees are applicable. Three issues associated with the selection of the funding method are:

1. Should the deficit be eliminated (fully funded) or frozen (funding interest on deficit only)?
2. Over what time period should the funding last?
3. Should the funding come from the fees of current residents only, from the fees of prospective residents only, or from some combination of both current and prospective residents?

The decision for each of these three questions must be based on management's assessment of the impact that an additional fee increase will have on the community's marketability and the resident's morale. With regard to the elimination or freezing issue, it is clearly more desirable to eliminate the deficit whenever possible. Similarly, shorter funding periods are preferable to longer ones. As mentioned previously, there are three sources of fees for funding the deficit: current residents only, prospective residents only, or some combination of the two groups. Methods using current residents are complicated by the fact that the current residents did not create the entire deficit. Past residents may have contributed to the deficit. Thus, it is difficult to argue that only the current group should bear the additional fee increase. Moreover, from a practical viewpoint, adjusting fees for the current group to eliminate the deficit while keeping new entrant fees in line may distort the overall fee structure (e.g., the actuarially adequate entry fees associated with the higher monthly fees may be much smaller than those currently offered). Thus, it is often advisable to fund such deficits from both current and prospective entrants.

An unlimited number of methods could be devised to fund an unfunded liability. Descriptions of the four alternative actuarial funding methods illustrated in Table 8–6 are given below:

One-time percentage increase. The one-time percentage increase required to eliminate a deficit is determined by dividing the unfunded liability by the present value of monthly fees. This method eliminates the deficit on the current valuation statement.

Additional percentage increase. The additional percentage increase in monthly fees required to eliminate a deficit is determined by estimating the increase in monthly fees (over and above the assumed inflation rate) required to raise the PVFR to cover the deficit. This amount will be greater than the amount required under the one-time percentage increase divided by the length of the funding period since future revenues are lost due to mortality of current residents. This method also eliminates the deficit on the valuation statement.

Flat dollar monthly surcharge. The flat dollar monthly surcharge required to eliminate a deficit is determined by dividing the deficit by the product of an n-year level dollar annuity times the expected number of surviving residents (closed-group) or total residents (open-group). The length of the annuity is the funding period. The closed-group approach will eliminate the deficit on the valuation statement. The open-group approach (which is used in Table 8–6) will show a deficit; however, the amount of the surcharge is smaller than that for the closed-group approach.

Deficit freezing. Deficit freezing can be achieved by applying the nonincreasing surcharge method over an infinite time period. The amount of the surcharge is determined by dividing the interest rate charge on the unfunded liability by the average population. This method is applied only on an open-group basis. The size of the unfunded liability is expected to remain constant in future years; however, it poses less of a financial problem since it becomes a relatively smaller portion of the aggregate assets as the latter increase for inflation.

Table 8–6 shows four methods of funding the deficits (and surpluses) that were estimated under the sensitivity analysis. The one-time percentage increase method shows that under the best case monthly fees could be reduced by 17 percent and that under the worst case they

TABLE 8-6 ———
Percentage Increase in Fees under Alternative Funding Options to Eliminate (or Freeze) Unfunded Liabilities Derived from Sensitivity Analysis

	Methods that eliminate unfunded liability			Method that freezes unfunded liability
Experiment	One-time percentage increase	Additional percentage over inflation for five years	Flat dollar monthly surcharge for 10 years	Flat dollar monthly surcharge
1 Baseline	0.0%	0.0%	$ 0	$ 0
2 +1% inflation	2.6	0.7	31	21
3 +2% inflation	5.4	1.3	70	47
4 −1% inflation	(2.4)	(0.5)	(26)	(18)
5 −2% inflation	(4.6)	(1.1)	(47)	(33)
6 +1% interest	(3.6)	(0.9)	(41)	(29)
7 +2% interest	(7.2)	(1.8)	(78)	(58)
8 −1% interest	3.7	0.9	44	28
9 −2% interest	7.5	1.8	93	57
10 +25% mortality	(7.0)	(1.7)	(176)	(52)
11 −25% mortality	9.2	2.2	114	77
12 +25% morbidity	3.1	0.8	35	23
13 −25% morbidity	(3.4)	(0.8)	(40)	(28)
14 +25% mortality −25% morbidity	(9.8)	(2.4)	(110)	(75)
15 −25% mortality +25% morbidity −2% inflation	12.8	3.0	155	105
16 +25% mortality −25% morbidity +2% inflation	(13.7)	(3.6)	(138)	(94)
17 −25% mortality +25% morbidity +2% interest	19.6	4.3	265	179
18 +25% mortality −25% morbidity −2% interest	(16.6)	(4.4)	(176)	(129)
19 −25% mortality +25% morbidity	20.9	4.6	271	167

would have to be increased by 21 percent. The increase under the additional percentage increase method, calculated to eliminate the deficit over five-year period, is slightly more than one fifth of the one-time percentage increase. The flat dollar monthly surcharge method was calculated to eliminate the deficit in 10 years. The deficit freezing method adds a surcharge that lasts in perpetuity and is 27 to 38 percent less than the 10-year flat dollar surcharge.

In summary, the appropriate method for funding a CCRC's deficit must consider the equity to current and prospective residents, the impact on residents' morale, and the effects on the CCRC's marketability. In some cases, it may not be possible or desirable to implement a closed-group funding approach, since an open-group method can permit all persons to pay the same monthly fees regardless of the year they entered the community. The authors' view is that any funding method should strive to eliminate the deficit within five years and that the burden should probably be shared between existing residents and new entrants.

TREATMENT OF EXPERIENCE DEVIATIONS

In the preceding analysis, inflation-related increases in monthly fees were sufficient to keep the community in actuarial balance. This section describes the methodology that can be used to determine the financial effects of variations in the underlying assumptions and the adjustments required to monthly fees to account for such variations. Experience deviations considered in this paper arise from variations in: (1) mortality rates, (2) morbidity rates, (3) inflation, and (4) interest earnings.

Experience deviations are referred to as actuarial gains or losses. An actuarial gain indicates that the expected experience for the current residents was more favorable, financially, than expected and fees can be increased at a lower rate than expected. An actuarial loss indicates that experience was worse than expected and fees must be increased more than expected to maintain actuarial balance.

Fee adjustments that eliminate experience deviations may require that the group equity concept (as described in Chapter 7) be violated, at least temporarily. It is not usually feasible or desirable to fund experience deviations from the fees of current residents only. Thus, new entrants' fees can be altered to help fund financial gains and losses. The examples presented in this section are based on open-group adjustments to fees (i.e., changes to current and prospective residents' fees). The first step in calculating the amount of the adjustment is to determine the financial (or actuarial) gain or loss.

Determination of Financial Gains or Losses

Financial gains or losses are determined by comparing the actual unfunded liability for a given year with the *expected* unfunded liability, as estimated from the previous year. The actual unfunded liability is determined by performing an actuarial valuation in the current year. The *expected* unfunded liability is determined by performing an actuarial valuation on the projected survivors from the prior year plus expected new entrants. If the actual unfunded liability exceeds the expected unfunded liability, the community experienced a financial loss. If the

166

reverse is true, the community experienced a financial gain. This calculation is expressed algebraically by:

$$FG/L_t = AUL_t - EUL_t$$

where

FG/L_t = Financial gain/loss in year t
AUL_t = Actual unfunded liability for year t
EUL_t = Expected unfunded liability for year t

Table 8–7 shows a five-year projection of unfunded liabilities and actuarial gains/losses based on one cash flow iteration generated by the

TABLE 8–7
Expected and Actual Net Aggregate Assets and Liabilities from Projected Actuarial Valuations and Calculation of Financial Gains and Losses *($000)*

	Actual values			Expected values			Financial losses (gains)
Fiscal year January 1,	Aggregate liabilities	Aggregate assets	Unfunded liability	Aggregate liabilities	Aggregate assets	Unfunded liability	
1983	—	—	—	—	—	—	—
1984	$62,572	$62,875	$(303)	$65,087	$65,075	$12	$(315)
1985	65,815	66,068	(253)	66,049	66,355	(306)	53
1986	70,370	70,156	214	69,597	69,835	(238)	452
1987	74,790	74,742	48	74,337	74,031	306	(258)
1988	79,187	79,196	(9)	78,926	78,851	75	(84)

stochastic population methodology described in Chapter 6. The unfunded liability in each year is determined by deducting aggregate assets from aggregate liabilities (column 2 minus column 3). The *expected* unfunded liability is calculated in a similar manner using the values in columns 5 and 6. No values are given for the community's first fiscal year, since at least one year's experience is needed to calculate experience deviations. In the second year, the actuarial valuation shows a negative unfunded liability, or actuarial surplus, of $303,000 (column 4). The expected unfunded liability is $12,000 (column 7).[6] Consequently, the year's experience generated a $315,000 financial gain (financial gains on this table are represented by negative values). The following two years generated financial losses of $53,000 and $452,000, while the last two years generated financial gains of $258,000 and $84,000. These results illustrate that, for a small group, there can be considerable variation in annual experience.

---

[6] The reason the expected unfunded liability is not zero is that, for this iteration, the actual distribution of new entrants (i.e., single, couple, and age mix) did not equal the expected distribution.

Methods for Amortizing Financial Gains and Losses

There are two methodologies for dealing with experience deviations: (1) the supplemental fee method and (2) the buffer fund method. The supplemental fee method spreads over a period of years the monthly fee adjustments required to fund deviations. Each year the experience deviation is calculated, and adjustments to amortize that year's gain or loss are then added to the sum of the remaining adjustments from prior years. The monthly fee in the current year is last year's monthly fee increased for assumed inflation plus (or minus) the supplemental monthly fees. Under the buffer fund method, fees for the current group of residents are increased by a factor to build up a contingency reserve that is statistically expected to cover potential variation over a fixed time period. Annual deviations are applied against the contingency reserve. Periodically, the reserves are recalculated and the fees adjusted to fund any shortfall between actual and required reserves.

Supplemental Fee Method. The supplemental fee method amortizes the actuarial gain and loss over a period of years. Implementing this method requires that management decide whether supplemental fees should be level (nonincreasing) or inflation-adjusted, and the time period over which the gain or loss is to be amortized. This method implicitly applies the amortization to the fees of both current and future residents.

The first-year results from Table 8–7 show an actuarial gain of $315,000. The level dollar decrease in monthly fees would be $19 ($315,000 ÷ 4.03735 × 12 × 350 residents). If the average monthly fee in the first year was $664, the appropriate monthly fee in the second year would be $711. This amount equals the initial fees increased for an assumed inflation rate of 10 percent ($730) and reduced by the amortization amount ($19).

The same procedure is used to determine the amortization amount in future years. Although Table 8–7 did not reflect changes in the unfunded liability due to any fee changes made to amortize prior years' gains and losses, the actuarial deviations given in column 8 would have been the same if annual fee adjustments had been applied. Table 8–8 compares average monthly fees under baseline assumptions with those required to eliminate the actuarial deviations shown in Table 8–7. Columns 2 and 3 present, respectively, the average monthly fees for the baseline assumptions and the percentage increase in fees. Columns 4 through 8 show fee changes (supplemental fees) for amortizing each year's actuarial gain or loss. The average monthly fees incorporating the amortization of experience deviations, which are the sum of baseline fees plus supplemental fees, are presented in column 9. For example, the average monthly fees in 1986 are $883 − $19 + $3 + $27, for a total of $894.

TABLE 8-8
Average Monthly Fees under Baseline Assumptions and Supplemental Monthly Fees to Amortize Financial Gains and Losses

Fiscal year January 1,	Baseline monthly fee	Percent change	Supplemental fees adjustments beginning in fiscal year:					Baseline monthly fee plus supplemental fees	Percent change
			1984	1985	1986	1987	1988		
1983	$ 664	—	—	—	—	—	—	$ 664	—
1984	730	10.0%	$(19)	—	—	—	—	711	7.1%
1985	803	10.0	(19)	$3	—	—	—	787	10.7
1986	883	10.0	(19)	3	$27	—	—	894	13.6
1987	972	10.0	(19)	3	27	$(15)	—	968	8.3
1988	1,069	10.0	(19)	3	27	(15)	($5)	1,060	9.5

This approach may seem somewhat cumbersome at first, due to the need to continually track remaining adjustments to amortize prior years' gains and losses; however, monthly fees should be combined as one fee when presented to residents. The separation is merely for management purposes, enabling it to set fees in a consistent and equitable fashion.

Buffer Fund Method. This approach actuarially estimates the potential variation in actuarial reserves (PVFE − PVFR) and the corresponding fee increases required to cover the variation associated with unfavorable experience. The buffer fund should cover risks associated with the misestimation of assumptions and with random deviations from the underlying assumptions. The liability values are selected so that the expectation of cumulative deviations exceeding this amount is relatively small (e.g., less than 10 percent). This amount, referred to as the liability for contingencies, would be recorded in the fund balance component of a valuation statement (in our example, this component was omitted). Monthly fees are typically used to fund this additional liability.

Calculating the buffer fund (liability for contingencies) requires two separate tasks. The first task is to generate the liability for estimation risk. Its value is determined from the results of the sensitivity analysis. The difference between the actuarial reserves from the sensitivity analysis and the baseline actuarial reserves are weighted by a set of subjective probabilities representing the actuary's relative belief in their occurrence. The liability is set equal to the sum of the weighted differences. In the example given in Table 8–9, the weights are 10

TABLE 8–9 _____
Liability for Contingencies

Estimation risk liability	$515,000
Percentage increase in baseline PVFR	1.7%

	Confidence level			
	75%	**90%**	**95%**	**99%**
Stochastic risk liability	$170,000	$260,000	$334,000	$506,000
Percentage increase in baseline PVFR	0.6%	0.9%	1.1%	1.7%

percent for the baseline valuation and 5 percent for the other experiments. The liability for estimation risk is $515,000. Monthly fees would have to be increased 1.7 percent ($515,000 ÷ $30,571,000) to fund this liability.

Calculating the stochastic liability requires that the potential variation in mortality, morbidity, inflation, and interest be analyzed. The stochastic risk liability presented in this chapter does not include inflation and interest variations. The risk associated with variations in inflation is minimal if both monthly fees and expenses are assumed to increase with inflation. This results in offsetting effects on the actuarial reserve and creates a sort of immunization of the community against inflation rate changes.[7] With regard to interest rate variation, the sensitivity analysis indicated that the actuarial reserves were relatively insensitive to interest rate changes. This fact, coupled with the difficulty of modeling future interest rates, indicates that a calculation of interest rate variation would be of minimal value.

The approach for determining the liability for stochastic risk requires that the distribution of the actuarial reserve for *current* residents be generated for the period over which the liability will be recalculated (five years in this case). The variation in this amount is compared to the expected difference between the PVFR and the PVFE for the same period. The value recorded on the valuation statement would be based on a specific probability that unfavorable experience will exceed that amount. The lower section of Table 8–9 contains stochastic buffer funds for the 75th, 90th, 95th, and 99th percentiles. The necessary increase in monthly fees to cover this liability is determined by dividing the liability by the PVFR. For example, the 99th percentile value would also be covered by a 1.7 percent ($506,000 ÷ $30,571,000) increase in monthly fees. New entrants' fees would also fund their respective liability for stochastic risk, an amount that would be added to the buffer fund in future years.

Fees would be increased for inflation under this approach, and periodically (i.e., every three to five years) the value of the buffer fund would be recalculated, with fees being adjusted to reflect the cumulative change. An alternative method for determining the recalculation of the buffer fund is to set a corridor such that if the buffer fund falls below a specific level, it would be recalculated at that time and fees increased to bring it up to the appropriate level. This approach (as opposed to predetermined periodic evaluations) allows management to react more rapidly to trends away from the underlying assumptions.[8]

---

[7] There is a risk that annual projections for inflation may be inaccurate and, therefore, that the immunization concept would not hold. The fee adjustments for this possibility should be covered by the estimation risk liability.

[8] The above description is based on a closed-group concept that strives to maintain entrant group equity. The stochastic risk liability calculated on an open-group basis will generate smaller values for this liability. By pooling the risk among several communities on an open-group basis, it may be possible to minimize the potential liability and effect a type of reinsurance scheme. The development of such a procedure is beyond the scope of this chapter.

Whenever the size of the buffer fund is reevaluated, the community's past experience with regard to mortality, morbidity, interest, and inflation should also be examined and used to adjust prior assumptions.

Summary

Actuarial valuations are the key component of the pricing methodology for CCRCs. Even if management initially charged fees that were in actuarial balance, it is not likely that these fees would remain in actuarial balance in future years since experience would deviate from the underlying assumptions. In order to avoid financial difficulties due to unfavorable experience deviations, an actuarial valuation generates the information needed by management to make appropriate fee changes.

In the discussion of the actuarial valuation methodology, the authors analyzed the impact of changes in underlying assumptions. This sensitivity analysis provides management with an estimate of the relative importance of various assumptions and allows it to assess the potential shortfall between fees and expenses for assumptions that may not be credible and to factor that information into its financial decisions. The authors also developed several methods for determining the required fee adjustments if the community is not in actuarial balance (i.e., the community has an unfunded liability under current pricing policies). For the cases where the imbalance is associated with experience deviations, two approaches were discussed to amortize the resulting financial gain or loss.

The closed-group valuation methodology described in this chapter represents a logical extension of the new entrant pricing theory presented in Chapter 7. If management wishes to charge inflation-constrained monthly fees, then the actuarial theory presented in these two chapters provides the appropriate tools to accomplish this goal. It is desirable that all CCRCs be priced so that their long-term financial position is sound, and actuarial valuations, whether open- or closed-group, represent a tool that can help to achieve this objective. The choice between an open-group valuation and a closed-group valuation depends on the community's age, management's philosophy, and the opinion of the financial analyst. The authors' recommendation is that new or maturing CCRCs employ closed-group valuations, though the open-group method may be acceptable for mature communities. Moreover, an actuarial valuation should be performed at least once every three years, and preferably on an annual basis. ∎

Chapter Nine

Cash Flow Statements and Case Site Analysis

■ The actuarial pricing methodology developed in the preceding two chapters generated fees that are adequate over the long run for a group of residents. Since present values are used in making this calculation, it is possible, though not likely, that a community could be in actuarial balance and yet have near-term cash flow problems. The third component of the financial valuation methodology, cash flow analysis, is used to determine whether an actuarially adequate pricing policy also meets the community's short-term cash expenditure obligations.

The purpose of this chapter is to explore the cash flow implications over a 20-year period of charging actuarially adequate fees. The cash flow projections are based on the stochastic projection methodology explained in Chapter 6, the fees developed in Chapter 7, and the expense assumptions presented in Appendix C. The chapter also includes the application of actuarial valuation, pricing, and cash flow projection methodologies to the six case studies.

CASH FLOW STATEMENTS

The methodology for developing a cash flow projection is straightforward. It requires that cash sources and uses be estimated annually, with the difference between the two being added to the preceding year's cash balance to generate the next year's balance. This process is repeated for each year of the forecast.

For many organizations, cash flow projections can be made simply by extrapolating current revenues and expenses into the future. In these cases, management's primary concern is the selection of appropriate assumptions, such as future inflation and interest. Since the future is uncertain, several projections might be made with alternative sets of assumptions.

Cash flow projections for CCRCs also require assumptions for future interest and inflation rates. However, such forecasts are further complicated by the dynamics of future population flows which have a direct impact on revenues and expenses. Thus, management must project apartment turnover and health care utilization as accurately as possible.[1] Since CCRCs are typically small (in numbers of residents), random deviations from the expected experience can also have a significant impact on cash flows, and the effects of such random deviations should be examined in a cash flow projection. Moreover, due to the deferred incidence of expenses (especially health care expenses) for a group of residents, cash flow projections over a short period of time may provide misleading information by showing a community to be cash rich when in reality its long-run financial status is questionable. Therefore, CCRC cash flow projections should be of sufficient length (e.g., 20 years or more) to uncover any hidden deficiencies in the current pricing policy.

Actuarial Cash Flow Projection

Table 9–1 shows a detailed cash flow projection for the hypothetical CCRC that has adopted actuarially adequate fees according to the real estate/actuarial approach.[2] Monthly fees, which are set to cover operating expenses, are assumed to increase *10 percent per year,* while entry fees, which are set to cover capital expenses, have a variable increase rate of from *2.6 percent to 10.0 percent* over the 20 years, with an average rate of increase equal to 5.5 percent. Interest income is derived by assuming a 12 percent return on investments. Operating expenses are assumed to increase at the same rate as monthly fees, or 10 percent. Capital expenditures include a level dollar debt service amount ($1,662,000) plus an amount for capital improvements (equipment replacement and refurbishment expenditures) that increases annually at 10 percent and is initially $270,000.[3]

---

[1] See Chapter 6 for a discussion of population projection methodology.

[2] This financial statement differs slightly from the standard CCRC Statement of Changes in Financial Position, which usually begins with the bottom line from the Statement of Revenues and Expenses and Changes in Fund Balance and removes noncash expenditures while incorporating capital expenditures not included in the income statement. The format in Table 9–1 has been chosen for pedagogic purposes and is similar to the income statement presented later.

[3] Admittedly, a new community would not need these expenditures during its early years. However, for convenience, it is assumed that such amounts are spent. In practice, the unused amounts would be reserved for future capital expenditures.

TABLE 9–1
Twenty-Year Projection of Statements of Changes in Financial Position Using Actuarial Fees ($000)

Fiscal year	Cash sources				Cash uses			Increase (decrease) in working capital	End-of-year cash balance
	Monthly fees = operating revenues*	Entry fees	Interest income	Total sources	Operating expenses	Capital expenditures	Total uses		
1983	$ 3,775	$ 0	$1,181	$ 4,956	$ 2,628	$1,932	$ 4,560	$ 396	$11,026†
1984	3,893	704	1,292	5,889	2,891	1,959	4,850	1,039	12,065
1985	4,043	823	1,411	6,277	3,180	1,989	5,169	1,108	13,173
1986	4,217	919	1,535	6,671	3,498	2,022	5,520	1,151	14,324
1987	4,383	1,085	1,667	7,135	3,848	2,058	5,906	1,229	15,553
1988	4,616	1,110	1,794	7,520	4,232	2,098	6,330	1,190	16,743
1989	4,939	1,311	1,944	8,194	4,656	2,141	6,797	1,397	18,140
1990	5,267	1,360	2,095	8,722	5,121	2,189	7,310	1,412	19,552
1991	5,636	1,471	2,255	9,362	5,633	2,242	7,875	1,487	21,039
1992	5,993	1,845	2,447	10,285	6,197	2,299	8,496	1,789	22,828
1993	6,481	1,895	2,644	11,020	6,816	2,363	9,179	1,841	24,669
1994	7,050	2,153	2,874	12,077	7,498	2,433	9,931	2,146	26,815
1995	7,688	1,994	3,090	12,772	8,248	2,510	10,758	2,014	28,829
1996	8,403	2,444	3,362	14,209	9,072	2,595	11,667	2,542	31,371
1997	9,148	2,583	3,653	15,384	9,980	2,688	12,668	2,716	34,087
1998	9,907	2,851	3,970	16,728	10,978	2,790	13,768	2,960	37,047
1999	10,948	3,085	4,333	18,366	12,075	2,904	14,979	3,387	40,434
2000	12,071	3,687	4,787	20,545	13,283	3,027	16,310	4,235	44,669
2001	13,341	3,439	5,242	22,022	14,611	3,162	17,775	4,247	48,916
2002	14,675	3,938	5,778	24,391	16,072	3,314	19,386	5,005	53,921

* These revenues include monthly fees from continuing care contractholders and per diem revenues from outside patients in the health care center.
† Assumed community has $10,630,000 in cash from original financing.

The projection shows for each year the increase in working capital, which is slightly less than $2 million after 10 years and slightly more than $5 million after 20 years. The cash balance increases from $11 million at the start to $54 million after 20 years. This amount, which may appear unduly large, is not an accumulation of profits.[4] The amount will be shown to be necessary to place the community in actuarial balance and represents a portion of the reserves required for future shelter and health care obligations for current residents. In fact, the ratio of the end-of-year cash balance to total sources is a constant 2.2 throughout the projection, indicating an equilibrium cash flow situation. It should be noted that the amount is expressed in terms of inflated dollars, based on a 10 percent inflation rate. In real terms (i.e., adjusting for inflation), the cash balance at the end of the forecast period is somewhat less than it was at the beginning ($8,016,000).

Ratio Analysis under Actuarial Fees

One methodology often used to interpret financial projections is ratio analysis. The ratios are constructed from data contained in an organization's financial statements. They are primarily used for purposes of comparison with ratios from similar organizations in the same industry. Also, they are frequently used in feasibility studies. The ratios include, but are not limited to, the debt service coverage ratio, the cash to annual debt service ratio, and the cash to debt ratio.

Table 9–2 contains three ratios for the hypothetical CCRC projected for 20 years. Normally, a debt service coverage ratio of 1.00 is considered good, since it indicates the relative ease with which a community will be able to meet its debt payments. The actuarial cash flows have excellent ratios, always greater than 1 and increasing to more than 2 within nine years.[5] The cash to annual debt service ratio, which measures the size of the reserves the community has to cover debt, is extremely high, starting in excess of 6 times debt service and increasing to more than 30 times. The third ratio, cash to remaining debt, measures the community's ability to retire the debt, a ratio of 1.00 being excellent. This ratio is achieved by the actuarially priced CCRC within five years.

Based on traditional ratio analysis guidelines, the cash flow projection associated with actuarial fees shows the community to be financially sound. In fact, such guidelines are greatly exceeded, and management might be led to believe that fee reductions are appropriate.

---

[4] All examples in this book are based on a 501(c)(3) nonprofit CCRC since 99 percent of all existing CCRCs are so structured.

[5] The ratios in the first years may be somewhat optimistic since an immediate fill-up was assumed for pedagogic purposes; during later years, however, the ratio is fairly realistic for an actuarially priced CCRC.

TABLE 9-2
Ratio Analysis of Actuarially Priced CCRC

Fiscal year	Debt service coverage ratio	Cash to annual debt service ratio*	Cash to debt ratio
1983	1.24	5.63	0.74
1984	1.63	6.26	0.81
1985	1.67	6.93	0.89
1986	1.69	7.62	0.97
1987	1.74	0.36	1.06
1988	1.72	9.07	1.14
1989	1.84	9.91	1.25
1990	1.85	10.76	1.35
1991	1.89	11.66	1.48
1992	2.08	12.74	1.62
1993	2.11	13.84	1.77
1994	2.29	15.13	1.96
1995	2.21	16.35	2.14
1996	2.53	17.88	2.37
1997	2.63	19.51	2.63
1998	2.78	21.29	2.92
1999	3.04	23.33	3.28
2000	3.55	25.88	3.73
2001	3.56	28.43	4.24
2002	4.01	32.44	4.88

* Excludes debt service reserve funds, which equal maximum annual debt service requirement.

However, this is not the case, as will be shown later. The drawback of ratio analyses is that, even though they may be useful for setting minimum standards, they are heavily dependent on a component that remains constant over time (debt service), whereas other elements are increasing for inflation.[6] This results in unusually high ratio values in future years. Therefore, taken alone, ratio analyses can present a misleading picture of the community's financial position.

The authors believe that the appropriate procedure for justifying substantial cash balances is to perform actuarial valuations on projected population censuses. The current cash balance plus any unfunded liability derived by an actuarial valuation is the appropriate size for the community's total cash reserves under the current pricing policy. To illustrate this procedure, actuarial valuations are performed on

[6] The ratios presented in Table 9-2 should not be taken as standards for all actuarially priced CCRCs. The level of debt has a direct impact on these ratios. This example was based on financing that covered slightly more than 50 percent of the total uses of funds. Higher financing percentages would result in lower ratios, but these would still be significantly higher than the guidelines typically used with ratio analysis. The development of ratio guidelines for CCRCs is an important topic for further research.

the beginning-of-year census from a single iteration of the stochastic cash flow model.[7] The results are presented in Table 9–3.

Aggregate assets are given in columns 2 through 5, and aggregate liabilities are given in columns 6 through 8. Liquid assets, which are primarily cash, start at $10 million and increase to slightly less than $40 million after 20 years. Note that the cash balance is $14 million less than the cash balance generated under the expected projection in Table 9–1. This means that, for this iteration, the community is expected to have an unfunded liability. The size of that unfunded liability is given in column 9. The total liquid assets that should be held by the community are given in column 10, which is the sum of columns 2 and 9. At the end of 20 years, the community should hold $52 million.[8]

This methodology confirms that the substantial cash balances that will be generated for an actuarially priced CCRC are needed to offset deferred obligations. By employing annual valuations, management can use the result to justify the need for fee changes to residents. While this technique may be easy to implement for a new community, there may be some difficulties in applying it to an existing CCRC, as discussed in the following section.

ACTUARIAL PRICING METHODOLOGY APPLIED TO CASE STUDIES

This section presents the results of: (1) an application of actuarial valuations to six actual communities, (2) an evaluation of the actuarial adequacy of fees for new entrants to these communities, and (3) the expected cash flow under each community's current pricing policy as well as under the fee modifications suggested by the actuarial valuation analysis. The six communities are different in age and characteristics but *are not* necessarily representative of the CCRC universe. Thus, the observations regarding the results of these communities *are not* necessarily applicable to other communities. Attempts to use the conclusions and recommendations with regard to these communities, or to make inferences from these results that are not explicitly stated by the authors, could lead to serious error. The purpose of this analysis is to illustrate the actuarial methodology for those who wish to conduct similar studies.

---

[7] A single iteration is used for purposes of simplicity since the valuation associated with the expected cash flow requires that multiple valuations be performed on each iteration and then averaged. The computer cost of this is quite high, and similar conclusions can be drawn from a single iteration.

[8] This amount is not equal to the expected cash flow of $54 million shown in Table 9–1 due to variances between the expected population demographics and the actual demographics for this iteration.

TABLE 9–3
Summary of Projected Actuarial Valuation Statements ($000)

Beginning of fiscal year	Liquid assets	AVFA	PVFR	Aggregate assets	Debt	PVFE	Aggregate liabilities	Unfunded liability	Target liquid asset total
1983	$10,630	$20,450	$ 30,571	$ 61,651	$15,000	$ 46,651	$ 61,651	$ 0	$10,630
1984	11,026	20,618	31,231	62,875	14,938	47,634	62,572	(303)	10,723
1985	11,767	20,791	33,510	66,068	14,868	50,947	65,815	(253)	11,514
1986	12,708	20,968	36,480	70,156	14,790	55,580	70,370	214	12,922
1987	14,007	21,148	39,587	74,742	14,703	60,087	74,790	48	14,055
1988	15,051	21,331	42,814	79,196	14,605	64,582	79,187	(9)	15,042
1993	22,257	22,447	66,199	110,903	13,909	96,704	110,613	(290)	21,967
1998	29,687	24,307	105,886	159,880	12,683	152,606	165,289	5,409	35,096
2003	39,600	27,316	172,705	239,621	10,522	241,251	251,773	12,152	51,752

AVFA = Actuarial value of fixed assets.
PVFR = Present value of future revenues.
PVFE = Present value of future expenses.

In an effort not to overburden the reader, the data generated by an actuarial investigation have been summarized in the tables contained in this section. Fee and contract provisions are presented in Table 9–4 for comparative purposes. The descriptions given for each portion of the analysis assume that the reader has a basic understanding of the methodologies explained in Chapters 7 and 8, and only the most important findings are discussed.

Actuarial Valuations of Case Studies

The baseline financial assumptions for each community were based on a review of their historical experience and their most recent financial statements. All financial assumptions are unique to the individual community except for long-term interest and inflation rates, which were selected to maintain consistency among all communities. The long-term inflation rate was assumed to be 8 percent, and the long-term interest rate was assumed to be 10 percent.[9] Aggregate liabilities for all communities include an estimate of the future financial aid requirements equal to 3 percent of the present value of future monthly fees. The present value of revenues associated with outside contributions is not reflected in the valuations since the goal of this analysis is to determine whether current fees are self-supporting (i.e., do not require subsidies).

Baseline valuation results are presented in Table 9–5. The asset section (rows 1 through 4) contains short-term assets, the actuarial value of fixed assets (AVFA), prospective assets, and aggregate (or total) assets. The liability section (rows 5 through 9) contains short-term liabilities, long-term liabilities, prospective liabilities, and aggregate (or total) liabilities. The unfunded liability, which is the difference between aggregate liabilities and aggregate assets, is given in the last row.

Reviewing the first row of this table, one finds considerable variation in the short-term asset values. The newest community, Case 4, has the largest short-term assets value of slightly under $7 million. This large value is expected due to the initial cash inflow associated with entry fees at the initial fill-up. The other communities hold between $2 million and $3 million in short-term assets, except for Case 5, which holds under $1 million. The value for Case 5 is out of line and may be indicative of an actuarial imbalance. Prospective assets as a percentage of aggregate assets (row 3 divided by row 4) range from 50 percent to 65 percent, with the new communities having smaller percentages. Pro-

---

[9] It should be noted that a 10 percent inflation rate and a 12 percent interest rate were used in the analysis presented in Chapters 7 and 8. Since the differential assumed here is also two percentage points, the results would have been quite similar if the 10 percent/12 percent assumptions had been used.

TABLE 9–4
Fee and Contract Characteristics of Case Studies

Characteristic	Case 1	Case 2	Case 3	Case 4	Case 5	Case 6
Entry fee range						
Minimum	$20,400	$33,265	$16,500	$33,900	$29,120	$24,950
Maximum	69,000	88,210	53,515	76,900	70,195	68,950
Weighted entry fee*	$36,511	$42,343	$25,023	$54,393	$44,453	$45,822
Monthly fee range						
Minimum	$ 660	$ 626	$ 666	$ 428	$ 426	$ 290
Maximum	1,423	1,460	1,444	1,033	914	720
Weighted monthly fee*	$ 784	$ 724	$ 797	$ 658	$ 519	$ 418
Meals included with standard fees	3	3	3	1	1	0
Death refund provisions included?	Yes	Yes	No	Yes	Yes	No
Period	12 months	3 months	N/A	84 months	84 months	N/A
Withdrawal/refund provisions included?	Yes	Yes	Yes	Yes	Yes	Yes
Period	50 months	50 months	100 months	84 months	84 months	60 months

* The weighted fee is an average of one-person fees weighted by apartment type.

TABLE 9–5 ————————————————————————————————————
Baseline Actuarial Valuation Statements *($000)*

Valuation component	Case 1	Case 2	Case 3	Case 4	Case 5	Case 6
1. Short-term assets	$ 2,552	$ 2,559	$ 2,786	$ 6,911	$ 670	$ 2,128
2. AVFA	12,573	13,251	15,020	18,981	10,624	9,447
3. Prospective assets	28,859	30,759	31,162	31,355	12,176	19,701
4. Aggregate assets	$43,984	$46,569	$48,968	$57,247	$23,470	$31,276
5. Short-term liabilities	$ 1,276	$ 1,168	$ 735	$ 566	$ 2,360	$ 525
6. Long-term liabilities	4,501	4,333	6,217	10,777	7,571	5,147
7. Prospective liabilities	40,552	43,969	34,520	41,678	19,584	26,849
8. Aggregate liabilities	$46,329	$49,470	$41,472	$53,021	$29,515	$32,521
9. Unfunded liability (8 − 4)	$ 2,345	$ 2,901	$(7,496)	$(4,226)	$ 6,045	$ 1,245

spective liabilities, which reflect only expenses for services promised in the continuing care contract, as a percentage of aggregate liabilities (row 7 divided by row 8) are over 80 percent for all the communities that are five years old or older and under 80 percent for the new communities (Cases 4 and 5). Cases 5 and 6 have a relatively small prospective liability since their contracts do not cover three meals per day and their expected health care utilizations are relatively low, thus understating the potential liability.[10]

Four communities have actuarial deficits or unfunded liabilities. The unfunded liabilities for Cases 1, 2, and 6 are fairly modest, ranging from $1 million to $3 million. The unfunded liability in these cases is less than 10 percent of the aggregate assets. Case 5 has an extremely large unfunded liability, slightly more than $6 million. This liability is more than 25 percent of the aggregate assets and will probably be associated with a near-term financial crisis[11] unless the fees are changed drastically, since the deficit is similar to an interest-bearing debt and will grow at 10 percent per year.

Two communities, Cases 3 and 4, show actuarial surpluses (i.e., negative unfunded liabilities). One of the communities is fairly old, and its surplus is partly due to a gain on the valuation of debt which was obtained at a substantially lower interest rate (5 percent) than the valuation interest rate. This may be the case for the valuations of many mature communities, which would make them more likely to be in actuarial balance even if their fees were not derived on an actuarial

---

[10] Refer to Chapter 5 for a discussion of the derivation of the mortality and morbidity rates for these communities.

[11] A definitive statement cannot be made until the adequacy of new entrants' fees has been examined.

basis. Of course, this hypothesis can only be verified by performing actuarial valuations on a much larger sample of CCRCs.

Table 9–6 presents the ratio of the unfunded liability to aggregate assets for an 11-experiment sensitivity analysis. This experimental de-

TABLE 9–6
Sensitivity Analysis of Variation in Ratio of Unfunded Liability to Aggregate Assets

Experiment		Case 1	Case 2	Case 3	Case 4	Case 5	Case 6
1	Baseline	5.3%	6.2%	(15.3)%	(7.4)%	25.8%	4.0%
2	1% inflation increase	6.4	7.9	(17.1)	(8.7)	27.1	4.1
3	1% inflation decrease	4.4	4.7	(13.3)	(9.6)	24.6	3.9
4	25% mortality increase	(0.2)	0.8	(18.0)	(11.0)	22.3	(0.3)
5	25% mortality decrease	13.0	13.5	(11.6)	(2.3)	31.0	10.3
6	25% morbidity increase	7.8	8.5	(14.5)	(5.9)	27.4	6.3
7	25% morbidity decrease	2.6	3.6	(16.1)	(9.0)	24.0	1.4
8	25% mortality increase and 25% morbidity decrease	(2.3)	(1.4)	(18.6)	(12.3)	20.9	(2.3)
9	25% mortality decrease and 25% morbidity increase	16.1	16.3	(10.6)	(0.3)	33.2	13.3
10	1% inflation decrease, 25% mortality increase, and 25% morbidity decrease	(3.1)	(2.5)	(20.2)	(14.2)	20.1	(2.9)
11	1% inflation increase, 25% mortality decrease, and 25% morbidity increase	17.6	18.5	(7.7)	(1.5)	35.1	13.7

sign reflects changes in the mortality, morbidity, and inflation rates. The best and worst case assumptions are contained in experiments 10 and 11, respectively. Cases 1, 2, and 6 show actuarial surpluses (i.e., negative ratios) under the best case assumptions even though the baseline valuation (experiment 1) generated an actuarial deficit. In no case did the variation in the ratios exceed 12 percentage points. This observation suggests that, even with substantial variations in assumptions, the continuing care concept is relatively stable.

Table 9–7 presents the fee adjustments under four funding methods to eliminate the unfunded liability associated with the baseline valuations. The funding methods are: (1) a one-time percentage increase, (2) an additional percentage increase over 5 years, (3) a flat dollar monthly surcharge for 10 years, and (4) a flat dollar surcharge to freeze the deficit.[12] In order to compare the flat dollar increase methods (3 and 4) with the percentage increase methods (1 and 2), percentage increases are derived for the flat dollar methods based on the weighted one-person monthly fees (refer to Table 9–4). These percentages are given in brackets under their respective flat dollar amounts. In Case 1, for example, the one-time percentage increase is 8.4%,[13] while the per-

---

[12] These methods are described in detail in Chapter 8.

[13] This percentage is adjusted for expected loss of future revenues associated with the financial aid liability.

TABLE 9–7
Funding Alternatives to Eliminate Baseline Unfunded Liability

Funding method	Case 1	Case 2	Case 3	Case 4	Case 5	Case 6
One-time percentage increase	8.4%	10.1%	(24.8%)	(13.9%)	51.2%	6.3%
Additional percentage increase (5 years)	2.2%	2.5%	(7.1%)	(3.7%)	10.7%	1.7%
Flat-dollar monthly surcharge (10 years)*	$77 [9.8%]	$78 [10.8%]	($225) [(28.2%)]	($119) [(18.1%)]	$321 [61.8%]	$30 [7.2%]
Flat-dollar deficit freezing*	$47 [6.0%]	$50 [6.9%]	($140) [(17.6%)]	($75) [(11.4%)]	$199 [38.3%]	$18 [4.3%]

* Values in brackets represent percentage change of single-resident fee for smallest one-bedroom unit.

centage increase of one-bedroom fees under the flat dollar monthly surcharge is initially 9.8 percent. However, this percentage will decrease under the flat dollar method because it remains constant while the underlying monthly fees (i.e., the portion not identified as a surcharge) increase with inflation.

The largest percentage increase is associated with Case 5, which also has the largest unfunded liability and requires a one-time increase of 50 percent in monthly fees to bring the community into actuarial balance. Such an increase is unlikely to be tolerable, as is the alternative of spreading the increase over five years, which would require an additional 10 percent plus the normal inflation increase. Alternative methods must be used to handle the extremely large deficit. This case illustrates the consequences of a small deficit that is left unfunded and allowed to grow. Cases 1, 2, and 6 require minor increases in fees to eliminate the actuarial imbalance if these increases are spread over five years. Monthly fees for Cases 3 and 4 could be reduced by more than 10 percent without jeopardizing the financial health of these communities.

Fee changes should not be based solely on the results of a valuation since it is generally desirable to charge both current and prospective residents the same monthly fees. It is likely that changes in current residents' monthly fees, as suggested by a valuation, will affect the actuarial adequacy of new entrants' fees. A community should examine new entrants' fees to determine whether they will reduce or increase the actuarial deficit and should make simultaneous and equal changes in the monthly fees of current residents and new entrants to eliminate the deficit. The results of such a pricing analysis of new entrants' fees are presented in the following section.

New Entrant Pricing Analysis of Case Studies

New entrant pricing analysis, which represents an actuarial valuation on an expected group of new entrants, determines the financial impact of that group on the next year's valuation statement. Table 9–8 contains the results of the pricing analysis using each community's current fees. The first row shows the present value of future revenues (PVFR) for an individual entrant weighted by the new entrant's characteristics with regard to age, sex, apartment type, and double occupancy. The PVFR is the sum of the entry fee plus the present value of future monthly fees (PVMF). All of the PVFRs are more than $100,000. The PVFEs, given in the second row, range from $80,000 to $140,000; the larger PVFEs are associated with newer communities, reflecting their higher construction costs. Row 3 shows the excess or deficiency of the PVFR over the PVFE, and row 4 expresses this difference as a percentage. For example, the PVFR for Case 1 is $146,082, and the PVFE is $140,248, which is $5,834, or 4.2 percent, redundant.

All of the communities except Case 5 have redundant new entrant fee structures. The implications for Case 5 are serious; not only is there a deficit for current residents, but new entrants add to this deficit. This is the worst possible situation for a CCRC. Cases 3 and 4 show the best possible situation; these communities have an overall surplus, and new entrants are expected to contribute to this surplus.

A redundant new entrant fee structure implies that each cohort group of entrants will automatically generate funds to help eliminate an unfunded liability. Thus, it may be possible to eliminate an unfunded liability from new entrants' fees only, without having to increase current residents' fees more than the community's inflation experience.[14] An estimate of the expected contribution that will be generated by the current year's entrants is given in row 5 of Table 9–8. The values in this row were determined by multiplying the excess of the PVFR over the PVFE (row 3) by the expected apartment turnover. Cases 2, 3, 4, and 6 all contribute more than $500,000 toward eliminating the unfunded liability, making it extremely tempting to use new entrants to fund deficits. Moreover, this unfunded liability contribution is expected to increase in future years if both entry and monthly fees are increased for inflation.

Although a fee structure may be adequate on a macro level, where all units are combined, specific fees for individual apartments and number of occupants may not be equitable. Actuarial pricing theory can also be applied to determine the equity of fees among specific apartment units and number of occupants. Table 9–9 shows the percentage redundancy (deficiency) for the most prevalent studio, one-bedroom, and two-bedroom units for one and two entrants. This table illustrates that even though fees may be adequate in the aggregate for a weighting of all apartment units, specific apartment units may show deficiencies.

---

[14] As was indicated in Chapter 8, this practice is not recommended.

TABLE 9–8

Comparison of the Present Value of Expected Revenues and Expenses for New Entrants in Fiscal Year 1982

Pricing statistics	Case 1	Case 2	Case 3	Case 4	Case 5	Case 6
PVFR* for typical entrant†	$146,082	$121,922	$109,502	$163,608	$127,419	$106,840
PVFE for typical entrant	140,248	104,554	98,984	137,417	133,149	82,063
Excess (deficiency) of PVFR over PVFE for typical entrant	$ 5,834	$ 17,368	$ 10,518	$ 26,191	$ (5,730)	$ 24,777
Percentage excess (deficiency) of PVFR over PVFE for typical entrant	4.2%	16.6%	10.6%	19.1%	(4.3%)	30.2%
Excess (deficiency) of PVFR over PVFE for expected group of entrants	$151,684	$503,672	$525,900	$680,966	($63,030)	$619,425

* PVFR = Entry fee plus present value of future monthly fees.
† Typical entrant refers to weighting of values by sex, age, apartment-type distribution, and double-occupancy percentage.

TABLE 9-9
Comparison of Percentage Excess (Deficiency) of PVFR over PVFE for Most Prevalent Apartment Units

Apartment type	Case 1	Case 2	Case 3	Case 4	Case 5	Case 6
Studio	(5.2)%	13.9%	17.5%	10.4%	(11.2)%	25.6%
One bedroom						
One person	7.8	29.8	27.6	30.2	2.2	42.5
Two persons	(5.7)	11.0	18.9	14.8	(7.3)	17.0
Two bedrooms						
One person	33.2	37.9	(7.3)	29.0	(6.0)	54.7
Two persons	2.8	20.1	(16.2)	15.8	(15.1)	29.2

The new entrant pricing analysis can be used to develop actuarially equitable fee differentials by apartment type and number of occupants. Moving to an actuarially equitable fee structure may require substantial changes in current fees, as indicated in Table 9-9. This table shows that for all cases, second-person fees (in the bedroom units) are inequitable with regard to first-person fees since their percentage excess (or deficiency) is less (or more) than the corresponding single-entrant values.

Cash Flow Projections for Case Studies

The next step in setting fees is to combine the fee changes suggested by the actuarial valuations and the new entrant pricing analysis to develop a consistent fee structure for both groups of residents that will eliminate any unfunded liability. Then the cash flows for this structure should be tested. The following discussion is based on the fee changes recommended on a macro basis (i.e., the percentage increase of all fees disregarding individual unit/occupancy inequities) to eliminate the unfunded liability and compares the 10-year cash flow projection of the recommended fees with the cash flow projection of the current fees. Adjustments to remove inequities among units are not explored in this analysis.

Table 9-10 contains the projected cash balance over the next 10 years where both current monthly and entry fees are increased with the inflation assumption. All of the communities except Case 5 are expected to have reasonable cash balances during the next 10 years. By the end of fiscal 1991, the cash balances for the five financially sound communities range from $15 million to $40 million. These amounts are all probably more than the amount required to be in actuarial balance since the fees of these communities for new entrants are redundant and are expected to generate excess cash. Case 5 is expected to have a

TABLE 9–10 ─────────────────────────────────
Ten-Year Expected Cash Flow Projection Based on Current Pricing Policies *($000)*

Fiscal year	Case 1	Case 2	Case 3	Case 4	Case 5	Case 6
1982	$ 1,422	$ 2,545	$ 652	$ 5,067	$(1,098)	$ 1,243
1983	1,518	3,249	2,797	6,615	(1,669)	1,796
1984	1,864	4,100	4,257	8,635	(1,434)	2,436
1985	2,359	5,178	5,934	11,059	(809)	3,406
1986	3,169	6,509	7,736	13,917	94	4,602
1987	4,311	8,023	9,909	17,586	(3,820)	6,011
1988	6,067	9,772	12,514	22,063	(2,238)	7,741
1989	8,264	11,883	15,657	27,320	316	9,809
1990	11,046	14,072	19,604	33,205	3,674	12,281
1991	14,733	16,747	24,215	40,221	8,031	15,286

negative cash balance in 6 of the 10 years; however, an $8 million balance is expected by the end of 10 years.

In order to eliminate any actuarial imbalance, the information generated from the actuarial valuation was combined with new entrant pricing analysis to develop a set of consistent changes in monthly fees for both current and prospective residents. Table 9–11 presents the sug-

TABLE 9–11 ─────────────────────────────────
Fee Adjustments to Eliminate Unfunded Liabilities

Fee changes	Case 1	Case 2	Case 3	Case 4	Case 5	Case 6
Percentage increase (decrease) in monthly fees in addition to inflation over next five years	1.1%	0.5%	(1.4%)	(3.7%)	5.3%	0.3%
Percentage increase (decrease) in entry fees in addition to inflation over next five years	(1.6)	(8.0)*	(6.0)	(2.0)	(4.4)†	(7.3)

* The actual derived decrease was 11.6 percent; however, the size of the decrease limited to the inflation assumption, so that the entry fees for any year will not be less than the entry fees for the prior year.
† Even though the community has a substantial deficit with regard to current residents, the mathematically adequate entry fees associated with the increased monthly fees (i.e., 5.3 percent more than inflation over the next five years) are less than the current entry fees. In this example, it was assumed that the deficit would be funded entirely from increases in the fees of current residents, and thus the entry fees were decreased. However, for a community having a deficit of this magnitude, the fees of both current residents and new residents would be used to eliminate the deficit, and a recommendation to decrease entry fees, although mathematically correct, would not be considered a practical alternative.

gested changes. These adjustments are assumed to be applied over the next five years. In Case 1, for example, monthly fees are to be increased an additional 1.1 percent over inflation for the next five years, and entry fees are to be raised 1.6 percent less than inflation over the same period. If inflation is assumed to be 8 percent, then monthly fees are to be increased 9.1 percent and entry fees are to be increased 6.4 percent.

The revised cash flow projections using actuarial fee adjustments are presented in Table 9–12. The cash balances at the end of 10 years are

TABLE 9–12 _____
Ten-Year Expected Cash Flow Projection Based on Actuarially Modified Fees *($000)*

Fiscal year	Case 1	Case 2	Case 3	Case 4	Case 5	Case 6
1982	$ 1,447	$ 2,567	$ 602	$ 4,909	$(1,049)	$ 1,251
1983	1,602	3,215	2,450	6,113	(1,498)	1,742
1984	2,040	3,911	3,443	7,534	(1,054)	2,243
1985	2,677	4,699	4,382	9,056	(120)	2,947
1986	3,690	5,571	5,132	10,655	1,239	3,745
1987	5,075	6,543	6,075	12,819	(2,149)	4,869
1988	7,107	7,653	7,272	15,509	54	5,869
1989	9,634	8,988	8,795	18,674	3,319	7,290
1990	12,806	10,329	10,830	22,140	7,500	9,006
1991	16,939	11,977	13,259	26,399	12,795	11,106

less than the cash balances using current fees (Table 9–10) for four of the six cases. In each of these cases, each new entrant cohort was expected to generate more than $500,000 in revenues over expenses during its stay in the community, thus placing the community in a surplus position at the end of the projection. Under the actuarial modifications, the reductions in accumulated cash range from 27 to 45 percent. These values should be close to the amounts required to be in actuarial balance; however, additional valuations should be performed to ensure that fee adjustments after five years are on track with the goal of actuarial adequacy.

Cases 1 and 5 generated higher cash balances under the actuarially modified fee structure as compared to their current fee structure. For Case 5, the fees were extremely inadequate and substantial increases were assumed. However, these increases were not enough to eliminate negative cash balances in the early years, and other alternatives (such as a moratorium on its debt payments or reduction in the level of its health care guarantee) would have to be explored in order to solve its financial problem. This case serves as an example of what could go wrong if a community consistently underprices its contract (as was indicated by the new entrant pricing analysis).

Summary

This chapter presented the cash flow associated with an actuarially balanced community. Such a community is expected to accumulate substantial cash balances, all of which are required to ensure that the community has assets to cover its deferred obligations. Typical ratio analysis will not justify the large cash balances, nor will current GAAP statements, which are the subject of the following two chapters, reflect the community's true actuarial position. The actuarial valuation is the tool required by management to make this justification, as illustrated in the text.

Except for Case 5, the authors found that relatively minor changes were required to bring the communities studied into actuarial balance. This result is significant in two respects. First, achieving an actuarially sound position is relatively easy for these communities, suggesting that communities based on a closed-group pricing methodology can offer marketable fees. Second, since four of the remaining five CCRCs have been in operation for at least five years and are close to being actuarially sound, the continuing care concept seems to be viable, provided that management employs proper financial planning methodologies. Of course, the validity of this statement can only be determined by performing the same financial studies on a number of older CCRCs and monitoring the financial course of those communities over a period of years. ■

Chapter Ten
Financial Reporting

■ The actuarial methodology for developing "actuarially adequate fees" presented in the preceding six chapters was not based on traditional accounting statements. Financial statements were not used because the correct method for determining the size of actuarial liabilities and of the corresponding fees for funding those liabilities requires *present value analyses* to equate future revenue and expense streams. It is not easy to incorporate this present value approach into traditional financial statements, whereas it is easy to incorporate it into the actuarial valuation methodology. However, it is important to determine the relationship between actuarially generated fees and the community's current financial position as reflected in its financial statements. Should these be inconsistent, appropriate modifications must be developed.

The impact of charging actuarially adequate fees on financial statements used by CCRCs is explored in this chapter and Chapter 11. This chapter presents an introductory discussion of basic financial statement preparation and the types of external reports generated by CCRCs. The goals of this chapter are to: (1) identify the financial statements prepared by CCRCs (and organizations in general) and describe their purpose, (2) explain the basis of preparation of these statements, and (3) discuss the points which limit the usefulness of the principal financial statements as management decision-making tools. This chapter presumes that the reader has little background in accounting and finance. The reader already knowledgeable in these areas may wish to go directly to Chapter 12, which presents recommendations regarding the statements that management should use to assess the current financial position of a community.

TYPES AND PURPOSES OF FINANCIAL STATEMENTS

This section describes four types of external financial reports used by continuing care retirement communities and then compares these reports to similar external reports prepared for organizations in general.

External versus Internal Reports

In the broadest sense, the financial reports generated by organizations can be divided into two categories: external reports and internal reports.

External reports are prepared for audiences external to the organization who have an interest in monitoring the organization's progress. Two key audiences are investors and regulators. These reports tend to be more standardized than internal reports because they are directed to a broad cross-section of individuals, some of whom have little or no understanding of the operations of the organizations whose reports they review. When management compiles the basic external reports, it generally has them reviewed by independent public accountants who are retained to express an opinion on the fairness of the statements and their conformance with generally accepted accounting principles (GAAP).[1]

Internal reports are designed for the use of management in carrying out its decision-making responsibilities. These "management tool reports" are not intended for external consumption and need not be prepared in accordance with dictates, principles, or rules set forth by any body external to management. The types of internal reports prepared by organizations vary with the type of business endeavor. One common set of internal reports consists of budget and budget variance reports. These reports require managers to estimate resource needs in advance, and on a periodic basis the reports identify actual resource use as compared with budgeted use. Another critical internal report is the cash flow projection. Cash flow statements are needed to monitor liquidity, predict peaks and valleys in an organization's cash balances, and identify how much cash can be expected to be generated from internal operations and how much will have to be supplied from other sources. This chapter does not consider internal reports.

There are at least three key differences between external and internal reports. The first difference applies to the level of standardization. External reports possess a degree of standardization as regards types of reports prepared, manner of presenting information, and manner of

---

[1] Typically, the governing body of an organization (its board of directors) retains the public accountants to review, independently, the statements of the organization.

ascertaining the values shown, while internal reports are highly individualized. Second, external reports are highly summarized, while internal reports may depict minute details. Finally, and perhaps the most important distinction, external reports provide summary data based on what has already happened on the assumption that the environment facing the organization in the past will exist in the future. Internal reports need not be constrained by this convention.

External Reports

The financial information made available by organizations for external audiences consists, typically, of the four documents listed below. The titles listed in the left-hand column are those commonly used by proprietary organizations. The right-hand column shows the terminology used by CCRCs to identify their financial statements:

Titles used by most proprietary firms	Titles used by CCRCs
1. Balance sheet	1. Balance sheet
2. Income statement	2. Statement of revenues and expenses
3. Statement of changes in owners' equity	3. Statement of changes in fund balance
4. Statement of sources and uses of funds	4. Statement of changes in financial position

Frequently, statements 2 and 3 are combined. Occasionally, the "sources and uses" statement is omitted.

Balance Sheet. The balance sheet is a summary financial statement prepared as of a given date. It depicts the organization's current wealth position in accordance with the accounting rules prescribed for the statement's preparation (these rules are discussed later). The left side of the statement lists all of the things owned by the organization that have a current "worth," referred to as assets. The right side of the balance sheet is divided into two parts—liabilities and fund balance. The items listed on the right side show who has a claim on the assets listed on the left side of the statement. Liabilities are listed before the fund balance because liabilities represent creditor claims. The fund balance represents the extent to which available assets exceed the claims of creditors. If liabilities exceed assets, the organization will show a negative fund balance, referred to as a deficit. The balance sheet does not specifically identify which assets belong to which creditors or owners. What it depicts is the relative claim on assets held by various creditor and owners.

Assets are usually shown in three groups—current assets, fixed assets, and intangible or other assets. The order in which assets are listed is from most liquid to least liquid. Current assets are shown first.

They are the most liquid and qualify as current assets because it is expected that all current assets not already in the form of cash will be converted to cash (i.e., "turned over") within the next accounting cycle (fiscal year). Cash, accounts receivable, and inventory are current assets. Assets within this group are listed in order of relative closeness to cash. For example, inventories follow accounts receivable because they typically become an account receivable before they become cash.

The next asset category, fixed assets, includes the plant and equipment used by the organization to produce goods and/or provide services. Such assets are long-term insofar as they will be utilized over more than one future accounting period. The portion of fixed assets "used up" during each accounting cycle is allocated to the appropriate accounting cycle by a depreciation charge. The final asset category includes "other assets." Such assets are usually a small portion of total assets and are often not physical assets. Most "other assets" would not have any value if the business were liquidated. Perhaps the most frequently encountered "other asset" is preopening and organization expense. This represents expenses incurred prior to opening which are established as assets (i.e., capitalized) and charged off as expenses, pro rata, over the time period benefited by the expenses.

Liabilities, the claims of creditors on the organization's assets, are shown in two categories—current liabilities and long-term liabilities. Accounts payable, taxes due, and the current portion of long-term debt constitute current liabilities. Long-term liabilities are made up of the organization's borrowings.

The fund balance identifies the amount of assets belonging to the owners of the organization. It is a residual figure insofar as it is the difference between assets and liabilities. The fund balance amount is a function of the asset and liability valuation practices employed by the CCRC.

The balance sheet provides a financial snapshot of an organization. It lists the stock of goods owned and owed at a given date. However, the balance sheet does not provide insight into how the organization attained its current position. For that, one must refer to other statements which tend to link successive balance sheets together. These are discussed later in this section.

The balance sheets prepared by other organizations are similar to those prepared by CCRCs. The differences found relate to the nature of a CCRC's business and to the nonproprietary ownership of most CCRCs. There are some differences in form and substance.

CCRCs often present separate balance sheets for various "funds." For example, one balance sheet may be prepared for the operating fund and another for the property fund. Some CCRCs prepare separate balance sheets for restricted and unrestricted funds.

The balance sheets prepared by most proprietary organizations do not refer to the excess of assets over liabilities as the fund balance. Instead, the difference between assets and liabilities is referred to as owners' equity. In investor-owned firms, owners' equity is segregated into two parts. Money supplied directly by owners is referred to as capital stock and paid-in-surplus, while the excess of prior years' earnings over dividends paid to owners is referred to as retained earnings. Regardless of the designation, this section of the balance sheet denotes the excess of assets over the claims of creditors whether or not the organization is operated for profit. In a sense, it represents the cushion of financial security available to the creditors of an organization.

The major substantive difference between the balance sheet of a CCRC and that of most other businesses relates to the liability side of the statement. It relates to the advance deposits of prospective residents and the entry fees paid by residents. These amounts, particularly in latter, are very sizable. They represent payments made by residents in advance of future services. They are earned in future years by the CCRC; until earned, however, the unearned balance is carried as a liability. The manner in which such fees are taken into earnings by a CCRC is subject to some discretion and is one of the most important accounting decisions facing CCRC management, as discussed later. Only a few firms, most notably life insurance companies, show liabilities that are similar in nature to those of CCRCs.

Statement of Revenues and Expenses. The statement of revenues and expenses depicts what has occurred over some specific time period (usually one year) rather than presenting information as of some specified date, as does the balance sheet. As such, it represents a "flow of activity" rather than a "stock of goods."

If one were to examine two balance sheets for a CCRC prepared one year apart, one would undoubtedly find some change in the fund balance reported in the successive statements. A key purpose of the revenue and expense statement is to explain the change in the fund balance from year to year. The revenue and expense statement provides the critical link between balance sheets. The balance sheet answers the question "What is the organization worth?" The revenue and expense statement answers the question "How much did the organization 'earn' this year?" However, it should be noted that the answers to both questions are only as good as the assumptions underlying the preparation of the statements.

The format of a statement of revenues and expenses is straightforward. The statement presents a listing of revenue items and expense items. Major revenue items are resident fees, investment income, amortized portion of entrance fees, and medical center collections, where applicable. The bottom line of the statement is usually referred to as excess of revenues over expenses (or vice versa).

The comparable statement prepared by most proprietary firms is called an income statement. (CCRCs, like most nonprofit entities, avoid proprietary-sounding statement names and account titles.) The largest revenue item found in most income statements is sales. Expenses are frequently grouped by type. Common expense categories, especially among manufacturing organizations, are cost of goods sold, administrative expenses, and general expenses. For-profit organizations usually show net income before and after federal income taxes.

Statement of Changes in Fund Balance. The third external report listed earlier was called the statement of changes in fund balance. Sometimes the purpose served by this statement is accomplished by extending the statement of revenues and expenses rather than showing a separate statement of changes in fund balance. Not all of the items that cause the fund balance to change during a year will be included in the "excess of revenues over expenses" figure discussed above. The fund balance of a typical CCRC is also impacted by such items as contributions, donated equipment, and transfers between funds. Such items cause an increase in assets and a corresponding increase in the fund balance to keep the balance sheet in balance. Since receipts of this kind cannot be considered "earnings," they are excluded from the statement of revenues and expenses. The transactions shown in the statement of changes in fund balance are unusual, nonrecurring items which typically do not arise from a firm's normal operations. A statement of changes in fund balance typically shows the beginning-of-year fund balance excess of revenues over expenses (or vice versa) followed by other transactions impacting on the CCRC's fund balance during the year but not reflected in the statement of revenues and expenses. A CCRC may have several such statements, depending on the number of separate funds maintained.

The corresponding statement issued by proprietary firms is called the statement of changes in owners' equity. Two key items often reflected in this statement are the receipt of cash for the issuance of additional shares of stock and the payment of dividends to shareholders. The format and purpose of the statement are exactly as described above.

Statement of Changes in Financial Position. The final statement included in the typical package of external reports is the statement of changes in financial position. "Financial position" is defined, for the purpose of this statement, as "net working capital." Net working capital is the difference between a CCRC's current assets and its current liabilities. Working capital is an important concept. It identifies the amount of money readily available to fund operations. A working capital ratio (i.e., current ratio) of 2 to 1 implies that an organization has $2 of relatively liquid assets for every $1 needed to meet its current needs. Working capital provides an important measure of a CCRC's liquidity and identifies the ability of the organization to take advantage of new opportunities or to weather bad times.

The statement of changes in financial position supplements the balance sheet. In a sense, it is like the statement of changes in fund balance. However, instead of explaining the change in the fund balance, the statement of changes in financial position explains the year's change in net working capital.[2]

The statement's format is straightforward. The first section lists the sources of working capital during the year. Key sources include excess of revenues over expenses (if any), entry fees received, donations, and interfund transfers. Excess of revenues over expenses has to be adjusted for deductions from revenue which do not require working capital funds during the year and for revenue items not adding to working capital funds during the year. A key item requiring adjustment is depreciation. Since depreciation reduces reported operating income, it must be added to the sources of funds because it does not require an actual expenditure of funds during the year.

The second section of the statement lists the uses of working capital. Key uses would be any operating loss incurred during the year, repayment of debt, and/or acquisition of fixed assets.

The difference between the sources and uses of working capital is then shown. It is usually labeled increase (decrease) in working capital. The net change in working capital has to be reflected in current asset and current liability account balances. The changes in these balances are shown as the third section of the statement of changes in financial position.

The external reports issued by proprietary firms typically include a statement that summarizes the change in working capital for the year. The statement is most often referred to as the statement of sources and uses of funds. In this statement, "funds" is defined as "net working capital." Regardless of the difference in name, the purpose and appearance of the statement are the same as those of the statement of changes in financial position, described above.

In summary, the external reports issued by CCRCs are consistent with those issued by other business organizations. The major distinctions are terminological and stem from the nonprofit sponsorship of

---

[2] Sometimes the statement of changes in financial position is limited to explaining the change in a CCRC's cash balance over only a year instead of serving the more comprehensive purpose discussed here.

most CCRCs. Examples of the external statements discussed above, as prepared by one CCRC, are included in Appendix E.

BASIS OF FINANCIAL STATEMENT PREPARATION

The previous section has described the purposes of external financial reports. In order to evaluate how well the various statements accomplish their intended purposes, it is necessary to understand the assumptions and conventions underlying statement preparation.

The role of the independent accountant is to verify that the financial statements prepared by management are based on generally accepted principles of accounting. After the independent accountant reviews (audits) the statements, an opinion is expressed on the fairness of the financial statement presentation in accordance with generally accepted accounting principles.

Accounting principles, whether generally accepted or not, cannot be applied in a vacuum. In other words, generally accepted accounting principles are applicable only when some other basic concepts or assumptions hold. Many persons confuse and/or fail to distinguish the underlying assumptions or basic concepts of accounting from generally accepted accounting principles.

Fundamental Concepts

One basic assumption is that the business venture being reported upon is viewed as an *entity* in its own right. It is viewed as distinct from those who furnish the capital to operate the *business,* and the statements prepared are those of the business entity, not the managers, the owners, or any other individuals concerned.

A second basic assumption is that the entity will continue to operate, that it is a *going concern.* The preparation of external financial reports rests on normal conditions and not on the assumption that the entity is to be liquidated, unless there is strong evidence to indicate that such is the case.

Accounting statement valuation is also based on the notion that the *cost* of acquiring an asset is the appropriate measure of the asset's worth. Cost is usually readily determinable and provides some objective evidence of an item's value—at least to someone at some time.

Another basic concept is that the production of revenue is the underlying reason for incurring cost. *Therefore, costs incurred should be properly matched against the revenues for whose production the costs were incurred.* This concept of proper *matching* of revenue and expense items is embodied in an accrual accounting system rather than in accounting done on a cash basis. Accrual accounting charges expenses to the time period in which associated revenues are recognized, regardless of when cash is distributed or received.

Other basic concepts or conventions important to accountants include the following:

Materiality: If disclosure of an item would probably influence the judgment of a reasonable person, it should be disclosed.

Conservatism: Uncertainties and risks should be given adequate consideration, and gains should not be anticipated.

Consistency: Principles and practices should be uniformly applied from one period to the next.

Full disclosure: Necessary information should be added to financial reports to prevent them from being misleading.

Principles of Accounting

Accounting principles are statements of accounting practice that arise from the basic concepts enumerated above. An accounting practice becomes a principle when it enjoys substantial "authoritative support." This support can come from various quarters: practices commonly found in business, statements of the Financial Accounting Standards Board (FASB) and its predecessor organizations, affirmative opinions of practicing and academic accountants, and so forth.

An example of a generally accepted principle of accounting is the principle that extraordinary gains and losses and nonrecurring items should be shown separately from usual operating results. This principle upholds the basic concepts of full disclosure and proper matching discussed above.

Generally accepted accounting principles are numerous. It is neither possible nor appropriate to state them all in this brief discussion.

Caveats Attending Interpretation of Reported Results

If a business enterprise is indeed a going concern, it follows that its financial condition and results of operation at any time, or for any short interval, will be impacted upon by past as well as future activities. The eventual results produced by a business cannot be measured accurately until liquidation. For a number of reasons, however, not the least of which is the assessment of taxes, results are reported periodically. Too often, individuals reading financial statements attribute too much finality to reported results. In fact, the financial results presented should be viewed as provisional, and any decisions based on the reports may have to be changed in light of future developments.

The assumption that recorded historical cost measures the value of assets implies a stable monetary unit. It follows that in periods of significant price movements, financial reports can present unrealistic asset and liability values and, as a result, inaccurate portrayals of fund balances, or owners' equity.

The meaning and application of accrual accounting have significant implications for interpreting reported financial results. The fact that there can be significant time lags between the receipt or disbursement of cash and the recognition of income or expense means that the income statement can present an unduly comfortable or uncomfortable picture of an organization's well-being. No matter how large an organization's income as reported under accrual accounting, it can face bill-paying problems if its cash receipts fall short of reported income. Conversely, an organization with large cash receipts in spite of operating losses may be lulled into a sense of complacency because of its ability to meet its cash requirements. In the long run, results reported on an accrual basis will be identical to net cash flow. Temporary imbalances between the two due to the existence of period accounting will evaporate over the life cycle of the organization.

Another noteworthy aspect of accrual accounting is that the matching process is one of allocation, not valuation. When the cost of fixed assets, for example, is apportioned over future periods by means of depreciation charges, the goal of the apportionment process is to allocate historical cost and not to estimate the current value or replacement cost of the portion of the productive asset consumed during the period under review.

Finally, many important features of an organization are not reflected in its financial statements. For an item to appear as an asset of an organization (and thus be included in the calculation of the fund balance or net worth), it must have been acquired for some consideration. This means that any potential infusions of resources from the organization's sponsor(s) or investors cannot be reflected, nor can the significant value attaching to the organization's human resources be included, in the organization's financial statements. Without some knowledge regarding these factors, it is impossible to gauge accurately an organization's true condition.

USEFULNESS OF BASIC FINANCIAL STATEMENTS FOR MANAGEMENT DECISION MAKING

The traditional external financial reports prepared by organizations typically are of limited use to the managers of such organizations for management decision making. This statement holds greater validity for managers of CCRCs than for managers of many other types of businesses. In the first place, CCRCs face more future contingencies outside their control than do most businesses. The analysis of resident mortality and morbidity rates is just beginning to reach the point where comfortable predictions can be made about turnover rates and future health care costs. Current per capita health care costs will often be significantly less than future per capita costs because of the maturation of the resident population, changes in methods of delivering health care to the aged, and general health care cost escalation. Changes in turnover rates impact sharply on the collection of entry fees which may have been counted upon heavily to finance needed capital improvements, retire debt, and so forth.

CCRC management has to recognize the deficiencies inherent in the financial results currently generated by the application of generally accepted accounting principles when setting fees—both entry fees and monthly fees—and planning future capital requirements. The reported income of CCRCs may overstate actual performance by a significant margin. Depreciation charges based on constant dollar assumptions, even if funded, will not produce enough money to replace equipment and buildings, let alone to provide capital funds for expansion. Even if cash equal to each year's depreciation is put into a restricted building and equipment fund and invested at a rate equivalent to the rate at which capital asset prices are appreciating, the funds set aside will be insufficient to replace the capital assets that require replacement. Inflation impacts the total price of an asset, not just the portion of the asset assumed to be used up during each accounting period. If entry fees and monthly fees are to provide funds for capital asset replacement, a capital charge based on constant dollar depreciation is inadequate.

Income may also be overstated because of too rapid amortization of entry fees. Typically, entry fees are taken into income over the life expectancies of residents.[3] This is *not* consistent with the matching concept discussed earlier, whereby revenues and related costs should be matched in the same period, regardless of the actual collection or disbursement of cash.[4]

There are two problems with this approach. Because those individuals who choose to live in CCRCs are required to make a sizable upfront deposit of funds, they may exhibit what insurance people refer to as adverse selection. If they expect to live a long life, they will view the size of the entry fee as an attractive price to pay for the promises made by the CCRC. The life expectancy rates used by accountants in recog-

---

[3] The 1981 CCRC survey showed that approximately 47 percent of CCRCs use amortization schedules based on the life expectancies of their residents.

[4] See Chapter 11 for a method of amortizing entry fees that is consistent with the matching concept.

nizing entry fees as income may be too optimistic inasmuch as residents may live longer than assumed in the mortality assumptions. One CCRC recently revised its life expectancy assumptions and, as a result, reduced 1981 revenues by $700,000. (Under the new assumptions, amortization of entry fees required $2,200,000 rather than the $1,500,000 reported.)

A second problem related to entry fee amortization deals with the question of whether or not entry fees should be amortized evenly over residents' life expectancies. Equal annual amortization implies that the expense of maintaining a resident, which an entry fee may be designed to support, at least in part, is constant from year to year. If this assumption holds, equal annual amortization can be justified. However, many of the costs of maintaining a resident increase with age. If the entry fee, as opposed to the monthly fee, is designed to underwrite some of the expenses that increase with age, the matching concept would seem to dictate other than equal annual entry fee amortization. If entry fees will be needed to support health care service costs, an amortization function that increases with age would seem more appropriate.

The discussion concerning depreciation and entry fee amortization has focused on the income statement consequences of current accounting practices. The balance sheet is also impacted by these practices. At any point, the fund balance measures the excess of CCRC assets over liabilities. This is a reliable figure only to the extent that all assets and liabilities are reflected in the balance sheet and shown at their appropriate value.

Past depreciation charges are reflected in the balance sheet as accumulated depreciation and reduce the carrying value of fixed assets by the amount of accumulated depreciation charges. The fund balance is also impacted by accumulated depreciation, since the fund balance represents the excess of assets over liabilities, and assets are reduced by accumulated depreciation. However, it can be argued that since depreciation represents an allocation of historical cost rather than a measure of replacement cost of assets used up in providing services, accumulated depreciation is an inadequate estimate of capital consumption for an ongoing business venture. If accumulated depreciation reflected more realistic estimates of capital consumption, a CCRC's fund balance would be reduced.

The discussion of depreciation is but one example of the deficiencies of historical cost, constant-dollar reporting. Other items included in an organization's financial statements are also impacted by price-level changes which are not reflected in reported results.

The fund balance is also overstated if the present value of the future costs of providing CCRC services exceeds the present value of future resident fees and the unamortized portion of entry fees. The deficit will have to be made up out of existing fund balances. Realistically, any such deficit should be reflected currently as a liability.

The level of summarization contained in the financial statements discussed in this chapter presents management decision-making problems. The financial operations of a CCRC's apartment complex are almost always combined with the operations of the health center. Hence, it is difficult to determine from reported results whether both activities are financially sound. Effective management requires the reporting of divisional and/or departmental results. In the case of a CCRC, costs and revenues should be allocated to major activity areas in order to set equitable and adequate fees as well as to maximize reimbursement from other parties that are responsible for making payment to the CCRC.

Summary

This chapter has identified the types and purposes of external financial reports prepared by business entities in general and by CCRCs in particular. The assumptions underlying the presentation of financial results have also been described, along with the implications of those assumptions as regards interpretation of reported financial results.

Some of the deficiencies of generally accepted accounting principles from the standpoint of management decision making were pointed out. Deficiencies result both from the principles themselves and from the application of those principles to CCRCs. It seems clear that improvements can be made in the financial reports of CCRCs even within the context of current generally accepted accounting principles. The implementation of such changes awaits appropriate experience, or what the accountant would refer to as "objective evidence."

However, even if more satisfactory financial reports are ultimately generated by CCRCs for the public, they will still be deficient as complete management decision-making tools. Appropriate data for decision making cannot be limited to information produced by the application of generally accepted accounting principles in the context of CCRCs. Actuarial assumptions, recognition of the time value of money, and greater detail must be incorporated into the data generation activity.

The following chapter deals with two of the problems noted above: (1) suggestions to improve the application of generally accepted accounting principles to CCRCs and (2) the development of a set of financial data more appropriate to management decision making. ∎

Chapter Eleven

Financial Management Statements

■ In the preceding chapter, several issues were raised regarding the limited usefulness of typical financial statements for management decision-making in a CCRC. The purpose of this chapter is to develop modifications to existing statements for improving their usefulness. This chapter, which focuses on income statements for CCRCs,[1] covers two types of statements. The first type comprises actuarial income statements based on the principles used to perform actuarial valuations. The second type comprises income statements prepared according to generally accepted accounting principles (GAAP).

INCOME STATEMENTS

An income statement reflects the results of an organization's operations during a one-year period on an accrual accounting basis (i.e., one that attempts to match revenues with expenses). The income statement, as opposed to the cash flow statement, attempts to reflect more fairly the results of prior years' operations by spreading the recognition of some cash receipts over future years in an attempt to match the incidence of expenses. If proper matching can be achieved, management could use the income statement (and the projected budget for the next year) as a guide to annual fee adjustments.

---

[1] These statements, which are also known as profit and loss (P&L) statements, are also referred to as statements of revenues and expenses by CCRCs.

In order to effect the matching of revenues and expenses for a CCRC, a statement is developed that compares budgeted monthly revenues and entry fee amortization with budgeted expenses. If, for the next year, budgeted revenues fall short of budgeted expenses, then revenues must be adjusted to eliminate the shortfall. This process is repeated annually, with revenues being adjusted to equal budgeted expenses. A disadvantage of using income statements as the primary basis for determining fee adjustments is that, if fees are not initially in actuarial balance, it may take several years before this deficiency flows through the income statement. Hence, income statements do not provide management with sufficient information on how to adjust fees in the current year to place the community in actuarial balance. This can only be determined from an actuarial valuation. Nevertheless, income statements, properly prepared, are useful for explaining how the community achieved its current financial position from its position in the prior year.

ACTUARIAL INCOME STATEMENTS

The term *actuarial income statements* is used to describe the theoretically correct management statements for CCRCs. Actuarial income statements are derived by applying the concepts underlying actuarial valuations for a CCRC. Revenues consist of monthly fees and the amortization of entry fees. The amortization of entry fees is determined such that the amortization amounts are expected to be equal to the difference between monthly revenues and total expenses during each resident's lifetime. Expenses consist of operating expenses and capital expenses, where capital expenses are set equal to the actuarial expenses associated with fixed assets.

Two issues associated with actuarial income statements are: (1) the development of correct methods for amortizing entry fees and (2) the calculation of actuarial expenses for fixed assets. Both of these issues require that imputed interest be recorded on the actuarial income statement. This procedure, while consistent with the present value methodology used to develop actuarial fees, is not consistent with generally accepted accounting principles. Statements that meet GAAP standards are discussed in the following section.

The basic premise of actuarially correct entry fee amortization schedules is that the annual amortization amounts should increase per life. This premise is a logical deduction from the actuarial pricing objective that limits increases in monthly fees to the inflation experience of the community. Since expected expenses will increase faster than inflation-constrained monthly fees (due to the increasing probability of higher health care costs as the resident ages), entry fee amortizations for surviving residents must necessarily be increased on a per life basis if they are to cover the difference between expenses and monthly fees. The exact pattern of this increase depends on the underlying assumptions for mortality, morbidity, and inflation.

Given that the entry fee amortization should be an increasing amount per life, it is relatively simple to develop the correct amortization schedule. The amount recorded on the actuarial income statement for a given year will equal a portion of the entry fee principal amount plus interest income on the unearned balance. In some cases, the unamortized balance may increase for a few years after entry, implying that total interest earnings on the unamortized balance may exceed the amount that should properly be amortized. This excess revenue (over what should be amortized) is not recorded on the actuarial income statement but is instead added to the unamortized entry fee balance used as the basis for determining the amortization amount in the following year. This means that, in order to generate an actuarial income statement, separate accounting for the unamortized entry fee balance must be maintained.

The second issue related to the development of actuarial income statements is the expenses associated with fixed assets. These expenses are based on the actuarial expense methodology described in Chapter 7, an approach that results in greater expenses than those generated by historic-cost depreciation.

The illustrative actuarial income statement presented in Table 11–1 is based on the cash flow projection associated with actuarially adequate fees (refer to Chapter 9 and Table 9–1) and is in exact actuarial balance throughout the projection.[2] Revenues consist of two components: monthly revenues and entry fee amortizations. Monthly revenues include the normal monthly fees paid by continuing care contractholders that are increasing with inflation plus per diem charges paid by outside patients in the health care center. Entry fee amortizations are derived by subtracting monthly fee revenues from total expenses.[3] No interest revenue is explicitly shown on this statement, since interest income is automatically included in the annual amount recorded for entry fee amortizations. Total revenues are increasing from nearly $5 million to nearly $20 million for this illustrative CCRC.

Total expenses, which include operating and capital expenses, range from nearly $5 million to nearly $20 million by the end of 20 years. Net income, equal to the difference between total revenues and expenses,

---

[2] Actually, projected valuations show the community to be in a slight surplus position; however, for pedagogic purposes, it is assumed that the surplus is negligible.

[3] In practice, a theoretically correct amortization schedule would be applied. Since it is somewhat complicated to develop such a schedule, a simpler approach was used to determine entry fee earnings in this example. Under this approach, entry fee amortization is set equal to the difference between total expenses and monthly revenues.

TABLE 11–1
Twenty-Year Projection of Actuarial Income Statements Using Actuarial Fees *($000)*

Fiscal year	Monthly revenues	Entry fee amortizations	Total revenues	Operating expenses	Capital expenses	Total expenses	Net income	Actuarial fund balance
1983	$ 3,775	$1,164	$ 4,939	$ 2,628	$2,311	$ 4,939	$0	$0
1984	3,893	1,349	5,242	2,891	2,351	5,242	0	0
1985	4,043	1,533	5,576	3,180	2,396	5,576	0	0
1986	4,217	1,726	5,943	3,498	2,445	5,943	0	0
1987	4,383	1,964	6,347	3,848	2,499	6,347	0	0
1988	4,616	2,175	6,791	4,232	2,559	6,791	0	0
1989	4,939	2,341	7,280	4,656	2,624	7,280	0	0
1990	5,267	2,550	7,817	5,121	2,696	7,817	0	0
1991	5,636	2,772	8,408	5,633	2,775	8,408	0	0
1992	5,993	3,066	9,059	6,197	2,862	9,059	0	0
1993	6,481	3,084	9,565	6,816	2,749	9,565	0	0
1994	7,050	3,281	10,331	7,498	2,833	10,331	0	0
1995	7,688	3,486	11,174	8,248	2,926	11,174	0	0
1996	8,403	3,697	12,100	9,072	3,028	12,100	0	0
1997	9,148	3,973	13,121	9,980	3,141	13,121	0	0
1998	9,907	4,335	14,242	10,978	3,264	14,242	0	0
1999	10,948	4,527	15,475	12,075	3,400	15,475	0	0
2000	12,071	4,762	16,833	13,283	3,550	16,833	0	0
2001	13,341	4,984	18,325	14,611	3,714	18,325	0	0
2002	14,675	5,292	19,967	16,072	3,895	19,967	0	0

is defined to be zero since fees for this CCRC are actuarially adequate and experience is assumed to follow the underlying assumptions. The actuarial fund balance is also zero throughout the projection.

While the actuarial income statement has the advantage for showing a fair financial picture of the community, it does not contribute information for setting fees beyond that generated by an actuarial valuation. One disadvantage of the actuarial income statement is that it requires an additional set of books to be maintained, since the community will undoubtedly continue to develop GAAP statements. Moreover, detailed accounting for interest earnings on fixed assets and entry fees must be monitored. Finally, the actuarial income statement is quite distant from GAAP statements, which are the accepted standards of comparison. Therefore, an approach that modifies GAAP statements to reflect a position reasonably consistent with the results of the actuarial income statement is desirable. Such an approach is discussed in the following section.

MODIFIED GAAP INCOME STATEMENTS

Because of the wide use of GAAP statements and because of the unique aspects of CCRCs, it is desirable that GAAP statements be modified in order to reflect more accurately the actuarial position of a community. Adjustments in statements that conform to GAAP standards are required in two areas: (1) the amortization schedules for entry fees and (2) expenses for fixed assets. In addition, the separation of statements by cost center (i.e., apartment versus health care) and the development of a separate health care reserve fund for continuing care contractholders would improve the picture presented by GAAP statements. Each of these topics is discussed in subsequent sections.

Entry Fee Amortization

The primary position adopted by the American Institute of Certified Public Accountants (AICPA) is that entry fees should be amortized in accordance with the future expenses they are to cover. However, because of the difficulty in determining these future expenses, the secondary position of the AICPA is that it is acceptable to amortize entry fees based on the resident's life expectancy, or in the case of refundable entry fees, in accordance with the refund provision. Not surprisingly, it is the current practice of many CCRCs to amortize entry fees on one of these two bases. These methods, however, earn entry fees too rapidly, because entry fees are completely earned prior to the death of all residents in the original entrant cohort. The resulting income statements will generate an overly optimistic view of the CCRC's financial position. Hence, using these statements to confirm pricing policies might lead to erroneous decisions. The following section presents income statements based on life expectancy amortizations to illustrate this problem.

Current Practice. The entry fee amortization methods commonly employed include: (1) the life expectancy method, (2) refund methods, and (3) immediate recognition. The life expectancy method is the most prevalent, being used by slightly less than 50 percent of all CCRCs. Under this method, an equal portion of the entry fee is recognized as revenue on the income statement. This amount is predetermined by dividing the initial entry fee by the life expectancy of the resident (or group of residents), and the same amount is amortized for a period equal to the life expectancy.[4]

Amortizations under the refund methods are based on the reduction in the amount to be refunded if the resident leaves the community. For example, if the resident is entitled to receive a refund of 80 percent of the original entry fee for withdrawal after one year in the community, then 20 percent of the entry fees would be recognized as income during the first year. This method is used by approximately 25 percent of all CCRCs. A few communities recognize all entry fee income immediately, and the amortizations under this approach are the same as the amount recorded on cash flow statements.

The general acceptance of the life expectancy method on GAAP statements is no doubt explained by the ease of its implementation, because the method does not adhere to the "revenue and expense matching" tenet as explained in Chapter 10. This approach does have a desirable characteristic in that amortizations increase on a per life basis (as is the case for the theoretically correct method), since the same dollar amount is earned each year, while the number of surviving residents from the original entry cohort decline over time. Entry fee amortizations become zero after the life expectancy period. Hence, there are no revenues to support the surviving residents (approximately equal to 50 percent of the original number of residents) and their associated expenses will be increasing, ranging from 20 to 40 percent of the total expected expenses at entry.

The impact of this premature entry fee earning is illustrated in the statement of revenues and expenses (or income statement) given in Table 11–2. The revenues in this example are based on a CCRC with

---

[4] The 1981 CCRC survey indicated that communities apply the life expectancy method on an individual basis three times more often than on a group basis. The individual application requires the community to develop amortization schedules for each resident, so that the total amortization is the sum of individual amounts. Group application of this method is done in one of two ways; either the life expectancy for the average age of the group is used or the individual life expectancies are summed and their average is used to amortize aggregate entry fees received from the cohort entrant group.

TABLE 11-2
Twenty-Year Projection of Statements of Revenues and Expenses Using Actuarial Fees and Group Life Expectancy Amortization of Entry Fees ($000)

Fiscal year	Operating revenues	Entry fee amortizations	Interest income	Total revenues	Operating expenses	Depreciation expense	Interest expense	Total expenses	Net income	End-of-year fund balance
1983	$ 3,775	$1,373	$1,181	$ 6,329	$ 2,628	$ 608	$1,600	$ 4,836	$1,493	$ 1,493
1984	3,893	1,436	1,292	6,621	2,891	630	1,593	5,114	1,507	3,000
1985	4,043	1,508	1,411	6,962	3,180	653	1,584	5,417	1,545	4,545
1986	4,217	1,590	1,535	7,342	3,498	679	1,575	5,752	1,590	6,135
1987	4,383	1,686	1,667	7,736	3,848	708	1,565	6,121	1,615	7,750
1988	4,616	1,785	1,794	8,195	4,232	739	1,553	6,524	1,671	9,421
1989	4,939	1,899	1,944	8,782	4,656	774	1,540	6,970	1,812	11,233
1990	5,267	2,021	2,095	9,383	5,121	812	1,525	7,458	1,925	13,158
1991	5,636	2,148	2,255	10,039	5,633	854	1,509	7,996	2,043	15,201
1992	5,993	2,309	2,447	10,749	6,197	900	1,490	8,587	2,162	17,363
1993	6,481	2,471	2,644	11,596	6,816	818	1,470	9,104	2,492	19,855
1994	7,050	2,248	2,874	12,172	7,498	861	1,446	9,805	2,367	22,222
1995	7,688	1,406	3,090	12,184	8,248	907	1,420	10,575	1,609	23,831
1996	8,403	1,563	3,362	13,328	9,072	959	1,391	11,422	1,906	25,737
1997	9,148	1,685	3,653	14,486	9,980	1,015	1,359	12,354	2,132	27,869
1998	9,907	1,861	3,970	15,738	10,978	1,077	1,322	13,377	2,361	30,230
1999	10,948	2,059	4,333	17,340	12,075	1,146	1,281	14,502	2,838	33,068
2000	12,071	2,262	4,787	19,120	13,283	1,221	1,236	15,740	3,380	36,448
2001	13,341	2,434	5,242	21,017	14,611	1,303	1,185	17,099	3,918	40,366
2002	14,675	2,659	5,778	23,112	16,072	1,394	1,127	18,593	4,519	44,885

actuarially determined fees. Column 3 contains entry fee amortizations based on the life expectancy associated with the average age of each cohort entrant group.[5] This statement shows that entry fee amortizations will increase almost 2 times in 20 years, from $1.4 million to $2.7 million. Since amortization amounts for the initial group of entrants cease at the end of their life expectancy (12 years), there is a drop in entry fee amortizations at that time (1994).

Depreciation (column 7) and interest (column 8) expenses replace capital expenditures on a cash flow statement to reflect more accurately the consumption of fixed assets. The excess of revenues over expenses (this item is referred to as net income in subsequent text and tables) is given in column 10 and shows a $1.5 million "profit" during the first year. This apparent profit increases to $4.5 million in 20 years. Judging from the GAAP income statement, management and other financial analysts might arrive at the erroneous conclusion that fees are too high and residents are being overcharged. Column 11 contains the end-of-year fund balance, equal to the cumulative total of excess revenues over expenses. For a nonprofit organization, this balance would be expected to be zero; however, it increases to $45 million after 20 years, implying that the community has a net worth equal to that amount.

Obviously, GAAP income statements present a misleading picture of the community's financial position. The GAAP accounting position is significantly different from the actuarial position, the latter having a $0 fund balance. Not only do GAAP income statements misrepresent the financial picture for a community using actuarial fees; they also overstate projections based on fees that are not actuarially sound. Table 11–3 shows the projected net income and fund balance using the four pricing policies discussed in Chapter 4—pay-as-you-go method, short-term cash balance method (or simply short-term method),[6] open-group method, and closed-group method—and life expectancy amortizations.

Net income for the pay-as-you-go method is negative for six years before becoming positive for the next six years. Since net income is increasing annually, management might feel that its pricing policy is appropriate even though monthly fees are required to increase substantially more than inflation. After the entry fees from the original group of

---

[5] Many communities using the life expectancy method base earnings on a rounded value for the life expectancy. This example does not round the life expectancy, and there are earnings in the fractional year (i.e., if the life expectancy is 13.5 years, then 7.4 percent is earned for the first 13 years and 3.7 percent is earned during the 14th year).

[6] This term is used to refer to the fact that a short-term outlook (i.e., five to seven years) was used to determine the adequacy of fees, as is done in many feasibility studies. It is *not* meant to imply that feasibility studies generate actuarially deficient fees.

TABLE 11-3

Comparison of Net Income and Fund Balances under Four Pricing Policies ($000)

Fiscal year	Pay-as-you-go fees		Short-term fees		Open-group fees		Closed-group fees	
	Net income	End-of-year fund balance	Net income	End-of-year fund balance	Net income	End-of-year fund balance	Net income	End-of-year fund balance
1983	$(426)	$(426)	$1,006	$1,006	$1,336	$ 1,336	$1,493	$ 1,493
1984	(647)	(1,073)	945	1,951	1,313	2,649	1,507	3,000
1985	(722)	(1,795)	892	2,843	1,304	3,953	1,545	4,545
1986	(555)	(2,350)	832	3,675	1,295	5,248	1,590	6,135
1987	(390)	(2,740)	736	4,411	1,258	6,506	1,615	7,750
1988	(274)	(3,014)	652	5,063	1,240	7,746	1,671	9,421
1989	7	(3,007)	634	5,697	1,298	9,044	1,812	11,233
1990	28	(2,979)	564	6,261	1,313	10,357	1,925	13,158
1991	44	(2,935)	471	6,732	1,316	11,673	2,043	15,201
1992	64	(2,871)	339	7,071	1,298	12,971	2,162	17,363
1993	277	(2,594)	386	7,457	1,471	14,442	2,492	19,855
1994	121	(2,473)	(22)	7,435	1,167	15,609	2,367	22,222
1995	(564)	(3,307)	(1,038)	6,397	206	15,815	1,609	23,831
1996	(458)	(3,495)	(1,155)	5,242	267	16,082	1,906	25,737
1997	(476)	(3,971)	(1,397)	3,845	221	16,303	2,132	27,869
1998	(535)	(4,506)	(1,705)	2,140	138	16,441	2,361	30,230
1999	(420)	(4,926)	(1,836)	304	262	16,703	2,838	33,068
2000	(337)	(5,263)	(2,000)	(1,696)	390	17,093	3,380	36,448
2001	(359)	(5,622)	(2,247)	(3,943)	462	17,555	3,918	40,366
2002	(436)	(6,058)	(2,545)	(6,488)	530	18,085	4,519	44,885

entrants have been amortized (fiscal year 1995), net income becomes negative again. The fund balance is negative for the entire projection. The income statement associated with short-term fees shows positive net income for 11 years. This statement, coupled with projected increases in cash flow for the eight years, does not give any indication of future problems if management continues with its current pricing policies. The projections based on open-group and closed-group fees also show a sound financial position. For the open-group method, net income is expected to be slightly more than $1.3 million during the first 11 years and is positive throughout the projection. For the closed-group method, net income increases to $2.5 million within 11 years. The fund balances by the end of 20 years accumulate to $18 million and $45 million for the open- and closed-group methods, respectively. Since the cash flows for these projections are also positive for each year, there is no way for management to identify the actuarial imbalance from GAAP income statements.

Theoretical Amortization Characteristics. The basic characteristics of the theoretically correct method of amortizing entry fees have already been described. These characteristics are derivatives of the revenue/expense matching tenet and the inflation-constrained monthly fee objective.[7] The first characteristic is that if members of a new entrant cohort are expected to survive beyond their life expectancy, then the amortization schedule should reflect earnings after that period. This characteristic will be referred to as earnings over the resident's *potential* lifetime. The second characteristic is that entry fee amortizations on a per life basis must be increasing since the expenses assumed to be covered by entry fees are also increasing. This characteristic is referred to as the *increasing-dollar per life* amortization schedule. It does not mean that if the earnings for a group of residents were traced over the residents' lifetime in the community, their aggregate amortization amounts would be increasing; what it means is that if annual amounts amortized were divided by the number of survivors, the earnings *per life* would be increasing.

The third and final characteristic is that if costs increase for changes in living status, then the amortization schedule should reflect the expected cost differentials weighted by the probability of change in living status. Hence, the per life amortization amounts will be increasing by more than the inflation assumption. This characteristic is referred to as the *cost differential adjustment.*

Given these characteristics, a theoretically correct amortization schedule consistent with GAAP (i.e., excluding imputed interest) can be developed. Certain trade-offs are necessary to generate a schedule

---

[7] If the inflation constraint objective were removed, it would be possible to set monthly fees so that entry fee earnings could be a level amount per life.

that can be easily implemented. The two questions that must be addressed are (1) whether the schedule should be implemented on a group or individual basis and (2) how the amortization amounts should vary if the community's experience does not match the underlying assumptions used to derive entry fees (referred to as adjustments for experience deviations).

If the amortization schedule is developed on a group basis, it must weight the ages and sexes of the cohort new entrant group. Aggregate amortization schedules are derived by amortizing the sum of the fees for a cohort group according to the group-based schedule. Individual implementation is more complicated, since this requires separate schedules that vary for age and sex as well as the number of occupants. The following discussion is based on a group amortization schedule. Also, it is initially assumed that experience follows the underlying assumptions, so there is no adjustment incorporated for experience deviations. This constraint will be removed in a later discussion.

Two new amortization methods are analyzed with regard to the three theoretically correct amortization characteristics. The first method, which was recently introduced, is described as a "level-dollar per life" amortization.[8] This means that the amortization amount per life is constant. The second method, developed by the authors, is characterized as an "increasing-dollar per life" method and generates in-

TABLE 11-4
Comparison of Expense-Matching Characteristics for Five Generic Methods of Amortizing Entry Fees on GAAP Income Statements

	Characteristics		
Method of amortization	Amortization over potential lifetime	Matches increasing expense pattern	Reflects higher health care costs
Immediate recognition	No	No	No
Refund	No	No	No
Life expectancy	No	No	No
Level-dollar per life	Yes	No	No
Increasing-dollar per life	Yes	Yes	Yes

creasing amortization payments per life over time. Table 11-4 presents a matrix comparison of these two methods, along with the immediate recognition, refund, and life expectancy methods, as they relate to the theoretically correct characteristics.

---

[8] Hershel D. Sosnoff and Jack E. Blumenthal, "Accommodation Fees: Have You Earned Them?" *American Health Care Journal*, January 1980, p. 23.

Level-Dollar per Life Method. This method spreads entry fee amortizations over the resident's potential lifetime. In essence, the amortization curve follows the expected survivorship curve, but this method does not address the other characteristics since it is derived from the assumption that amortizations on a per life basis should be level and there is no adjustment for a change in living status. Although some CCRCs may initially set entry fees to cover "bricks and mortar" (implying constant earnings), it is doubtful that these communities have been able to adhere to this policy, since nearly all communities increase entry fees for inflation. Therefore, this method generally would not be appropriate except for a few isolated cases, yet it does eliminate the concern over a premature cutoff of entry fee amortization.

A comparison of the percentage of the original entry fee that is amortized annually under the level-dollar per life method with the amortization percentage under the life expectancy method is given in Table 11–5. These percentages are based on an age-75 female entrant.

TABLE 11–5
Entry Fee Amortization Schedules for Age-75
Female Entrant

		Amortization method		
Year (t)	Age (x)	Life expectancy	Level-dollar per life	Increasing-dollar per life
0	75	7.364%	7.364%	2.509%
1	76	7.364	7.268	2.774
2	77	7.364	7.154	3.061
3	78	7.364	7.018	3.369
4	79	7.364	6.858	3.695
5	80	7.364	6.669	4.035
6	81	7.364	6.447	4.381
7	82	7.364	6.190	4.725
8	83	7.364	5.893	5.053
9	84	7.364	5.556	5.350
10	85	7.364	5.178	5.596
11	86	7.364	4.760	5.771
12	87	7.364	4.305	5.851
13	88	4.267*	3.821	5.815
14	89	0.000	3.318	5.649
15	90	—	2.812	5.349
16	91	—	2.322	4.927
17	92	—	1.865	4.408
18	93	—	1.457	3.830
19	94	—	1.108	3.233
20	95	—	0.821	2.656
25	100	—	0.127	0.679
30	105	—	0.009	0.077
35	110	—	0.000	0.001

* This percentage represents earnings for expected survivorship for fractional year.

Entry fee amortizations are determined by multiplying the percentage given in this table by the original entry fee. Columns 3 and 4 show that the life expectancy and level-dollar per life methods amortize the same percentage in the first year, but thereafter the level-dollar amortization declines.[9] The decline reflects a decreasing number of survivors in future years (dividing the percentage by the number of survivors will generate a constant amount). The level-dollar per life method amortizes 84 percent of the entry fee at the end of 14 years (life expectancy); the remaining 16 percent is amortized over the next 21 years.

Increasing-Dollar per Life Method. This method incorporates the concept of amortization over the resident's potential lifetime as well as increasing amortization amounts per life based on the annual cost differential for the probability of survival in the health care center. In order to develop an amortization schedule employing these characteristics, assumptions must be made on the rate of increase and the additional cost differential for living in the health care center. Table 11–5 contains the amortization percentages for a schedule based on a 10 percent per year rate of increase and a 1.75 ratio of health care to apartment costs. In practice, the assumptions for these two values should be based on the community's pricing philosophy regarding expenses to be covered by entry fees and their rate of increase, and may vary according to a specific community's experience. The increasing-dollar per life method shows substantially less amortization during the first year than do the other two methods (2.509 percent compared with 7.364 percent). Beginning in the 11-th year, the increasing-dollar per life amortizations exceed the level-dollar per life amortizations. Aggregate amortizations for a group of entrants increase for 13 years despite a decreasing number of survivors. At the end of 14 years, 62 percent of the original entry fees has been amortized.

Figure 11–1 graphically illustrates entry fee amortization schedules under three GAAP amortization methods for a group of entrants who paid a total of $10 million in entry fees. This figure shows that amortization amounts under the increasing-dollar per life method initially start at $250,000 and increase for 13 years before declining. Amortization amounts under the other two methods, life expectancy and level-dollar per life, are at their highest right after entry.

Comparison of Income Statements. In order to determine the financial impact of these alternative amortization schedules, the community's income was projected using each method. Table 11–6 presents net income and the end-of-the year fund balance for the life expectancy

---

[9] These percentages are based on the assumption that deaths occur at the end of the year. This is done for pedagogic purposes only, and implementation of this method for an actual case would reflect a percentage that assumed midyear deaths.

216

FIGURE 11-1 ――――――――――――――――――――――――――――――――――――
Annual Entry Fee Earnings under Three GAAP Amortization Methods

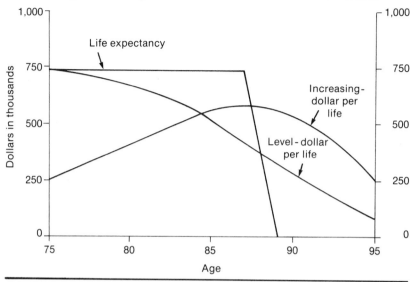

TABLE 11-6 ―――――――――――――――――――――――――――――――――――――
Comparison of Net Income and Fund Balances for Three GAAP
Amortization Schedules *($000)*

	Net income			End-of-year fund balance		
Fiscal year	Life expectancy	Level-dollar per life	Increasing-dollar per life	Life expectancy	Level-dollar per life	Increasing-dollar per life
1983	$1,493	$1,492	$ 658	$ 1,493	$ 1,492	$ 658
1984	1,501	1,482	693	3,000	2,974	1,351
1985	1,545	1,485	747	4,545	4,459	2,098
1986	1,590	1,487	809	6,135	5,946	2,907
1987	1,615	1,462	846	7,750	7,408	3,753
1988	1,671	1,455	913	9,421	8,863	4,666
1989	1,812	1,524	1,058	11,233	10,387	5,724
1990	1,925	1,552	1,167	13,158	11,939	6,891
1991	2,043	1,572	1,272	15,201	13,511	8,163
1992	2,162	1,578	1,346	17,363	15,089	9,509
1993	2,492	1,787	1,621	19,855	16,876	11,130
1994	2,367	1,936	1,820	22,222	18,812	12,950
1995	1,609	2,045	1,980	23,831	20,857	14,930
1996	1,906	2,243	2,192	25,737	23,100	17,122
1997	2,132	2,408	2,354	27,869	25,508	19,476
1998	2,361	2,540	2,458	30,230	28,048	21,934
1999	2,838	2,913	2,785	33,068	30,961	24,719
2000	3,380	3,398	3,191	36,448	34,359	27,910
2001	3,918	3,880	3,613	40,366	38,239	31,523
2002	4,519	4,422	4,077	44,885	42,661	35,600

method and the two alternative methods. A comparison of the net income for the three methods (columns 2 through 4) shows similar amounts for the life expectancy and level-dollar per life methods. The level-dollar method *does* eliminate the drop in income associated with the cessation of amortization amounts from the initial cohort of entrants under the life expectancy method. At the end of 20 years, the difference in net income under the two methods is less than 2 percent. On the other hand, net income for the increasing-dollar per life method is less than half that of the other two methods during the first year. Net income for this method increases constantly for 20 years and is approximately 10 percent less than net income under the life expectancy method at the end of 20 years.

The fund balances for the life expectancy and level-dollar methods are also similar. In fact, at the end of 20 years, they are within $2 million of each other. The increasing-dollar fund balance is $9 million less than the life expectancy fund balance at the end of 20 years. While the increasing-dollar per life method does offer substantial improvements over the other two, all three methods are distant from the true actuarial position of the hypothetical CCRC. This means that additional modifications are in order—either a more drastic reduction in entry fee amortizations or corrections in the other elements of the income statement, such as an alternative to cost-basis depreciation. The methodology for dealing with gains and losses is described before these modifications are considered.

Gains and Losses. The implementation of the preceding amortization schedules is accurate if experience exactly follows the underlying assumptions. This situation is unlikely to occur, and management may wish to adjust its amortization schedule to reflect the variations. Gains and losses will also occur if the utilization assumptions are changed and/or if the residents' contracts are altered. The methodology for dealing with experience deviations can be applied to any of the five types of amortization schedules. It requires that the methods be applied on an individual basis rather than a group basis (i.e., separate entry fee amortization schedules are developed for each entrant based on his or her age and sex, and the total amortization amounts for a given year are a weighted sum of the individual amounts).[10] Thus, as the experience of the community unfolds, the amortization schedules reflect deviations away from the expected survivorship and transfer patterns.

---

[10] This methodology is explained in more detail in David L. Hewitt, "Actuarial Amortization of Entry Fees for Life Care Communities," *1981–82 Proceedings of the Conference of Actuaries in Public Practice,* pages 506–23. This paper presents an application of the gain and loss methodology using the life expectancy earnings method.

Depreciation

In an inflationary environment, historic-cost depreciation does not fairly reflect the consumption of fixed assets. Therefore, an income statement using historic-cost depreciation would overstate net income and show an overly optimistic financial picture. An even more important concern is that if a community funds the depreciation expense, it will not generate sufficient revenues to replace fixed assets even if interest earnings on the funded depreciation expense are included. An alternative method for depreciating fixed assets is replacement-cost depreciation. The pros and cons of this procedure are discussed extensively in the accounting literature, and it is not the purpose of this section to determine whether this procedure is reasonable from a GAAP viewpoint. However, replacement-cost depreciation is a useful method for preparing internal statements that will better represent the community's financial position. A description of the two methods for expensing fixed assets is given below.

Under historic-cost depreciation, the cost of the asset is expensed over its assumed useful lifetime. Thus, if a building cost $15 million and is expected to last 40 years, the historic-cost depreciation expense would be $375,000 for each of the 40 years. Replacement-cost depreciation is based on the premise that the depreciation expense is derived from the replacement value of the asset each year. Thus, if the building is assumed to appreciate in value at an inflation rate of 10 percent, the depreciation expense would be $375,000 in the first year, $412,500 (375,000 × 1.1) in the second year, $453,700 (412,500 × 1.1) in the third year, and so forth.[11]

Table 11–7 shows an income statement that implements both replacement-cost depreciation and increasing-dollar per life entry fee amortizations (revenues are based on actuarial fees). This statement shows that net income never exceeds $1 million, and the fund balance at the end of 20 years is only $13 million, or $2 million more than the actuarial statement fund balance. The inclusion of replacement-cost depreciation appears to eliminate some of the discrepancies associated with GAAP income statements. However, it should be pointed out that the implementation of this procedure is less straightforward than it seems to be in the example. One of the major issues is the appropriate inflation measure for determining depreciation expenses. There must be controls on the inflation assumption since it could be used to manipulate the financial picture presented by a community. A second issue is that a community would have to keep two sets of financial statements, one based on historic-cost depreciation and the other on replacement-

---

[11] This is a rather simplified example; in practice, midyear adjustments would be made and the actual depreciation expense would be the average of beginning- and end-of-year asset values.

TABLE 11-7

Twenty-Year Projection of Statements of Revenues and Expenses Using Actuarial Fees, Increasing-Dollar per Life Amortization, and Replacement-Cost Depreciation *($000)*

Fiscal year	Total revenues	Depreciation expense	Total expenses	Net income	End-of-year fund balance
1983	$ 5,495	$ 608	$ 4,837	$658	$ 658
1984	5,806	691	5,174	632	1,290
1985	6,165	783	5,548	617	1,907
1986	6,561	887	5,961	600	2,507
1987	6,966	1,005	6,417	549	3,056
1988	7,438	1,137	6,922	516	3,572
1989	8,028	1,285	7,480	548	4,120
1990	8,625	1,451	8,098	527	4,647
1991	9,267	1,638	8,780	487	5,134
1992	9,933	1,848	9,535	398	5,532
1993	10,725	1,741	10,027	698	6,230
1994	11,625	1,937	10,881	744	6,974
1995	12,555	2,154	11,822	733	7,707
1996	13,614	2,395	12,859	755	8,462
1997	14,708	2,663	14,002	706	9,168
1998	15,835	2,961	15,261	574	9,742
1999	17,287	3,291	16,648	639	10,381
2000	18,930	3,658	18,177	753	11,134
2001	20,713	4,066	19,862	851	11,985
2002	22,671	4,518	21,718	953	12,938

cost depreciation, because it is unlikely that third-party reimbursement agencies would allow replacement cost to be used as a basis for determining expenses.

Health Care Reserve Fund

One of the unique characteristics of continuing care retirement communities is that they combine residential units with nursing care beds. This often leads to a combined financial statement for both of these cost centers. Such a combination may be confusing. During the early years of the community, when the health care beds are occupied by outside residents who pay full costs and the community experiences the rich cash flow associated with the initial entry fees, it may be difficult for management to determine whether the continuing care fees are building up the proper health care reserves. Due to this robust financial position and no cost center separation, management may depress monthly fees while health care utilization is low, thus having to raise fees more than inflation as health care utilization matures.

A method for eliminating this potential confusion is to develop separate statements for the apartment and health care centers, with fees allocated proportionally to cover apartment-related expenses and health care–related expenses. If an actuarial pricing analysis has been performed, this separation is a by-product of the fee structure. The portion of fees allocated to health care expenses can be credited to a third statement, a health care reserve fund, which would be debited for 100 percent of the per diem costs for health care utilization by continuing care contractholders. The amount debited from the health care reserve can be reflected as revenues for the health care center statement. In addition to revenues from the health care reserve fund to cover per diem costs, the health care center can have as revenues fees from outside patients. Completing the system, the apartment center statement can show monthly fees and entry fee amortizations for those funds designated for residential costs.

The size and cash flow of a health care reserve must be carefully monitored by performing annual actuarial valuations to determine whether the reserve is at the proper level. The size of the reserve may seem excessive, since it should greatly exceed health expenses for any one year. Once the community's health care utilization matures, the growth in the reserve should match inflation, but prior to that time it should increase faster than inflation. The advantage of this approach is that if for any reason the community chooses to modify or cease offering continuing care contracts, it would have the necessary funds identified to cover its contractual obligations to its existing continuing care contractholders.

Summary

This chapter discussed the usefulness of income statements for assessing the financial position of a CCRC. Income statements were developed to rectify the major problem inherent in the cash flow statement (i.e., revenues not matching expenses). An actuarial income statement was developed amortizing entry fees in the theoretically correct fashion and requiring that interest be imputed for revenues and expenses associated with investments in fixed assets. This statement presented a fairly realistic financial picture; however, it was seen that even if the actuarial statement is consistent with the actuarial valuation methodology, it does not solve the problems associated with GAAP statements. Three issues discussed in this chapter were: (1) the method for amortizing entry fees, (2) the depreciation of fixed assets, and (3) fund accounting for health care costs.

The major issue was the manner in which entry fees were amortized. A method was developed that better matched revenues with expenses by amortizing entry fees over the resident's potential lifetime and increasing earnings per life to match the ever-increasing gap between expenses and inflation-constrained monthly fees. It was found that this method, in combination with replacement-cost depreciation, painted the most realistic picture of the community's financial position, but even this method did not capture the true picture.

In summary, the appropriate tools for setting fees are the combination discussed in Chapters 7 through 9: actuarial valuations, new entry pricing analyses, and cash flow projections. These tools tell management where its pricing policy will lead the community, as opposed to where the community has been. Income statements and the budgeting process can be improved to reflect more fairly the community's actuarial position, but they are not sufficient for explaining the reasons for fee increases since they only tell the community where it has been, not where it is going. ■

Part Three

Legal Analysis

Chapter Twelve ⎯⎯⎯⎯⎯⎯
Status of Current Legislation

■ The purpose of this chapter is to provide a descriptive analysis of existing formal legal regulation of continuing care retirement communities. This material will serve as the foundation for the authors' normative analysis. The discussion is divided into three parts, based on three different types of formal legal responses to CCRCs:

> *Detailed state regulatory schemes:* The first part discusses the responses of nine states and at least one organization—detailed regulation of CCRCs.[1]

> *Limited state regulatory schemes:* The second part discusses the responses of at least three states—selected regulation of one or two of the problems of the continuing care retirement community industry susceptible to legal regulation.

> *Nonregulation:* The third part discusses the responses of the remaining thirty-six states, the District of Columbia, and the federal government—virtually total inaction. Included in this part are comments on proposed, but as yet unenacted, legislation and judicial attitudes toward CCRCs.

⎯⎯⎯⎯⎯

[1] The footnotes used throughout this chapter contain references to several state statutes and model acts; however, copies are not included. Appendix F contains information on where the reader can obtain copies of statutes and model acts. In order to summarize this information and to simplify comparisons over state lines, comparative charts are included.

EXTENSIVE STATE REGULATORY SCHEMES

This is perhaps the most important and complex part of this chapter. Regardless of whether one prefers that states adopt comprehensive regulation, selective regulation, or no regulation at all, the experience of the states that have adopted comprehensive regulatory schemes will be a valuable data base.

Ten comprehensive statutes will be explained, discussed, and contrasted in this section: those of Arizona, California, Colorado, Florida, Indiana, Maryland, Michigan, Minnesota, and Missouri[2] and the model legislation proposed by the American Association of Homes for the Aged (AAHA).[3]

There are obviously a number of ways to impart the form and content of these 10 statutes. In order to maximize the key aims of providing an exhaustive, yet comprehensible, background on the current status of legal regulation of CCRCs, the following organizational scheme has been selected. This section is broken down topically, with each topic being one type of regulation typically found in a comprehensive state legislative scheme (e.g., definition, reserve requirements, and rights of resident organization). Within each topic, the type of regulation is described and the advantages and disadvantages of that form of regulation are noted.[4] An explanatory discussion of how each of the above 10 statutes deals with each element follows.

DEFINITION OF ENTITY TO BE REGULATED

It is apparent at this point that the institutions variously referred to as life care, continuing care, living care, perpetual care, residence and

---

[2] Work on this chapter concluded in spring 1982, and, therefore, the chapter includes no reference to legislative or regulatory action thereafter. For example, Illinois adopted comprehensive legislation following completion of the chapter. As a result, its legislation is not analyzed herein.

[3] In addition to the AAHA model act, Life Care Services Corporation, a proprietary continuing care management company, has promulgated a model act that can fairly be classified as comprehensive legislation. That statute, however, has nothing in any of its individual sections that is not fully discussed later in this section, and, therefore, it is not included as one of the statutes discussed therein.

In brief, the Life Care Services Corporation model act contains a typical definition of continuing care; provides for comprehensive registration of all facilities; requires an annual report; has an independent revocation proceeding; provides for substantial disclosure; mandates both an entrance fee and a reserve fund escrow; grants a lien to residents that is filed by the administering agency before registration or subsequently; contains a full investigative, rehabilitative, and liquidation procedure; and provides for civil and criminal penalties for violation of the act.

[4] These advantages and disadvantages were developed by the authors, following thorough collaboration with the study's Advisory Committee and other experienced professionals in the continuing care field. Nevertheless, no value judgments are made in this chapter as to whether any particular type of regulation should be adopted. Such judgments are reserved to Chapter 13, which was drafted following receipt and analysis of the Wharton School survey.

care, and life lease are anything but homogeneous. Various communities differ significantly in substance, depending on the respective termination rights of the community and the resident, the amount of services and medical care covered under the contract at no or a nominal extra charge, and the financing arrangements between the resident and the community.

Given the diverse characteristics of separate CCRCs, if a state wants to regulate continuing care, it must first determine which type of CCRC it wants to regulate, and then it must draft a definition that ensures that all of these types of communities will be brought under the scope of the statute.

California's definition appears to have avoided most of the typical pitfalls:

> "Life care contract" means a contract to provide to a person for the duration of such person's life or for a term in excess of one year, nursing services, medical services, or health-related services, board and lodging and care as necessary, or any combination of such services for such person in a facility, which is conditioned upon the transfer of property. Such transfer may include a payment of an entrance fee to the provider of such services or the payment of periodic charges for the care and service involved, or both such payments, and includes continuing care agreements.[5]

Note that this definition includes terminable continuing care agreements explicitly, as well as all types of financing arrangements between the resident and the community. Michigan's definition has also apparently caused few problems.[6]

Arizona's definition is similar to California's,[7] but most facilities within Arizona have stopped charging entrance fees altogether, thereby avoiding regulation, raising their periodic fees, and, therefore, moving closer to becoming fee-for-service providers.[8] Maryland's definition[9] and Minnesota's definition[10] appear susceptible to the same problems faced by Arizona, though the statutes are still too new in these states to tell.[11] Similarly, the AAHA definition[12] and the Indiana

---

[5] California §1771(i).

[6] Michigan §§554.803(5)–(6).

[7] Arizona §20–1801(5).

[8] Ohio Nursing Home Commission Memorandum from Paul Wallace to Catherine Hawes (October 18, 1978).

[9] Maryland §7(b).

[10] Minnesota §80.D.02(2).

[11] Colorado's statute also appears to be susceptible to this problem. Colorado §12–13–101(6).

[12] AAHA §2(a).

Definitions

Arizona: Contract to provide for a person for life or for a term in excess of one year medical services and board and lodging conditioned on payment of an entrance fee in addition to or in lieu of periodic payments.

California: Contract to provide for a person for life or for a term in excess of one year medical services and board and lodging conditioned on payment of an entrance fee in addition to or in lieu of periodic charges, including continuing care agreements.

Colorado: Care provided under a contract for life of an aged person, including health care, board, and lodging.

Florida: Furnishing of nursing care, shelter, and food upon payment of an entrance fee. Continuing care shall include only life care, care for life, or care for a period of one year or more.

Indiana: Contract to provide for a person for life or for a term in excess of one month medical services, board, and lodging conditioned on payment of an entrance fee in addition to or in lieu of periodic payments.

Maryland: Furnishing for money, care or shelter to an individual over age 60 under a contract which (1) requires 12 or more months of care to another to be paid in advance, (2) provides for care for more than one year, or (3) provides for life care.

Michigan: Three-part definition covering only life care and care for more than one year. Labels the former "life interest" and the latter "long-term lease."

Minnesota: Furnishing to an individual board and lodging together with medical services pursuant to a written agreement effective for the life of the individual or for a period in excess of one year.

Missouri: Furnishing shelter, food, and nursing care to an individual for life or for a term of years. Care for a term of years defined to include care in excess of one year and an agreement for continuing care for an indefinite term.

AAHA: Agreement for the payment of an entrance fee and/or periodic charges in exchange for living accommodations, medical care, and related services, which is effective for the life of the individual or for a period in excess of one year.

---

definition,[13] because they do not expressly include mutually terminable agreements, might cause problems.

Florida provides an example of the hazards of improper definition of the institutions to be regulated. The earliest Florida legislation applied only to institutions using total-fee-in-advance or assignment-of-all-assets methods of financing[14] and only to contracts for life or for a term of years.[15] In 1978, Florida expanded its definition beyond fixed-fee arrangements[16] by expressly including terminable continuing care contracts within the definition of "care for a term of years."[17] New Florida

---

[13] Indiana §1.

[14] Fla. Stat. Ann. §651.02(4) (West 1972).

[15] *Id.* §651.02(3). Colorado's statute is similar. Colorado §12–13–101(6).

[16] Fla. Stat. Ann. §§651.011(6), (8) (West Supp. 1978).

[17] *Id.* §651.011(7); *see id.* 651.011(2). This is the model followed by the new Missouri statute and should cause no problems. Missouri §1(1), (2).

legislation, though including the expanded definition of "care for a term of years,"[18] deleted any reference to that phrase in its definition of continuing care.[19] Thus, it was possible that Florida's new statute did not apply to communities offering mutually terminable continuing care contracts that need not last for more than one year. Florida is now amending its statute again, and it is expected that this definitional problem will be resolved.

Two further illustrations of definitional problems can be found in states that apparently tried to prohibit life care arrangements. New York's nursing home regulations prohibit any "residential health-care facility" operator from accepting prepayment for "basic services" for more than three months[20] or from entering into any contract for "life care."[21] This language has been construed to mean that CCRCs are prohibited in New York;[22] yet it may not apply to communities that offer terminable contracts and earmark prepaid entrance fees for capital expenditures rather than basic services. Indeed, at least 11 facilities in New York purport to offer continuing care contracts.[23] Similarly, Pennsylvania's nursing home regulations provide that such facilities "shall not require or permit a patient to assign his assets to the facility in return for a life care guarantee,"[24] yet continuing care retirement communities that use mutually terminable contracts are common in that state.[25]

PREOPENING PROCEDURES: CERTIFICATION

All nine states and the AAHA model act require some sort of preliminary registration and certification by a relevant state authority before

[18] Florida §651.011(7).

[19] Florida §651.011(2).

[20] N.Y. Code of Rules & Regulations, tit. 10, §730.2(f) (1979); *see id.* §415.1(f), §420.1(f).

[21] *Id.* §730–3(b); *see id.* §414.16(b).

[22] See, e.g., Brown, *An Appraisal of the Nursing Home Enforcement Process,* 17 Arizona L. Rev. 304, 350 (1975).

[23] *See* AAHA, *Directory of Members* 50–61 (1982). These may be contracts that were in existence before promulgation of the present regulations.

[24] 28 Pa. Code §201.38 (1979). The confusion surrounding this regulation arises from the failure to define "life care" and the use of the word *assets* without any modifier. Does it mean *any* assets, thus apparently prohibiting continuing care, or *all* assets, thus apparently prohibiting only assignment-of-all-assets contracts? *See* Jenkins, *Life Care Contracts—Problems?,* Concern. February–March 1976, at 27, 30.

[25] *See* N. Adelman, *Director of Life Care Communities,* 2d ed. (Kennett Square, Pa.: Kendal Crosslands, 1980); and Howard E. Winklevoss and Alwyn V. Powell, *1982 Reference Directory of Continuing Care Retirement Communities* (Philadelphia: Human Services Research, Inc. (1982).

Certification

Provisional certification

Arizona: None.

California: None.

Colorado: None.

Florida: Required application with attachments. Then can collect entrance fees and enter into feasibility study.

Indiana: None.

Maryland: None.

Michigan: None.

Minnesota: None.

Missouri: None.

AAHA: None.

Certification

Arizona: Cannot sell contract without certification.

California: Cannot sell contract without certification.

Colorado: Cannot sell contract without certification.

Florida: Required for operation.

Indiana: Cannot sell contract without certification.

Maryland: Cannot sell contract without certification.

Michigan: Cannot sell contract without certification.

Minnesota: Cannot sell contract without filing (self-executing statute).

Missouri: Cannot sell contract without certification.

AAHA: Cannot sell contract without certification.

Financial information required

Arizona: Balance sheets, income statements, and projected income statements.

California: Past three years' balance sheets and income statements plus five-year projections.

Colorado: Certified financial statements and projected income statements for at least a five-year period.

Florida: Use of proceeds statements plus balance sheet and income statement. Also, computation of debt service requirement and information on plant equipment and property.

Indiana: Financial statements of the provider prepared in accordance with generally accepted accounting principles.

Maryland: Certified statement of applicant's financial condition.

Michigan: Balance sheet, use of proceeds statement, and feasibility study.

Minnesota: Balance sheet and income statements. Projected income statement for next year.

Missouri: Comprehensive financial statements with specifics varying depending on whether the CCRC is new or old. Also, statement of reserve and escrow provisions.

AAHA: Certified financial statements and income statements. Projected income statements for next year.

Renewals, revocations, etc.

Arizona: Annual filings, but certification valid until revocation.

California: Annual filings, but certification valid until revocation. Independent revocation procedure.

Colorado: Annual renewal procedure. Independent revocation procedure.

Florida: Annual renewal procedure. Independent revocation procedure.

Indiana: Annual filings, but certification valid until revocation. Independent revocation procedure.

Maryland: Annual renewal procedure. Independent revocation procedure.

Michigan: Annual renewal procedure. Independent revocation procedure.

Minnesota: Annual filings, but certification valid until revocation. Independent revocation procedure.

Missouri: Annual renewal procedure. Independent revocation procedure.

AAHA: Annual filings, but certification valid until revocation. Independent revocation procedure.

---

the beginning of operations. Failure to comply with these requirements can result in civil or criminal penalties.

This element of regulation involves an attempt by the state to screen "unacceptable" operators out of the continuing care industry. The notion is that, based on some sort of comprehensive application complete with required submissions, the state will be able to determine the financial stability and capacity, the sincerity, and the integrity of a prospective continuing care operator. Prospective certification, coupled with annual monitoring and various enforcement provisions, is the major mechanism by which the states currently regulating in detail supervise the financial stability of the continuing care industry.

Thus, the purpose of such certification is to ensure compliance with whatever standards the governmental agency decides to impose. The key problems are whether the states have isolated proper standards, whether the information they request helps them to evaluate financial stability, and whether the responsible state agency has the time, inclination, or expertise to evaluate that information properly. Given some skepticism about the efficacy of government certification programs, it has been suggested that private accreditation might eventually replace such systems.[26]

As mentioned above, all 10 statutes require that the provider be certified before the execution of any continuing care agreement. Florida requires each provider to apply for a provisional certificate of authority.[27] Florida requires prospective continuing care operators to

---

[26] Governmental reliance on a private accreditation system would not be unprecedented. For purposes of Medicare certification, the federal government usually requires no more of hospitals than that they meet standards set by the Joint Commission on Accreditation of Hospitals. *See* 42 U.S.C. §1395bb (1976). Also, the Council on Developmental Disabilities is a private accreditation program for facilities for the handicapped. A private accreditation program for continuing care retirement communities is in the final planning stages in the New Jersey/Pennsylvania area.

[27] Florida §651.031.

submit advertising, organizational information, construction data, and financial information to the state. The state then issues a provisional certificate that entitles the provider to collect deposits from prospective residents, so long as they are kept in escrow, and to undertake the feasibility study required for permanent certification.[28]

The Arizona, California, Colorado, Indiana, Maryland, Michigan, Minnesota, Missouri, and AAHA statutes simply provide that a continuing care operator may not sell or offer to sell a continuing care contract until a certificate of authority is granted.[29] Applications for certification, complete with the required attachments, are made to the appropriate state departments. The most important attachments are actual and projected financial statements,[30] a copy of the contract to be used,[31] services provided under the contract and charges for services not provided under the contract, and ownership and financial responsibility disclosure statements.[32]

The Colorado, Florida, Maryland, Michigan, and Missouri statutes provide for annual renewal of the certificate of authority after required financial forms are filed and specific statutory requirements are met.[33] The Arizona, California, Indiana, Minnesota, and AAHA certificates are valid until revoked, but annual reports similar to the financial filings in the other states are still required.[34] All the states except Arizona have specific, detailed procedures for revocation and/or suspension of certificates of authority.[35]

---

[28] Florida is presently considering amending its provisional certification requirements to mandate submission of a preliminary feasibility study before the proposed community is permitted to collect any deposits.

[29] Arizona §§20–1802–1803; California §1770(a); Colorado §12–13–102(1); Indiana §3(a); Maryland §9; Michigan §554.807; Minnesota §80D.03; Missouri §3; AAHA §3. The amended Minnesota statute is somewhat unique in the continuing care field. It is a completely self-executing legislative scheme. Thus, CCRCs are not *registered* under the act; they are required to file a disclosure statement with the county clerk meeting the requirements of section 80D.04. Similarly, there is no annual report to an administering agency—there is, however, an annual filing required. Finally, the administering agency and court step in only upon violation of a statutory provision.

[30] The states require balance statements, income statements, and statements of use of proceeds in varying combinations.

[31] The provisions that must be in the contract vary from state to state and will be discussed below.

[32] The Arizona, California, Colorado, Missouri, and AAHA statutes are the most advanced in this area. *See* Arizona §20–1802(B); California §1771.8(d)–(e), (h)–(k); Colorado §12–13–102; Missouri §4; AAHA §4(a)–(y).

[33] Colorado §12–13–108; Florida §§651.026(l), (8); Maryland §22; Michigan §§554.821–.822; Missouri §5(2).

[34] Arizona §§20–1803(B), –1807; California §§1782.5, 1783; Indiana §8(a); Minnesota §80D.12; AAHA §7(a).

[35] California §1784; Colorado §12–13–105; Florida §§651.026(8), .105, .114, .125; Maryland §22; Michigan §554.817; Minnesota §80D.12; AAHA §7.

LEGAL REGULATION OF FINANCIAL STATUS

Escrow Provisions

The basic policy behind escrow provisions is the view that an extra protection is needed for the residents' investments. Mandated escrow provisions might be viewed as tacit acknowledgments of the inadequacy, at least in certain instances, of disclosure, certification, and enforcement of other regulatory provisions. A disadvantage of mandated escrow provisions is that such provisions, by definition, direct capital into relatively stagnant bank accounts or other relatively unproductive uses of money, thereby depriving the residents of the full value of their money, in that some part of their investment is not working as efficiently for them as it might.

It is important to note, therefore, that escrow provisions must represent a delicate balance between these two policies. On the one hand, all of the community's reserves should not be in escrow because, though that maximizes protection of resident investment, it limits the community's capacity to put money to work for the residents. On the other hand, it might be advisable to require some funds to be placed in escrow at some time (for example, when the residents could not monitor the funds themselves), in order to ensure some protection of resident payments.

There are at least three different types of escrow requirements, representing to some extent different views on the outcome of the balancing process between the competing policies suggested above:

Entrance fee and deposit escrow until the resident moves into the community, at which time all funds are released to the operator.

Entrance fee escrow maintained even after residence is established because of a legal or self-imposed standard requiring a certain amount of funds, ranging from relatively small amounts to the full value of all resident payments to the community, to be kept in escrow.

General fund escrow of varying levels imposed on a perpetual basis by a bonding authority or bank holding a mortgage on the property.[36]

In the first category, Arizona, California, Colorado, Indiana, Michigan, Minnesota, and Missouri all require the maintenance of an escrow account for all entrance fees and deposits received before the resident occupies his or her unit.[37] The AAHA statute authorizes the regulatory

---

[36] Although this third form of escrow is fairly common, because it is largely a matter of private contract, it need not concern us in this chapter.

[37] Arizona §20–1804; California §1773.5; Colorado §12–13–104; Indiana §6; Michigan §554.810(b); Minnesota §80D.05; Missouri §10. *See also* 22 Cal. Code §84204.

Escrow Provisions

Arizona: Entrance fee escrow until occupancy for new units. Complicated formula for release of funds. Also requires a reserve fund escrow equal to aggregate principal and interest payments due on first mortgage over next 12 months.

California: Entrance fee escrow until occupancy for new units. Simple formula for release of funds. Also requires a reserve fund escrow equal to aggregate interest, principal, and lease payments due over next 12 months if there is no contractual provision for adjusting monthly fees.

Colorado: Entrance fee escrow until occupancy for new units. Complicated formula for release of funds. Also requires a reserve fund escrow equal to 65 percent of all large initial payments. This reserve is to be amortized over the first five years of residence, but at no time is the reserve to fall below 35 percent of the original requirement.

Florida: Entrance fee escrow required until certification and obtaining of long-term financing. Also requires a reserve fund escrow equal to aggregate of one half of the principal interest and lease payment due over the next fiscal year.

Indiana: Entrance fee escrow until occupancy for new units. Complicated formula for release of funds.

Maryland: Entrance fee escrow required until certification.

Michigan: Entrance fee escrow until occupancy for new units. Special provision authorizing state to require an escrow of a reasonable amount when financial conditions become precarious.

Minnesota: Entrance fee escrow until occupancy for new units. Complicated formula for release of funds. Also requires a reserve fund escrow equal to aggregate of principal and interest payments on first mortgage due over next 12 months.

Missouri: Entrance fee escrow until occupancy of new units. Complicated formula for release of funds. Also requires a reserve fund escrow equal to 50 percent of any entrance fee paid by the first occupant of the unit. This reserve is to be amortized and "earned" at the rate of 1 percent each month. But the reserve never can fall below 150 percent of the annual long-term debt, principal, and interest payments of the provider.

AAHA: Authorizes the department to require an entrance fee escrow until occupancy. Complicated formula for release of funds.

---

department to require an entrance fee escrow but does not mandate it.[38] Adopting a slightly different balance, Florida and Maryland require an escrowing of entrance fees and deposits until the operator is certified.[39] Michigan falls even further down the scale by granting the Corporations and Securities Bureau the discretion to require an escrow deposit of a "reasonable amount when the facility's economic condition is precarious."[40]

Arizona, California, Colorado, Florida, Minnesota, and Missouri all mandate some type of reserve fund escrow, as well as the entrance fee

---

[38] AAHA §6.

[39] Florida §651.031(4), (6); Maryland §11(c)–(d). Florida's requirement also mandates maintenance of escrow until long-term financing has been attained.

[40] Michigan §554.816.

escrow described above.[41] This kind of escrow requirement is of the second type noted above, and will be discussed in more detail in the next section.

Release of funds from the escrow account can be either very simple or extremely complicated. For example, California's entrance fee escrow is released when the facility is 50 percent completed and 50 percent subscribed to.[42] But the Arizona, Colorado, Indiana, Minnesota, Missouri, and AAHA statutes have complicated formulae governing release of the escrow funds, depending on whether the unit is new or old and, if new, depending on the stage of construction or financing.[43]

Reserve Funds

Six statutes—all of the statutes with the exception of Indiana's,[44] Maryland's, Michigan's, and AAHA's—mandate the maintenance of financial reserves. The major policy argument in favor of reserves is that, at least in theory, the maintenance of "adequate" reserves provides a financial buffer to help the CCRC survive through difficult financial times. In particular, adequate reserves protect communities from the low rates of turnover typical early in their existence, from actuarial miscalculations and aberrations, and from subsequent unexpectedly low turnover or unpredictably high inflation rates or costs.

On the other hand, arguments exist against mandatory reserve funds. Good financial and actuarial planning should go a long way toward obviating the need for such requirements. Again, as with escrow provisions and depending on investment limitations imposed on reserve funds, mandating reserve funds might well prejudice the future financial stability of the community by preventing funds from being put to their optimal use. Finally, even assuming the desirability of requir-

---

[41] Arizona §20–1806; California §1774.4; Colorado §12–13–107; Florida §651.035; Minnesota §80D.06; Missouri §7.

[42] California §1773.5.

[43] Arizona §20–1804(A)(2); Colorado §12–13–104; Indiana §6; Minnesota §80D.05; Missouri §10; AAHA §6.

[44] Indiana's statute contains unique provisions in place of a reserve requirement. Sections 13 through 18 of the Indiana statute establish a Retirement Home Guarantee Fund, a concept first suggested in Comment, *Continuing Care Retirement Communities for the Elderly: Potential Pitfalls and Proposed Regulation,* 128 U. Pa. L. Rev. 883 (1980). The purpose of the fund is to protect the interests of the residents if the CCRC goes into bankruptcy. A $100 fee is assessed on each CCRC resident entering into a continuing care contract. Indiana §13. That fund is then available for distribution to residents of CCRCs upon the meeting of certain conditions. Indiana §16. There are a number of exemptions from participation in the fund, including the tax-exempt status of the provider. Indiana §19.

Reserve Funds

Size

Arizona: Total of interest and principal payments due over the following year on account of any first mortgage or other long-term financing of the facility.

California: Total of interest, principal, and rental payments due during the next year (same as Arizona plus rental payments). Also, a requirement that reserve be sufficient to cover the obligations assumed under continuing care agreements, as calculated through the use of state-approved mortality tables.

Colorado: 65 percent of the amount of any advance payment made by all residents. Straight-line amortization over a five-year period. At no time can reserve fall below 30 percent of the original requirement.

Florida: Amount equal to one half of the aggregate amount of all principal and interest payments due during the fiscal year on any mortgage or other long-term financing on the facility, including taxes and insurance and leasehold payments.

Indiana: None. Has a Retirement Home Guarantee Fund instead.

Maryland: None.

Michigan: None.

Minnesota: Amount equal to the total of all principal and interest payments due during the next 12 months on account of any first mortgage or on account of any other long-term financing of the facility.

Missouri: Requires a reserve fund escrow equal to 50 percent of any entrance fee paid by the first occupant of the unit. This reserve is to be amortized and "earned" at the rate of 1 percent each month. But the reserve never can fall below 150 percent of the annual long-term debt, principal, and interest payments of the provider. In addition, each CCRC must establish a reserve equal to at least 5 percent of the facility's total balance of contractually obligated move-out refunds at the close of each fiscal year.

AAHA: None.

Investment limitations

Arizona: Must be placed in "escrow," but the principal of escrow account may be "invested," apparently without limitation, with the earnings and up to one sixth of the principal payable to the provider. Principal released to the provider must be repaid within two years.

California: The former reserve requirement must be placed in escrow, but the funds can be invested with the same limitations as apply to the second type of reserve. These limitations allow investments in bank deposits, first mortgages, approved bonds and stocks, real estate, and furniture and equipment of the community. Twenty-five percent must be in cash and listed bonds and stocks. If the community has at least half of its contracts on a monthly basis, only 5 percent need be in these liquid investments.

Colorado: Reserves must be held in bank accounts, first mortgages, real estate, or furniture of the community. At least 10 percent must be in bank accounts and listed bonds or stocks.

Florida: Subject to general investment limitations imposed on insurance companies with provision for emergency release of funds to the provider.

Indiana: None. Has a Retirement Home Guarantee Fund instead.

Maryland: None.

Michigan: None.

Minnesota: Must be placed in "escrow," but the principal of the escrow may be "invested," apparently without limitation, with the income and one twelfth of the principal payable to the provider.

Missouri: Must be placed in "escrow," but can be held in federal government or other marketable securities, deposits, or accounts insured by the federal government.

AAHA: None.

ing reserve funds, the calculation of a uniform level of reserves to be applied to all CCRCs might well be difficult.

Thus, as with the policy debate covering escrow provisions, the decision whether to adopt reserve requirements involves balancing sharply competing policies. This balancing takes place on two different levels in the reserve debates. First, one must determine the level of reserves that is necessary or desirable. Second, one must determine the investment limitations to be placed on whatever level of reserves is selected.

As noted above, Arizona, California, Colorado, Florida, and Minnesota all have some form of reserve requirements.[45] Each of these statutes has varying requirements covering both the size of the reserve and investment regulation. These distinctions are presented in tabular form in the accompanying chart and need not be repeated here. However, the following two general points should be noted. First, with respect to the size of the mandated reserves, the statutes typically tend to look to the basic commitments of the community over a 12-month period. This approach is not universal, but, as the recent Florida amendments make clear, it is a growing trend. The other type of approach would involve setting reserves based on net worth requirements established by the state. Such reserve requirements necessarily rest on the assumption that the liquidation value of the facility's real estate and equipment counts as part of the reserve. Second, with respect to investment limitations, the lower the level of required reserves in any statute, the stricter the limitations on investment tend to be.

Bonding Requirements

Before discussing the policy arguments underlying a bonding requirement in the continuing care industry, it is necessary to distinguish between two types of bonds. The first, referred to herein as a *fidelity* bond (or fidelity insurance), is obtained by the community in order to cover losses due to the dishonesty or negligence of employees handling money of the residents. The second, referred to as a *surety* bond, is obtained by the community as a substitute for, or in addition to, the reserve requirements just discussed.

The policy arguments that need to be discussed here apply basically to the second form of bonding requirements. Bonds (or insurance) covering the fidelity of employees are common in all industries in which the money of third parties is routinely handled by employees.

The notion of surety bonds insuring the financial stability of a CCRC is more novel and controversial. Theoretically, bonds, like reserves, can provide a financial buffer to aid the community through difficult financial times or to protect it against unfavorable actuarial experience.

---

[45] Arizona §20–1806; California §§1774.4, 1775; Colorado §12–13–107; Florida §651.035; Minnesota §80D.06; Missouri §7.

Bonding Requirements

Arizona: None.

California: Agency may require a bond in any reasonable amount when necessary to protect the residents. Fidelity bond also required.

Colorado: None.

Florida: None.

Indiana: A community may replace entrance fee escrow requirement with a letter of credit.

Maryland: None.

Michigan: Agency may require a bond in any reasonable amount when necessary to protect the residents.

Minnesota: None.

Missouri: None.

AAHA: A community may replace entrance fee escrow requirement with a surety bond.

Theoretically, bonds are even better than reserves in that they provide this buffer without tying up funds in unproductive uses such as bank accounts. But surety bonds, even if obtainable, would probably be extremely expensive. Finally, as with reserves, administrative problems are involved in determining the size of a surety bond for individual communities.

The California, Indiana, Michigan, and AAHA statutes all require, or authorize the administering agency to require, the filing of fidelity or surety bonds under certain circumstances. California and Michigan authorize the administering agency to require a surety bond in any reasonable amount necessary to protect the residents of the community.[46] California also requires the bonding of agents and employees who handle substantial sums of money.[47] The AAHA and Indiana statutes allow a community the option of securing a surety bond or a letter of credit in lieu of maintaining its entrance fee escrow.[48] Finally, and worthy of note, Florida and Colorado have removed their old surety bond requirements in their new statutes.

Fee Regulation

An intrusive form of regulation is direct setting of fees by the state, or supervision of fee-setting by the state. Such fee regulation might be

---

[46] California §§1773, 1773.5; Michigan §554.816.

[47] California §1774.

[48] AAHA §6(e); Indiana §11.

modeled after the detailed regulation of rates commonplace in the insurance industry.[49]

The assumption behind direct fee regulation is that one cannot "trust" operators to charge the "correct" fees. They might charge too much, thus gouging the residents. Or they might charge too little, thus guaranteeing financial collapse of the community in time. Therefore, the argument runs, the state should regulate the setting of fees in order to ensure the "proper" fee and maximum protection.

There are some serious contrary policies. First, even assuming the validity of the assumptions, the administrative problems involved in fee-setting are substantial. Second, and more telling, in terms of its objectivity and motivation, the state may be no better suited to set fees than continuing care operators, and possibly far worse suited.

None of the statutes under discussion has any fee-setting provisions.

LEGAL REGULATION OF RELATIONSHIPS BETWEEN RESIDENTS AND THE COMMUNITY

Financial Disclosure to Residents

The basic assumption behind full disclosure to prospective and current residents is that, by making such disclosure, the community informs all residents and the state about the past, present, and future financial condition of the facility, thereby rendering the residents better able to protect themselves without any additional regulatory intrusions. Further, it is assumed that full disclosure protects the community from making mistakes because of the premise that the state administering agency now possesses complete information. Proponents of full disclosure, therefore, may be heard to say that "we should let the market work" by equalizing bargaining power and that such equalization occurs through the providing of information.

Problems exist, however, with relying on disclosure as the only form of regulation. Even giving information might not equalize bargaining power between residents and operators—the information must be comprehensible. Because, by its nature, financial information is complex, disclosure of only raw financial data may not be effective in its major goal of equalizing bargaining power. Further, if, because of age or educational background, residents are inherently weaker bargaining partners than operators, disclosure will not equalize bargaining power. Thus, the efficacy of disclosure is linked to the validity of the assump-

---

[49] *See* R. Keeton, *Basic Text on Insurance Law,* 557–67 (1971).

Financial Disclosure to Residents

Arizona: Furnish copy of latest annual report to prospective residents before signing of contract.

California: Furnish financial statements to prospective residents before signing of contract.

Colorado: Furnish copy of latest annual report to prospective residents before signing of contract.

Florida: Allows public inspection of reports filed with the state. Must post a summary of latest examination report and latest annual report in facility. Disclosure of same to prospective residents.

Indiana: Allows public inspection of reports filed with the state. Furnish copy of latest annual report to prospective residents before signing of contract.

Maryland: Allows public inspection of filings.

Michigan: Allows public inspection of filings.

Minnesota: Detailed financial disclosure to prospective residents before signing of contract.

Missouri: Furnish copy of latest annual report to prospective residents before signing of contract. Annual disclosure.

AAHA: Detailed financial disclosure to prospective residents before signing of contract. Annual disclosure.

---

tion that lack of information is the sole or a major cause of the disparity in bargaining power.

All 10 statutes have included some form of disclosure within their detailed regulatory schemes. The disclosure provisions can be divided into three basic types:

Florida, Indiana, Maryland, Michigan, and Minnesota allow general public inspection, on request, of financial statements and annual reports filed with the administering agency.[50] Such a right is available to prospective residents, current residents, and the general public.

Arizona, California, Colorado, Florida, Indiana, Minnesota, Missouri, and AAHA require that continuing care providers furnish copies of specified disclosure material of varying content to all prospective residents or their advisers before the execution of the contract.[51] Of these statutes, the Minnesota and AAHA lists of required disclosure are the most comprehensive, including such

---

[50] Florida §651.091(1); Indiana §7(b); Maryland §10(f); Michigan §554.840; Minnesota §80D.04. Actually, because the Minnesota statute is completely self-executing, the disclosure material is filed with the county recorder and is available for public inspection in that office.

[51] Arizona §20–1802(G); California §1779.3(a); Colorado §12–13–102(7); Florida §651.091(4); Indiana §7(a); Minnesota §80D.04; Missouri §4(8); AAHA §4.

information as identity and background of the provider; identity of the manager; description and location of the property and facility; description of all services, fees, and health and financial conditions required for acceptance and termination; certified financial statements; and future income statements.

The Florida, Missouri, and AAHA statutes provide for annual disclosure statements to current residents.[52]

Given its disclosure orientation, the AAHA statute is a model of what a disclosure statute should be. The authors commend sections 4 and 5 of that statute to the reader, especially the breadth of the disclosure, the requirement for narrative descriptions in addition to raw financial data, and the requirement that the disclosure form be on file with the state. In this regard, the Minnesota provision on understandability of the disclosure statement is also pertinent.[53]

Form and Contents of the Contract

A regulatory provision governing the contents of the continuing care agreement would, like regulations mandating full disclosure, attempt to equalize bargaining power between providers and prospective residents. By regulating the form of contracts (e.g., size of print and plain English requirements) and the content of agreements (e.g., fees, refunds, and termination provisions), the state can, in a relatively unintrusive way, mandate that the agreement reached and signed between the community and the resident contain some basic protections for the resident and approximate a contract that would be reached between negotiators of equal bargaining strength. Further, regulation of certain substantive terms has the incidental benefit of reducing uncertainty and, therefore, simplifying much of the contract litigation surrounding continuing care.

Contrary policy arguments against regulation of the form and contents of continuing care agreements include (1) the potential administrative difficulties, and (2) the possibility that state regulation in this area would have to be quite complete for fear that certain communities would include in their contract only the provisions required by the statute.

The discussion of how the 10 statutes under consideration deal with this element of regulation will be divided into several parts. Two initial comments are necessary. First, the AAHA, Indiana, and Minnesota statutes are the only statutes that do not regulate the form or contents of the continuing care agreement, although certain aspects of content

---

[52] Florida §651.091(3); Missouri §4(8); AAHA §5.

[53] Minnesota §80D.04(4).

are addressed in the disclosure form provisions.[54] Second, four of the statutes require that the community's contract be submitted to and approved by the responsible regulatory agency.[55]

Increasing Certainty. Two sections of the Florida statute that may forestall litigation require that the contract contain a provision governing increases in fees[56] and that no resident be permitted to waive his statutory rights.[57] California, Colorado, Florida, and Maryland all have general, albeit detailed, requirements that clauses be included covering the rates of the community, the manner in which rates can be changed, the cost and duration of the services to be provided, and the health and financial conditions each resident must meet to remain in the community.[58]

Refunds. Refund provisions vary substantially. Only Florida, Maryland, Michigan, and Minnesota specifically require that the contract grant a right of full refund to a resident who dies before taking occupancy.[59] More generally, the Florida statute requires that all refund terms be clearly stated in the contract,[60] adding that the contingency of death after occupancy must be addressed.[61] California's refund regulation requires only a refund of entrance payments, less a reasonable processing fee and the reasonable value of services provided, within 10 days of cancellation,[62] but it does not attempt to deal with the contingency of death.[63] Maryland's statute mandates coverage of refunds and the contingency of death.[64]

---

[54] AAHA §4; Indiana §4; Minnesota §80D.04. The Missouri statute also contains substantial regulation of the contract form in its disclosure provisions. *See* Missouri §4.

[55] *See* California §1778; Colorado §12–13–113(2); Florida §651.026(5); Maryland §§10(a)(b), 10(d)(2). Indiana, Minnesota, and Missouri require submission of contracts, but not approval. *See* Indiana §4; Minnesota §80D.04(1); Missouri §4. Again, because of the self-executing nature of Minnesota's statute, the "submission" of the contract is to the county clerk for recording.

[56] Florida §651.055(1)(i). *See also* Maryland §§13(8)–(9).

[57] Florida §651.065.

[58] California §1779; Colorado §12–13–114; Florida §651.055; Maryland §13. The California guidelines for fee increases are generalized. Further, they authorize CCRC changes in fee policy with prior state agency approval. *See* 22 Cal. Code §84331.

[59] Florida §651.055(5); Maryland §80D.04(3); Michigan §554.810(a); Minnesota §80D.04(3)(b).

[60] Florida §651.055(1)(g). Refunds must be made within 120 days and must be on a pro rata basis with no more than 2 percent per month of residence deducted from the entrance fee.

[61] *Id.* §651.055(1)(h). The contract may provide for retention of the entrance fee by the community on the resident's death and must provide for the contingency of the death of one resident in a two-resident apartment.

[62] California §1779.8(a).

[63] *Id.* §1779.8. *See also* Michigan §§554.810(i),(e).

[64] Maryland §§13(6)–(7).

Resident Termination Rights. Regulation of resident termination rights is also diverse. Arizona, California, Florida, and Missouri mandate a 7-day cooling-off period before occupancy, during which the resident may cancel the contract with no penalty;[65] Minnesota has a similar 10-day cooling-off period;[66] and Colorado has added a new 60-day cooling-off period.[67] In Florida, after the initial 7-day period, the resident must be permitted to withdraw on 30 days' notice.[68] Arizona and Minnesota have no comparable provision. California allows cancellation of the contract without notice or cause by either party within the first 90 days; thereafter, 90 days' notice is required from the party that wishes to terminate.[69] Michigan does not limit resident termination rights, but the amount of refund varies with the time of cancellation.[70]

Dismissal. California and Colorado permit contracts that provide for dismissal of residents with or without cause; in the event of such a dismissal, however, they mandate a refund of the difference between the amount paid by the resident and the cost of his care.[71] Florida's strict regulation allows dismissal of residents by the community on 30 days' notice,[72] but only for a good cause.[73] Maryland allows the cancellation of the agreement on 60 days' notice, but only for good cause.[74] Michigan's statute is somewhat unique: it provides that residents dismissed without good cause are entitled to immediate refunds specified in the contract, but that continuing care providers may mitigate potential damage suits by placing these residents in adequate alternative facilities.[75] Unless the provider supplies alternative accommodations, however, it must give 30 days' notice before cancellation.[76] The Colorado and Missouri statutes simply require that the contract contain the terms under which either the provider or the resident may terminate the contract.[77]

---

[65] Arizona §20–1802; California §1779.8(a)–(b); Florida §655.055(2); Missouri §4(7). *See* California §1779(f); Michigan §554.819.

[66] Minnesota §80D.04(3)(a).

[67] Colorado §12–13–102(5).

[68] Florida §651.055(1)(g). *See* Maryland §16.

[69] California §1779(d)–(f). California also requires each contract to be accompanied by a notice explaining all rights of cancellation. *Id.* §1779(e)–(f).

[70] Michigan §554.810(c)–(d). *See id.* §554.810(e).

[71] California §1780; Colorado §12–13–105. The Colorado statute authorizes tax-exempt CCRCs to make refunds on other bases if such schedules are set forth in the contract. Colorado §12–13–105(2).

[72] Florida §651.055(1)(g).

[73] *Id.* §651.061. Good cause will not be found simply because of an inability to pay monthly fees, at least until the entrance fees have been exhausted as well.

[74] Maryland §15.

[75] Michigan §554.810(2).

[76] *Id.* §554.810(3).

[77] Colorado §12–13–102(2); Missouri §4(4)(13).

Contract Regulation

Submission to state

Arizona: No.
California: Submit and approve.
Colorado: Submit and approve.
Florida: Submit and approve.
Indiana: Submit only.
Maryland: Submit only.
Michigan: No.
Minnesota: Submit only.
Missouri: Submit only.
AAHA: No.

Detailed requirements

Arizona: No.
California: Yes.
Colorado: Yes.
Florida: Yes.
Indiana: No.
Maryland: Yes.
Michigan: No.
Minnesota: No.
Missouri: No.
AAHA: No.

Refunds

Arizona: Not addressed.
California: Must have refund of admission fee less reasonable expenses within 10 days of cancellation. Does not deal with contingency of death.
Colorado: Must have refund of difference between amount paid in and amount used for care of the resident. Special provision for tax-exempt CCRCs.
Florida: Full refund if resident dies before occupancy. All refund provisions must be stated in contract. Must be within 120 days and on a pro rata basis. Contingency of death must be addressed.
Indiana: Not addressed.
Maryland: Full refund if resident dies before occupancy. All refund provisions must be stated in contract. Contingency of death must be addressed.
Michigan: Full refund if resident dies before occupancy.
Minnesota: Full refund if resident dies before occupancy.
Missouri: Not addressed.
AAHA: Not addressed.

Rights of Self-Organization

The policy behind giving residents the right to self-organization is that, at its core, the community is for the residents. By giving them a voice and a role in its governance, one is, in effect, charging the residents with partial responsibility for ensuring that the community functions

Rights of Self-Organization

Arizona: None.

California: Regulations grant right to form a residents' association.

Colorado: None.

Florida: Right of self-organization, plus required quarterly meetings between management and residents.

Indiana: None.

Maryland: None.

Michigan: One resident as advisory member of board of directors.

Minnesota: None.

Missouri: One resident as member of board of directors.

AAHA: None.

smoothly and efficiently. Like disclosure, therefore, this element of regulation is designed to put in the hands of the residents the power and information to safeguard their own interests.

There are some contrary attitudes. One reason given for opposing this type of regulatory provision is that, if the residents' role in the governance of the community is such that they gain effective control of the community's operations, the facility's tax-exempt status might be in jeopardy. Our survey, however, has disclosed no examples of this potential problem.

A second objection to granting residents rights of self-organization applies only to the issue of whether it should be mandatory that residents sit on the facility's board of directors. It is contended that residents sitting on a board of directors might be unable to execute their responsibilities properly due to a sense of emotional, rather than administrative and financial, responsibility. For example, residents on a board might hesitate to raise rates or might tend to negotiate lower increases because of their concern for the reaction of their fellow residents (because they will continue to live in the community).

Only the Florida, Michigan, and Missouri statutes recognize any right to resident self-organization.[78] Michigan simply requires that one resident serve as an advisory member on the facility's board of directors.[79] Missouri's new statute requires that at least one member of each facility's board of directors be a regular paying resident of the CCRC.[80] Florida grants residents the right of self-organization, the right to be

[78] California's new regulation for residential facilities for the elderly grants residents the right to form a residents' association. *See* 22 Cal. Code §87614.

[79] Michigan §554.812.

[80] Missouri §8.

represented by individuals of their own choosing, and the right to engage in concerted activity for the purpose of keeping informed or for mutual aid or protection.[81] Florida also requires quarterly meetings (if requested by residents) between management and residents to discuss income, expenditures, financial problems, and proposed changes in policies or services.[82]

Advertising Regulation

Another attempt to cut down on misinformation on the part of residents, is direct regulation of the form and contents of advertising by CCRCs. Indeed, advertising regulation is a basic antifraud protection common in many industries. The purpose of such regulation is to ensure that any advertising put out by a continuing care operator does not intentionally or negligently mislead a prospective resident. Among the bases for objections to this policy are a general reluctance to meddle in what is basically a private matter, as well as the argument that existing truth-in-advertising rules and regulations already adequately cover this element of regulation. There is also an administrative cost involved that some say is not worth the incidental benefit gained.

California, Florida, Maryland, and Michigan all mandate that a copy of all advertising and promotional literature be filed with the state before publication or dissemination.[83] In Colorado and Florida, the mention of any other organization in the literature or advertising must be accompanied by a statement of the extent of that organization's financial responsibility for the community.[84] The California, Indiana, and Missouri statutes require only that the statement of financial responsibility be filed with the proper agency.[85] The Michigan legislation grants the administering agency the discretion to promulgate regulations governing the form and contents of advertising.[86] Maryland prohibits distribution of "prohibited" advertising, but does not define that term.[87]

---

[81] Florida §651.081.

[82] *Id.* §651.085.

[83] Florida §651.095; Maryland §10(a)(10); Michigan §554.82b(2). California's requirements appear only in its regulations. *See* 22 Cal. Code §84555.

[84] Colorado §12–13–116; Florida §651.095(3).

[85] California §1789; Indiana §4(8); Missouri §4(4)(8). The California regulations, however, require submission of advertising material to the administering agency. *See* 22 Cal. Code §84555.

[86] Michigan §554.826(1).

[87] Maryland §18(b).

Advertising Regulation

Arizona: None.

California: If any third party is mentioned, must file a statement of its financial responsibility with the state. Violation is a misdemeanor and can lead to revocation of certificate. Regulations require filing.

Colorado: If any third party is mentioned, must include statement of its financial responsibility for the community. Violation is a misdemeanor.

Florida: Filing. If any third party is mentioned, must include statement of its financial responsibility for the community.

Indiana: A statement of financial responsibility by any affiliated charitable organization must be on file with the state.

Maryland: "Prohibited" advertising must not be distributed; term not defined.

Michigan: Filing. Agency can promulgate regulations on contents.

Minnesota: None.

Missouri: A statement of financial responsibility by any affiliated charitable organization must be on file with the state.

AAHA: None.

Lien Provisions and Preferred Claims

This element of regulation, the last in this section, differs qualitatively from the other elements discussed above. While the four preceding elements of regulation are designed to equalize the informational position of residents and providers, this element is designed to provide a modicum of financial protection for the residents should the community fail.

Definitionally, a *lien* gives the residents something beyond their contracts to sue on. Most critically, a filed lien gives the residents *priority* over subsequent claimants even if the community goes under 10 years after the filing. A *preferred claim* is, in essence, a special lien used only in liquidation proceedings.

Thus, the policy of giving liens and preferred claims to residents is that they shield residents from total financial loss. An incidental benefit of giving residents such an interest in the property of the community, is that doing so might limit excessive encumbrances on the property by subordinating subsequent creditors' claims to the interests of the residents.

There are several contrary policies. First, the residents' liens will invariably be subordinated to existing encumbrances such as first mortgages. Such encumbrances are usually the largest obligations of a CCRC, thereby cutting dramatically into the residents' rights. Second, the existence of residents' liens or preferred claims inevitably increases the cost of borrowing to communities by lowering the priority

---

Lien Provisions and Preferred Claims

Arizona: Lien as a precondition to certification. Subordinated to prior recorded encumbrances and may be subordinated to later recorded encumbrances.

California: Liens where necessary to secure performance of the continuing care contract. Subordinated to prior recorded liens.

Colorado: Liens as a precondition to certification. Subordinated to prior recorded liens and may be subordinated to later recorded liens.

Florida: Preferred claim to residents on liquidation, but prior recorded liens retain their priority.

Indiana: None.

Maryland: None.

Michigan: None.

Minnesota: Lien comes into existence when facility begins operation. No subordination at all.

Missouri: None.

AAHA: None.

---

of subsequent creditors. Third, such residents' interests may make certain borrowing impossible, thus limiting communities' expansion plans. Finally, under the new bankruptcy code, liens and preferred claims may well be invalid as statutory liens. That legislation allows the bankruptcy trustee to avoid any statutory lien[88] that first becomes effective against the debtor (the community), *inter alia,* when its financial condition fails to meet a specified standard[89] or when a third party levies to make the lien effective.[90] If a lien is created through administrative action when necessary for the protection of the residents, both of these provisions are implicated;[91] if a lien is created by administrative action at the time of certification, only the latter applies.[92] In both cases, however, the lien is suspect and would defeat the major purpose of the provision.

The statutes at issue here use two types of lien provisions. The California statute provides for a lien when necessary to secure performance of the continuing care agreements.[93] The Arizona and Colorado statutes, on the other hand, require that a lien be filed as a condition to certification.[94] Minnesota's self-executing statute provides that a lien

---

[88] A statutory lien is defined as a "lien arising solely by force of a statute on specified circumstances or conditions." *See* 11 U.S.C. §101 (38) (Supp. II 1978).

[89] *Id.* §545(1)(E).

[90] *Id.* §545(1)(F).

[91] This is the case in California and Colorado.

[92] This is the case in Arizona and Minnesota.

[93] California §1772. The California lien attaches only to real estate.

[94] Arizona §20–1805; Colorado §12–13–106.

Responsible Agency

Arizona: Department of Insurance. No advisory council.

California: Department of Social Services. Eight-member advisory board.

Colorado: Department of Insurance. No advisory board.

Florida: Department of Insurance. Seven-member advisory council.

Indiana: Department of Securities.

Maryland: Office of Aging. No advisory board.

Michigan: Corporation and Securities Bureau of the Department of Commerce. No advisory board.

Minnesota: None.

Missouri: Division of Insurance.

AAHA: Left to option of states. No advisory board.

exists on all real personal property of the CCRC from the time the facility is first occupied by a resident.[95] All of these states except Minnesota subordinate the lien to first-mortgage liens,[96] and Arizona and Colorado allow the administering agency to subordinate the lien to certain later recorded liens.

There are also two forms of preferred-claim provisions. Florida gives a preference to resident claims, but the priority of duly recorded liens is retained on liquidation.[97] California, on the other hand, apparently grants an absolute preference to resident claims in the event of liquidation.[98]

STATE ADMINISTRATION OF THE STATUTE

Responsible Agency

At a policy level, not much can be said about this particular issue. Basically, the goal is to ensure that the responsible agency has both the expertise and the interest to administer whatever regulatory program one develops. Many of the statutes resort to advisory councils to aid the appropriate agency in administering the program. Of significance is Minnesota's approach to this issue. Because that state's statute is wholly self-executing, there is no need for any day-to-day administer-

---

[95] Minnesota §80D.08.

[96] This is probably a drafting error by the Minnesota legislature. Unless the residents' lien is subordinated to first-mortgage liens, no bank will give any mortgage and no investment bank will underwrite any bond. The deletion of the provision explicitly subordinating the residents' lien in this manner is probably an oversight.

[97] Florida §651.071.

[98] California §1777.

ing agency. This appears to be a unique approach in the continuing care field, and the Minnesota experience should, therefore, be interesting to observe.

The attached chart depicts the way in which the 10 statutes have dealt with the issue.

Investigative, Enforcement, and Rehabilitative Powers

Most of the policy arguments on this element of regulation pertain to the degree of power, and not to the need for some power. No matter what form a regulatory scheme takes, and regardless of whether it is by government or private sources, enforcement is essential. And investigation and audit are essential adjuncts to the enforcement power.[99] The policy debates, therefore, center mostly on the scope of the investigative, enforcement, and rehabilitative powers that need to be granted, and, more specifically, on the nature of the enforcement and rehabilitative powers that need to be granted. These arguments are mostly apparent and self-explanatory and therefore need not be explored here.

Investigation. The investigative powers granted by each of the statutes are slightly different. In Arizona, continuing care examiners with the same power as that of insurance examiners are authorized to conduct inspections as often as may be necessary.[100] Michigan grants a limited power to investigate when mandatory records or annual reports are incomplete,[101] as well as a more structured and general investigative authority to protect against other violations of its statute.[102] Indiana, Maryland, and AAHA all authorize this latter general investigative power, including a subpoena power.[103] Florida grants a general examination authority to be exercised from "time to time."[104] Colorado authorizes the administering agency to conduct an examination as often as it deems necessary for the protection of the residents.[105] In contrast, California permits the administering agency to conduct inspections at any time[106] but allows the agency to rely on an annual audit

---

[99] The Missouri legislature apparently disagrees, as that state's recent legislation contains no enforcement power. This is particularly curious because of the statutory authorization to revoke certificates of authority. *See* Missouri §5(2). One cannot help but speculate about how, without investigative and enforcement powers, the administering agency will revoke a certificate of authority to operate.

[100] Arizona §20–1809.

[101] Michigan §554.823.

[102] *Id.* §554.833.

[103] Indiana §22; Maryland §71; AAHA §9.

[104] Florida §651.105(1).

[105] Colorado §12–13–110.

[106] California §1781.

in lieu of inspection.[107] Because the Minnesota statute is wholly self-executing, there is no administering agency and therefore no investigating authority.

Enforcement. Enforcement mechanisms also vary from statute to statute. Colorado, Florida, Indiana, Maryland, Michigan, and AAHA all authorize injunctive relief against violations or threatened violations of any provision of the legislation.[108] Indiana, Michigan, and AAHA also authorize the administering agency to seek a cease and desist order.[109] As an important additional sanction focused specifically on the performance of administrators, all of the statutes except that of AAHA provide either civil or criminal penalties (or both) for violations of the statute by individuals.[110]

Rehabilitation. In what is perhaps the most controversial of these mechanisms, Arizona, California, Colorado, Florida, Indiana, Maryland, and Minnesota all authorize the administering agency to assume the management of continuing care facilities in certain specific situations in order to rehabilitate communities in serious financial trouble.[111]

The California rehabilitation procedure, probably the most detailed, is triggered when a CCRC fails to file its annual report and the Department of Social Services has reason to believe that "the provider is insolvent, is in imminent danger of becoming insolvent, is in a financially unsound or unsafe condition, or that its condition is such that it may otherwise be unable to fully perform its obligations pursuant to life care contracts."[112] The facility is first allowed to propose a plan to correct the deficiencies.[113] Next, in case of an emergency that threatens immediate closure of the facility, or if no approved plan is forthcoming, the administering agency may petition a court for appointment of an administrator.[114] The administrator has broad powers, including total power over all property, equipment, and funds and the power to perform all the duties of the original provider.[115] The statute provides for

---

[107] *Id.* §1782.

[108] Colorado §12–13–117(1); Florida §651.125(3); Indiana §23; Maryland §20; Michigan §554.834; AAHA §10.

[109] Indiana §23; Michigan §554.828; AAHA §10.

[110] Arizona §20–1811 (misdemeanor); California §1788 (misdemeanor); Colorado §12–13–117(2) (misdemeanor); Florida §§651.108, 651.125(1), 651.13 (administration fines, felony, and civil penalties); Indiana §9 (misdemeanor); Maryland §18(c) (misdemeanor); Michigan §554.836 (fine and imprisonment); Minnesota §§80D.13, 80D.16 (civil and criminal liability).

[111] Arizona §20–1808; California §§1790–1790.6; Colorado §12–13–109; Florida §651.114; Indiana §21; Maryland §20(b); Minnesota §80D.11.

[112] California §1790.

[113] *Id.*

[114] *Id.* §1790.1.

[115] *Id.* §1790.4.

Investigative, Enforcement, and Rehabilitative Powers

Arizona: Examiners can conduct examinations as needed. Misdemeanor to violate. Rehabilitative authority.

California: Inspections authorized at any time, but annual audit can be relied on instead. Misdemeanor to violate. Rehabilitative authority.

Colorado: Examinations when necessary. Injunctive relief. Misdemeanor to violate. Rehabilitative authority.

Florida: General examination authority. Injunctive relief. Felony and civil penalties for violations. Rehabilitative authority.

Indiana: General investigative authority plus subpoena power. Injunctive relief. Cease and desist orders allowed. Misdemeanor to violate. Rehabilitative authority.

Maryland: General investigative authority. Injunctive relief. Misdemeanor to violate. Rehabilitative authority.

Michigan: Limited power to investigate when records are missing plus general investigative authority. Injunctive relief. Cease and desist orders allowed. Fines and imprisonment for violation.

Minnesota: Self-executing statute. Civil and criminal penalties for violation. Resident-initiated rehabilitation and liquidation procedure.

Missouri: None.

AAHA: General investigative authority plus subpoena power. Injunctive relief. Cease and desist orders allowed. No penalties for violation.

---

termination of the intrusion when the defect is cured,[116] as well as for liquidation or dissolution of the provider if rehabilitative efforts fail.[117]

The Minnesota statute, owing to its self-executing character, has a unique triggering mechanism for its rehabilitation/liquidation provision. If any CCRC fails to meet its reserve requirements, if any provider has been or will be unable to meet its obligations, or if any provider files for relief from its creditors, then any *resident* can petition a court for an order directing the appointment of a trustee.[118] The court can then appoint a trustee who will attempt to rehabilitate or liquidate the facility.[119] There is no involvement of any state administrative agency at any point in the proceedings.

LIMITED STATE REGULATORY SCHEMES

The second set of state responses after detailed regulation is selective, specific regulation of certain aspects of the continuing care industry. Six states have adopted legislation falling short of detailed regulation

---

[116] *Id.* §1790.5.

[117] *Id.* §1790.6.

[118] Minnesota §80D.11(1).

[119] *Id.* §80D.11(1), (4).

and, in most cases, isolating one of the more serious problems of continuing care, and attempting to eliminate that problem without imposing a full-scale regulatory program.

MEDICAID AND PUBLIC ASSISTANCE REGULATIONS

Connecticut[120] and Illinois[121] have enacted statutes limiting the eligibility of life care residents to receive public assistance or Medicaid. These statutes are usually implicated in the following situation: Over time, or even immediately after payment of the entrance fee, residents qualify for public assistance because of their reduced net worth and the resultant reduced income stream. They, therefore, apply for Medicaid benefits, often at the behest of the provider, and all such benefits are turned over to the community.

In Connecticut, a life care resident (life care is not defined) is eligible for assistance only if: (1) care under the contract commenced before April 3, 1957; (2) the operator is a charitable institution; (3) the applicant is a resident at the time of application; (4) the consideration paid for the resident's care has been exhausted, assuming a rate of $75 per month; and (5) the income of the provider is insufficient to permit continued performance of the agreement.[122]

Under the Illinois statute, a person maintained in a private institution qualifies for aid only if he has not purchased care or, if he has, only if his payment has been wholly consumed. A regulation of the Illinois Department of Public Aid explains that a "resident that has an agreement for life care . . . shall be considered not in need of public assistance on the basis that he has a resource to meet his needs."[123] The difference between the statute and the regulation is quite significant: the statute appears to say that any life care resident who lives longer than expected will be eligible for aid because the entrance fee would

---

[120] Conn. Gen Stat. Ann. §§17–116, 17–316 (West 1958).

[121] Ill. Ann. Stat. ch. 23, §3–1.5 (Smith-Hurd 1971); Ill. Dept of Public Aid Rules & Regulations, art. 8, rule 8.02.02, cited in *Cornue* v. *Department of Pub. Aid,* 64 Ill. 2d 78, 81, 354 N.E.2d 359, 361 (1976).

[122] This statute may ultimately be declared invalid under the supremacy clause of the Constitution. *Rowland* v. *Maher,* 176 Conn. 57, 404 A.2d 894 (1978), held a related statute unconstitutional as contrary to the federal policy that the only legitimate ground for withholding Medicaid is actual unavailability of assets. The court stated in dicta that §17–116 was unconstitutional to the extent that it "deprives a person holding a life care contract of medical assistance on any ground other than actual availability of assets." *Id.* at 63, 404 A.2d at 895.

[123] Ill. Dept. of Public Aid Rules & Regulations, art. 8, rule 8.02.02, cited in *Cornue* v. *Department of Pub. Aid,* 64 Ill. 2d 78, 81, 354 N.E.2d 359, 361 (1976).

have been "wholly consumed"; the regulation explicitly negates this interpretation.[124]

REFUND REGULATIONS

Only one state has chosen to regulate refunds of entrance fees in isolation. Oregon has enacted legislation requiring that any such fees or transfers of property made before or during the first six months of occupancy must be refunded to any resident who withdraws from the facility within the first six months of occupancy.[125] One should note that this statute covers only a small part of the refund problem, as death is not normally considered equivalent to withdrawal, and the statute applies to withdrawal only during the first six months of residence.

PROHIBITION

Although not strictly selective regulation, two state attempts to outlaw the institution of life care are relevant in this regard. As noted above, New York[126] and Pennsylvania[127] have apparently attempted to prohibit the offering of life care contracts. As also noted above, neither effort appears to have been successful owing to definitional difficulties.

PROPRIETARY/NONPROFIT DISTINCTION

As part of its detailed regulatory program, Michigan incidentally prohibits proprietary operators from entering into "pure" life care agreements.[128] To the authors' knowledge, no other state has taken this step.

This provision, based on the notion that profit seeking has an adverse effect on the quality of care and services, attempts to eliminate the opportunity to profit from continuing care operations. Regardless of one's views on the desirability of such a policy, a provision excluding proprietary operators would not effectively advance this aim. First,

---

[124] The Illinois Supreme Court upheld both the statute and the regulation in *Cornue. See Reynolds* v. *Department of Pub. Aid,* 26 Ill. App. 3d 933, 326 N.E.2d 109 (1975). These decisions, however, were based on construction of the statute and the regulation and did not involve consideration of federal constitutional limitations.

[125] Or. Rev. Stat. §91.690 (1977).

[126] N.Y. Code of Rules and Regulation, tit. 10, §§730.2(F), 730.3(b) (1979). See id. §§414.16(b), 415.1(F), 420.1(f).

[127] 28 Pa. Code §201.38 (1979).

[128] Michigan §554.805(5).

the policy is too broad in that it would exclude desirable proprietary operators from the industry.[129] Second, it is too narrow in that it could easily be circumvented. A person who wishes to operate a continuing care retirement community for profit can establish a nonprofit "front," thus satisfying the statutory provision. The front could then, in effect, distribute "profits" to the providers through contracts between the nonprofit entity and for-profit entities that the provider owns or controls—most obviously, a management service company hired to run the community.[130] Such legal self-dealing arrangements are extremely effective tools for breaking the "nondistribution constraint" traditionally associated with nonprofit organizations.[131]

REMAINING RESPONSE: NONREGULATION

The third potential state response following detailed and selective regulation is the most common of our three sets of responses. The response of nonregulation has been "adopted" by 36 states, the District of Columbia, and the federal government. Notwithstanding the simplicity of the nonregulation response, some comments are necessary.

THE STATES

It is unfair to say that 36 states have done nothing to regulate CCRCs. Several states have considered or are currently considering legislation to regulate the continuing care industry. Illinois[132] and Massachusetts have considered such legislation in the past; New Jersey[133] and Penn-

---

[129] Because of the tax consequences, it is questionable how successful a proprietary CCRC could be. Without the tax advantages in the treatment of receipt of entrance fees, it is unclear whether continuing care is a desirable vehicle for proprietary operators.

[130] *See* Hansmann, *The Role of Nonprofit Enterprises,* 87 Yale L.J. 835, 838 (1980).

[131] *See* Comment, *Continuing Care Communities for the Elderly: Potential Pitfalls and Proposed Regulation,* 118 U. Pa. L. Rev. 883, 896 (1980).

[132] Following preparation of this chapter, a comprehensive statute regulating CCRCs went into effect in Illinois. As a result of timing difficulties, no discussion of that new legislation occurs in this work.

[133] New Jersey has definitely not yet enacted any form of continuing care legislation. On May 14, 1981, however, Assemblyman Snedeker introduced comprehensive legislation concerning the continuing care industry.

The provisions of Bill No. 3359 may be summarized as follows: (1) administering agency is the state Department of Health; (2) standard definition of continuing care, complete with the potential problems discussed in this chapter; (3) requirement that only nonprofit entities may offer continuing care agreements similar to the Michigan provision; (4) general antifraud provision; (5) requires obtaining a certificate of authority before selling any continuing care contract—procedure for certification involves submission of application form complete with typical attachments, including financial data and

sylvania[134] are currently considering such legislation; and discussions are taking place in Ohio that could lead to proposed legislation. Other states have, in all likelihood, considered similar legislation in the past, but the information sources disclosing such matters are scattered and unreliable.

The dearth of state regulation clearly is not a result of lack of interest in the problems of the elderly: all 50 states and the District of Columbia require the licensing of traditional nursing homes. In fact, the 54 state agencies charged with regulation of nursing homes comprise the largest contingent of such agencies in the entire field of health care regulation.[135]

In some states in which the legislature has not acted to regulate continuing care, the state judicial system has been pressed into service. It is important to note, however, that judicial regulation of continuing care is, definitionally, quite different from legislative regulation. Private litigation usually arises after the damage occurs—damage that, in the case of continuing care, may often be irreparable. No judicial

---

full disclosure; (6) annual renewal and reporting requirements; (7) independent revocation of registration procedure; (8) detailed regulation of the contents of the continuing care agreement, including a seven-day cooling-off period and mandatory arbitration of disputed claims between residents and the community; (9) one resident must be permitted to sit on each facility's board of directors; (10) filing of a financial plan for the community, which could lead to the discretionary imposition of an escrow or bond requirement; (11) advertising regulation; (12) public inspection of all documents filed including the disclosure statement; (13) full investigative and injunctive powers, including subpoena power and authority to seek cease and desist orders; and (14) civil and criminal liability for violations.

[134] Pennsylvania is actively considering the possibility of enacting some form of legislation regulating the continuing care retirement industry. Early in 1981, the state Senate adopted Senate Resolution No. 32, which established a task force "to investigate nonprofit corporations providing for retirement homes and retirement communities." The task force produced a bill proposed in 1982 which has been amended and introduced as Senate Bill No. 1270 (Session of 1982). The provisions of this bill may be summarized as follows: (1) standard definition of continuing care, complete with the problems discussed in this chapter; (2) complete certification provisions; (3) provisions governing annual disclosure; (4) provisions authorizing revocation of certification of authority; (5) advertising regulation; (6) detailed reserve requirements; (7) reserve fund escrow provision; (8) provision granting residents a subordinated lien; (9) entrance fee escrow provision; (10) regulation of the form and contents of continuing care contracts; (11) provision establishing an advisory council; (12) provision granting residents rights of self-organization; (13) rehabilitation and liquidation procedures; (14) regulation of conflicts of interest on the board of directors; and (15) civil and criminal penalties for violations of the statute.

Finally, the Pennsylvania House has also been considering legislation governing the continuing care field. House Bill No. 2348, introduced on March 22, 1982, can be summarized as follows: (1) an insufficient definition section; (2) administration vested in the Department of Insurance; (3) complete certification provision; (4) disclosure provisions; (5) reserve provision; (6) audits required every three years; (7) civil and criminal penalties; (8) injunctive relief; (9) rehabilitation and liquidation authority; and (10) provision on suspension of registration.

[135] Department of Health, Education, and Welfare, *Health Resources Statistics: Health Manpower and Health Facilities*, 328, 473, 479–80 (1976–77).

mechanism exists to head off the potential dangers of improper financial and actuarial planning that inhere in the process of continuing care. The bulk of the litigation involving CCRCs has focused on the relatively narrow issues of contract terminations, refunds, and the fee/service structure of community operators. Through a narrow focus on the case-by-case equities, and often with reference to vague notions of public policy, state courts have apparently added to the financial uncertainties of continuing care. Although the results of litigation have been generally predictable, the inherent unpredictability of cases in equity and the dearth of clear statements of law have also had two effects: the potential plaintiffs are encouraged to litigate the particular facts of their grievances, and communities are prevented from planning intelligently. Instead, they must devote a substantial amount of resources to countering the threat of costly litigation.

Continuing care litigation may be divided for analytical purposes into suits by residents, which generally are successful, and suits by heirs of residents, which generally are not. This chapter is not the place to enter into a comparative analysis of the case law.[136] Suffice it to say that, should a state opt to legislate a comprehensive regulatory program, one of the goals of the state might well be a reduction of the litigation uncertainty.

THE FEDERAL GOVERNMENT

With the exception of standard Medicare and Medicaid certification regulations for nursing facilities in CCRC, the federal presence in the field is virtually nonexistent. Several congressional committees and federal agencies have, from time to time, expressed interest in the problems of continuing care, but none has yet addressed them directly.[137]

In 1977, Representatives William Cohen and Gladys Spellman introduced legislation that would have required continuing care providers subject to federal jurisdiction[138] to disclose financial information to all current and prospective residents and to maintain minimum cash reserves.[139] The bill required that the contract between the community

---

[136] For a summary discussion of the extensive continuing care case law, see Comment, *Continuing Care Communities for the Elderly: Potential Pitfalls and Proposed Regulation,* 128 U. Pa. L. Rev. 883, 903–09 (1980).

[137] *See id.* 902.

[138] Such communities would have had to have been engaged in interstate commerce, to have received Medicare or Medicaid reimbursement, or to have been constructed with federal assistance.

[139] H.R. 4170, 95th Cong., 1st Sess. (1977). The Cohen/Spellman bill was in response to a proposal introduced by Representative Claude Pepper, which would have prohibited any residential health facility operator from accepting prepayment for basic services for more than three months.

and the resident (1) provide for full written financial disclosure, (2) include a full description of charges and services, (3) make clear that the contract granted no property rights, (4) contain assurances that all fees would be spent on patient care and related expenses, (5) specify termination conditions, and (6) provide for an annual audit. Each community would have been required to maintain financial reserves sufficient to meet its obligations. Payments to facilities under construction would have had to be held in escrow. The bill died at the end of the 95th Congress and has not been reintroduced. ■

Chapter Thirteen
Evaluation of Legislative Options

■ Chapter 12 reported on the formal legal positions of the states and the federal government vis-à-vis the continuing care industry. It contained a comprehensive review of existing legislation, court decisions, administrative regulations (where available), proposed legislation, and draft model statutes. Every attempt was made to keep the presentation contained in that chapter as neutral as possible; it was the authors' intent that no value judgments be drawn in that initial analysis.

In sharp contrast to the material in Chapter 12, this chapter draws many value judgments. These judgments are the views of the authors, reached after thorough collaboration with many persons familiar with and experienced in the continuing care field.

It will be readily apparent that this study has not proposed its own suggested model legislation. It was the authors' judgment that the typical state legislature considering implementation of legislation regulating the continuing care industry is blessed with an abundance of legislative options. Chapters 12 and 13 are designed to inform the typical state legislator—not to confuse him or confront him with additional complicating statutory language. Thus, it is the authors' hope that these chapters can serve as a catalyst for discussion in this area.

Foremost among our judgments is the conclusion that legislation at the state level will be appropriate in many states. The rationale underlying this conclusion cannot be explained in general terms; rather, the conclusion can be justified only through analysis of the value judgments drawn with respect to each element of regulation. It should not be surprising, therefore, that this chapter is again organized according to the various elements of regulation identified in the previous chapter.

This chapter contains a series of value-laden conclusions as to whether each of the identified elements of regulation has any place in state legislation. Some of these conclusions are based on no more than the authors' analysis of competing policy considerations. Others are based on more traditional types of legal analysis. Whenever appropriate, the authors have drawn on the study's results and based the conclusions on current practice in the continuing care industry.

It has been the authors' experience that each element of regulation fits relatively neatly into one of three categories:

1. First, some elements of regulation definitely belong in any state statute regulating the continuing care industry.
2. Second, some elements of regulation present much closer questions based on one's value judgments and analyses. In these cases, it was felt that some states might want to adopt such sections, while other states might prefer not to or might prefer alternatively phrased sections.
3. Third, certain elements of regulation should not be included in any enlightened state statutory scheme.

This chapter, therefore, contains an analytic commentary on which elements of regulation the authors have concluded to be appropriate in state legislative schemes. Reasonable persons can differ over the conclusions and opinions expressed in this chapter. It is for this reason that we have provided the underlying analysis for our conclusions as well as alternative proposed statutory provisions. In the final analysis, of course, each individual state must decide what form, if any, its legislative regulation of the continuing care industry will take.

One value judgment is implicit in all that follows. As noted above, the authors have concluded that legislation at the *state* level is appropriate. We have chosen this option in full recognition of the reality that, in order to comprehensively regulate the continuing care industry nationwide, it requires 51 independent legislative enactments, whereas an option involving *federal* legislation would involve the legislative action of only one Congress.

We made this choice for three reasons. First, because of the detail required and the nature of the subject matter, the type of regulation envisioned appears more suited to state administration than to federal supervision. Second, CCRCs are still relatively new, and, at least at present, it would be advantageous to encourage the variety of legislative programs that would develop at the decentralized state level. Third, a jurisdictional problem exists whenever the federal government attempts to regulate essentially local institutions.

This last point can best be explained by reference to H.R. 4170, the federal legislation introduced in 1977 by Representatives William Cohen and Gladys Spellman. That legislation regulated only ''federally assisted continuing care institutions,'' which was defined to include communities that offered long-term care to the elderly and engaged in interstate commerce, received Medicaid or Medicare reimbursement, or were constructed with federal assistance. It is the authors' judgment that too many communities might structure their organization so that they would not fit within this definition and would thereby be exempted from regulation should only a federal statute be enacted. This conclusion is reinforced by the history of the continuing care industry in Arizona and Florida, detailed in Chapter 12, where certain communities structured themselves so as to fall outside the definition of the regulated entity in the statutes of those two states and, therefore, escaped regulation.

DEFINITION OF ENTITY TO BE REGULATED

Based on the first comprehensive survey of continuing care retirement communities, it is known that the institutions variously referred to as life care, continuing care, living care, perpetual care, residence and care, and life lease are anything but homogeneous. Communities differ significantly in substance, depending on the respective termination rights of the community and the resident, the amount of services and medical care covered under the contract at no or a nominal extra charge, the length of the contract, and the financing arrangements between the resident and the community. Given the diverse characteristics of separate CCRCs, it is absolutely essential to draft a definition to ensure that all types of CCRCs will be brought within the scope of the statute.

Given the authors' conclusion that legislation will be appropriate for adoption in many states, it should not be surprising that we consider the definitional section of the CCRC statute to be an absolute necessity—that is, the definitional element of regulation clearly falls within the first category described in the introduction. A proper definition should include all contracts that last for more than one year or for the life of the resident (including mutually terminable continuing care contracts); that provide (either on-site or contractually) shelter and various health care services; that provide for either a payment of an entrance fee or periodic payments, or a combination of the two; and that are not completely based on a fee-for-service theory of payment (i.e., if there is *any* prepayment). In this way, the problems experienced in Arizona, Florida, New York, and Pennsylvania, which were discussed in the preceding chapter, can perhaps be avoided.

PREOPENING PROCEDURES: CERTIFICATION

This element of regulation involves an attempt by the legislating authority to screen "unacceptable" operators from the continuing care industry. The theory behind certification requirements is that some sort of comprehensive application process, complete with required submissions, will enable the regulatory agency to determine the financial stability, capacity, sincerity, and integrity of prospective and existing continuing care operators. Such prospective certification, coupled with annual monitoring and various enforcement provisions, is the major mechanism used to supervise the financial stability of the continuing care industry by the states that have adopted comprehensive statutes.

As noted earlier, all statutes reviewed in the preparation of the study contain relatively extensive registration and certification provisions. Failure to comply with these provisions can result in the imposition of civil and/or criminal penalties. Similarly, there is some current discussion of the possibility of developing local, state, regional, or national self-accreditation programs. For example, seven communities in Pennsylvania, New Jersey, and Maryland have been attempting to establish such an accreditation program.[1] Such self-accreditation programs have worked efficiently to varying degrees with hospitals, nursing homes, mental hospitals, and schools.[2] Governmental reliance on a private accreditation system would not be unprecedented. For purposes of Medicare certification, the federal government usually requires no more of hospitals than that they meet standards set by the Joint Commission on Accreditation of Hospitals.[3]

It is the conclusion of the authors that certification requirements should be classified within the first category of regulatory elements discussed in the introduction—that is, they should definitely be adopted by all states implementing continuing care legislation. Yet, this conclusion is tempered by a unique twist that, to the authors' knowledge, has not been proposed in any other analysis to date. We urge that all legislation provide a mechanism whereby the administrator of the responsible agency in each state shall approve private self-accreditation programs that meet certain specified standards—some of which are provided in the uniform legislation and some of which must be developed through regulatory processes. Once a self-accreditation program has been approved by the administrator, all CCRCs that receive accreditation from that program should be exempted, in large part,

---

[1] See Kendal-Crosslands Annual Report for the Year April 1, 1978 to March 31, at 6, 1979.

[2] See National Center for Health Statistics, Office of Health Research, Statistics, and Technology, Public Health Service, Department of Health, Education, and Welfare, Health Resources Statistics: Health Manpower and Health Facilities, 300 (1976–77).

[3] See 42 U.S.C. §1385bb (1976). In the JCAH, there are four organizations with arguably conflicting goals and interests that offset one another's parochial interests in the setting of policy, while all members of a CCRC self-accreditation program would have homogeneous views. But the analogy still has substantial value.

from the statutory certification procedures.[4] Finally, the legislation should require reapproval of each accreditation program at periodic intervals, such as every five years.

Legislative provisions on certification should contain two independent types of provisions. First, they should include provisional certification procedures to be applied only to new prospective operators who have not yet acquired the necessary facilities or land or who have not yet begun construction of a CCRC. Such operators should be required to submit advertising, organizational information, a statement of proposed location and size, and at least a preliminary feasibility study demonstrating the future viability of the facility. After review of these submissions, the responsible agency should have the authority to issue a provisional certificate that entitles the applicant to collect deposits from prospective residents, to pursue contractual commitments with contractors, and to start out on the path toward permanent certification. It is the authors' opinion that, definitionally, the exemption discussed above for members of approved self-accreditation programs cannot apply to this type of provisional certification (as a prospective provider could not yet be a member of any approved accreditation program).

Second, all CCRCs presently operating in each state, as well as all new communities following the provisional certification procedure, should be required to apply for and receive permanent certification in order to sell or offer to sell continuing care contracts. Applications for certification should be developed by the responsible administering agency. A number of attachments to the application should be required, including a copy of the contract being used by the community, ownership and financial responsibility disclosure statements, a copy of the disclosure statement required for distribution to residents elsewhere in the statute, and a series of actual and projected financial statements.

The authors take the position that once a certificate of authority to operate is issued by the administering agency, it should remain perpetually valid, subject to the revocation procedures provided for elsewhere in the statute. Notwithstanding this conclusion, we would require the filing of annual reports, consisting of current financial statements as well as notification of any changes from information on file with the administering agency. We believe that, in this way, all the benefits of certification could be achieved while minimizing the admin-

---

[4] This option in CCRC legislation is modeled after the similar exemption procedures discussed above in the federal Medicare program. The major differences between this accreditation exemption and the JCAH program are that our exemption is not complete, as is JCAH accreditation, and that our accreditation program need not be national in scope, as is JCAH accreditation. The same type of exemption is discussed elsewhere in this chapter as well *See, e.g.,* pp. 275–78.

istrative burdens. Finally, members of approved self-accreditation programs should be required to file these annual reports with the responsible administering agency. This requirement is included to ensure that there is one central repository for all relevant information on each CCRC operating in any state.

LEGAL REGULATION OF FINANCIAL STATUS

Escrow Provisions

The basic view underlying escrow provisions is that some extra protection is needed for the residents' investment beyond disclosure, certification, and enforcement of other regulatory provisions—at least in certain instances. The objection to mandated escrow provisions is that, by definition, they direct capital into relatively stagnant bank accounts or other relatively unproductive uses of money, thereby depriving residents of the full value of their money, in that some part of their investment is not working as efficiently for them as it might.

Two basic approaches to escrow requirements could be used. The first approach would be to require an entrance fee and deposit escrow until the resident moves into the community, or until some other point in time, at which point all funds are released to the operator. The second approach would be to require general escrow funds of varying levels on a perpetual (or sometimes more limited) basis. This second requirement is typically imposed by a bonding authority or bank holding a mortgage or lien on the property.[5]

The Arizona, California, Michigan, and Minnesota statutes all require the maintenance of an escrow account for all entrance fees and deposits received before the resident occupies his or her unit. The AAHA statute authorizes the regulatory department to require an entrance fee escrow, but does not mandate it. Florida and Michigan require an escrowing of entrance fees and deposits only until the operator is certified. Finally, Michigan grants the administering agency the discretion to require an escrow deposit of a "reasonable amount when the facility's economic condition is precarious."

The existing state statutes approach in varying ways the issue of when funds should be released from the escrow account. For example, California's statute permits the entrance fee escrow to be released when the facility is 50 percent completed and 50 percent subscribed. The Arizona, Minnesota, and AAHA statutes, however, have more

---

[5] Chapter 12 also discussed the notion of an entrance fee escrow, which is an account maintained even after residence is established because of a legal or self-imposed standard requiring a certain amount of funds, ranging from relatively small amounts to the full value of all resident payments to the community. This type of fund escrow, classified herein as a reserve fund escrow, is discussed in the "Reserve Funds" section of this chapter.

complicated formulae governing release of the escrow funds, depending on whether the unit is new or old and, if new, depending on the stage of construction or financing.[6]

Against this background, the authors have reached the judgment that some type of escrow provision is a mandatory element of regulation. In reaching this result, which is not viewed as punitive, we found it helpful to isolate three different types of problems that entrance fee escrow requirements could arguably ameliorate:

First, a totally unscrupulous operator could commit fraud by absconding with the residents' entrance fees. Of course, this type of fraud could theoretically occur at any point in the life of a CCRC. It is the authors' judgment, however, reflected in the balance that we have struck between competing policies, that the likelihood of this type of fraud is greatest before the resident occupies his or her unit. Additionally, special protections might be advisable in the case of an operator who has not yet constructed his facility, but is collecting entrance fees.

Second, in the case of a new CCRC, the use of an entrance fee escrow is one mechanism to ensure that the community is in a position to meet the expectations of the promoter. A primary assumption made by the developer of any community is that the operator of a new community can attract a certain number of residents at a certain price to "buy in" to that facility. By forcing a CCRC to hold all of its entrance fees in escrow until a certain percentage of its capacity is subscribed to, one can statutorily ensure the accuracy of this crucial assumption.

Third, an escrow requirement could be used to help ensure the financial stability of the CCRC. Thus, it could be argued that any community maintaining a certain level of "cash" would be financially stable and secure.[7]

Balancing all of these considerations has led the authors to the conclusion that two different types of entrance fee escrows should be required by statute. First, all entrance fees, including refundable deposits in excess of 5 percent of the then-existing entrance fee for the

---

[6] Arizona's statute provides one example of this type of complex formula. If the entrance fee paid is for a unit that is currently occupied, it will be released when the unit becomes available for occupancy by the payor. If the entrance fee is for a new unit, however, it is released when three requirements are satisfied: (1) construction is substantially complete, and an occupancy permit has been issued; (2) commitment has been secured for long-term financing; and (3) aggregate entrance fees added to the proceeds from long-term financing total 90 percent of the total cost of the facility plus 90 percent of the money necessary to fund start-up losses. Ariz. Rev. Stat. Ann. §20-1804(A)(2) (Supp. 1979).

[7] This is presumably the theory underlying reserve fund escrows. The authors have concluded that it is more appropriate to account for this theory in the "Reserve Funds" section of this chapter.

unit requested, paid to *existing* and *operating* communities for occupied units before the resident takes occupancy, should be held in a cash escrow account.[8] With this type of escrow account, all funds should be released to the community on the day that the unit becomes available for occupancy by the resident.

Second, state legislation should require that entrance fees and refundable deposits paid to *new* communities before their construction or opening be held in a cash escrow account.[9] For the purposes of this section, any escrow required by a bonding authority or bank holding a mortgage on the community or its property, for either construction or permanent financing, should be considered to count against the requirements of the statute. Thus, the statute's escrow requirement should be concurrent with any escrow requirements established as a result of private contract. For funds held in this second type of escrow account, the entrance fee should be released in whole when all of the following conditions are satisfied:

The CCRC becomes 50 percent subscribed through receipt of entrance fees from a sufficient number of residents to fill 50 percent of the community.

Commitments have been secured for both construction and long-term financing. Further, any conditions that must be met to activate those commitments before disbursement of funds thereunder, other than completion of the construction or closing of the purchase of the community, must be satisfied.

Aggregate entrance fees received by or pledged to the provider plus anticipated proceeds from any long-term financing commitment plus funds from other sources in the actual possession of the provider must equal not less than 100 percent of the aggregate cost of constructing or purchasing, equipping, and furnishing the community, plus not less than 100 percent of the funds necessary to fund start-up losses of the community.

The most controversial aspect of this proposed statutory requirement—the release formula for the entrance fee escrow in a new community—represents a delicate balance among the various options discussed above. On the one hand, the proposed approach would make these funds available to the operator as soon as is practicable in a policy sense. On the other hand, in order to protect the residents from

---

[8] The term *cash escrow account* should be a defined term in the statute. Essentially, it should include any bank or similar company account specifically identifiable as an account held by the individual for the benefit of the community.

[9] This was an extremely difficult judgment for the authors to reach because of the difficulty it will create for small, church-related providers who may depend on the use of the entrance fees to fund their predevelopment costs. But the risk to residents—and the CCRC industry—and the capability of these providers to generate predevelopment costs by charging nonrefundable deposits tipped the balance. In this way, prospective residents' funds that are, in reality, at economic risk are identified clearly as such.

fraud and to ensure the integrity of the assumptions in the feasibility study, funds would not be released to the provider until it has received substantial commitments from potential residents and from sources of both short- and long-term funds.

The apparent harshness of the third requirement should be ameliorated, at least in part, by the statutory provision that the statute's escrow requirements be concurrent with, and not additional to, any escrow accounts entered into as a result of private contract. Because of the private market protective mechanisms that will come into play, no additional protection appears necessary to residents once the statutory requirements have been satisfied. Thus, the bank or bonding authority releasing funds to the provider under construction or permanent financing commitments should be policing the hopeful operator to protect against fraud. The interest of such entities in seeing the community's construction completed is as powerful as that of the potential residents. Because these lenders or financiers are sufficiently sophisticated to protect the interests of the residents, admittedly for different reasons, no additional statutory protection is necessary at this point.

Reserve Funds

As noted in Chapter 12, the major policy argument in favor of reserves is to ensure that the CCRC can provide the services associated with the deferred liabilities for which it has contracted with its residents. Applications of sound principles of actuarial science to determine liabilities associated with CCRCs, thereby resulting in the establishment of actuarially sound reserves, could be the most significant contribution of this study to the continued viability of the continuing care industry. Thus, the maintenance of actuarially sound reserves by all CCRCs should serve as the best protection residents can expect, both in terms of the sound financial planning that such a practice would bring to the continuing care industry and in terms of the inherent early warning signaling device that such a procedure would produce.[10]

---

[10] The Report on the Feasibility of the Trustee's Plan to Reorganize Pacific Homes concludes that "one of the key ingredients to the long term viability of an organization is the maintenance of adequate cash reserves." That report concludes that there should be reserves of two types: operational and future liabilities. The report explains its reasoning as follows:

> Operational reserves are maintained to cover normal operating expenses. These protect against unforeseen drops in occupancy or in slow payment from the residents. This reserve should be at least thirty to forty-five days of cash operating expenses.
>
> Future liability reserves are set up to provide for future replacement of property, plant and equipment, protect against emergency capital expenditures, and maintain reserve against potential future liability due to the contract residents. While there is no widely agreed upon level for this amount, it should probably be at least six months' operating expenses.

For the reasons explained later, the authors accept the report's statements on operational reserves but reject its conclusions on future liability reserves.

Residents expect and are entitled to a basic guarantee that their community will retain the essential financial wherewithal over the years to provide the services to which it has committed itself contractually, without the need to have monthly fees increase faster than inflation. This would appear to be a desirable goal of a CCRC, as discussed in Chapters 7 and 8. The goal implies that the community's current assets plus the present value of future inflation-constrained monthly fees must be at least as large as the community's current liabilities plus the present value of future expenses. Moreover, because future inflation-constrained monthly fees will fall short of future expenses (because of increased health care utilization as individuals age), the difference must be made up from current assets (or reserves) for the concept to work. Thus, the basic contractual guarantee can be provided only through the maintenance of sound actuarial reserves.

As will be recalled from a review of Chapter 12, the existing statutes tend to regulate both the level of reserves necessary or desirable and the investment limitations to be placed on whatever level of reserves is selected. Six of the 10 statutes studied contained some form of reserve requirements. The most typical regulations of size tend to look to the basic commitments of the community over a 12-month period and require that the amount necessary to meet those commitments be held in a cash or quasi-cash reserve. California also has a general requirement that the reserve be sufficient to cover the obligations assumed under continuing care contracts, as calculated through the use of state-approved mortality tables. Colorado requires that 65 percent of the amount of any advance payments made by all residents be held in a reserve to be drawn upon on a straight-line basis over a five-year period. Finally, with respect to investment limitations, the lower the level of required reserves in any statute, the stricter the limitations on investment tend to be.

The authors do not consider it advisable to specify in the cold type of this book the appropriate level of reserves for all communities, as has been done in other analyses of actual and proposed legislative schemes. It is our expectation that the discussions in this book will prompt the actuarial, continuing care, and accounting professions to research, test, and develop meaningful methodologies for evaluating the long-term financial soundness of individual CCRCs. Although these issues are explored in Chapters 7 and 8 along with a methodology for evaluating a community's actuarial position, no specific recommendation for legislative language is made here on the theory that something of this significance must await substantial additional field research.

Notwithstanding the lack of a specific recommendation, the authors feel strongly that mandating actuarially sound reserves is the best long-term legislative solution. We are simply reluctant to make a definitive prescription as to actuarial reserves and liquid asset requirements at this stage of the research, because of the risk that such a standard would be either too harsh or too weak, given the limited scope of this study.

Bonding Requirements

As was pointed out in Chapter 12, it is necessary to distinguish between two types of bonds. The first, referred to herein as a *fidelity bond,* is obtained by the CCRC in order to cover losses owing to the dishonesty or negligence of employees handling residents' money. The second, referred to as a *surety bond,* is obtained by the community as a substitute for, or in addition to, the reserve requirements just discussed.

Current practice in the continuing care industry is relatively consistent and easy to discern. Although only the California statute requires a fidelity bond for agents and employees who handle substantial sums of money, bonds covering the fidelity of employees are common in all industries in which the money of third parties is routinely handled by employees, including the CCRC industry. Ironically, although several state statutes require, or authorize the administering agency to require, the filing of surety bonds under certain circumstances, the authors are not aware of a single instance in which a CCRC obtained a surety bond to ensure its financial stability.

The authors have reached a mixed conclusion on this element of regulation. With respect to fidelity bonds, we are unpersuaded that it is necessary for states to include a statutory provision mandating all CCRC operators to obtain fidelity bonds for their employees. Recognizing, however, that certain states might feel more comfortable with such a provision, we have classified this element of regulation in category two as an optional section. With respect to surety bonds, however, we have concluded that no such provision is advisable in any state regulatory scheme. This element of regulation therefore falls within category three.

This conclusion was based on a number of considerations. First, surety bonds would not appear to be obtainable given the current experience. Second, even if obtainable, surety bonds would probably be prohibitively expensive. Third, the surety bond might have a poor incentive effect on the community's management; in short, it is arguably better to run a community well than to rely on a surety bond. Fourth, there are difficult administrative problems involved in determining the size of a surety bond for individual communities. Finally, the entire theory of reserves is that communities maintaining an actuarially sound reserve will have no need for further intrusive regulation of economic and financial status. Imposing a bonding requirement in addition to the reserve requirement would be superfluous.

Fee Regulation

The ultimate in intrusive regulation is direct setting of fees by the state, or supervision of fee-setting by the state. Such fee regulation might be modeled after the extensive regulation of rates commonplace in the insurance industry.

It is the authors' firm conclusion that no such fee regulation provision is appropriate in any state legislative scheme. Not surprisingly, all current existing and proposed pieces of legislation concur in this judgment, and do not contain fee regulation provisions. This element of regulation has, therefore, been placed in the third category noted in the introduction.

The appropriate setting of fees by CCRC operators is both complicated and essential to the welfare of the residents. It is recognized that operators might set fees too high, thereby gouging the residents, or that they might set fees too low, thereby attracting residents away from financially stable communities and ensuring the collapse of their own communities. And the frequent comparisons that have been made between the continuing care industry and the insurance industry are also noted. But the solution to this complex and crucial problem is not, and never will be, fee regulation by the state. Simply stated, there is no evidence that the state is any better suited for the fee-setting function than are CCRC operators. Indeed, the high administrative costs involved in such an apparatus would appear to disqualify the states automatically.

The search for solutions to the problem of correct fee-setting has led the authors to a more obvious answer. The fastest and most efficient way in which to improve the setting of fees for CCRCs is to improve the information base upon which such decisions are made. An improved information base, coupled with appropriate consultations with knowledgeable experts, will do more to improve the reliability of fee-setting decisions than will any state involvement in the fee-setting procedure. The goal of improving the information on which CCRC operators base their decisions was, of course, a major consideration in the decision to go forward with this research.

LEGAL REGULATION OF RESIDENT RELATIONSHIPS WITH THE COMMUNITY

Financial Disclosure to Residents

The basic rationale underlying full financial disclosure to both prospective and current residents is that, by making such disclosure, the community informs all residents about the past, present, and expected future financial condition of the facility, thereby rendering the residents better able to protect themselves without any additional regulatory intrusions. Thus, financial disclosure equalizes bargaining power between otherwise "ignorant" residents and "sophisticated" providers. The notion is that residents will not move into financially precarious CCRCs and will agitate to improve such communities once they reside there. For this reason, CCRCs will not risk allowing their financial condition to deteriorate, because this can lead to total collapse arising from a refusal of residents to move in.

Underlying the remainder of this chapter, which suggests the advisability of a comprehensive statute going beyond disclosure, is the judgment that problems exist with relying solely on disclosure to protect resident rights. Just giving information might not equalize bargaining power between residents and providers—the information must also be comprehensible. Because, by its nature, financial information is complex, disclosure of only raw financial data is probably not effective in its major goal of equalizing bargaining power. Further, if, because of age or educational background, residents are inherently weaker bargaining partners than operators, disclosure will not necessarily equalize bargaining power. Thus, the efficacy of disclosure is linked to the validity of the assumption that lack of information is the sole or major cause of the disparity in bargaining power.

Finally, the assumption that operators will not allow their facilities to deteriorate for fear of not attracting new residents requires close examination. Even if this were the case in most communities, the size and unrecoverable nature of each resident's investment in a CCRC might give rise to a more substantial obligation on the part of the state to safeguard the continued viability of CCRCs. In short, the authors have reached the judgment that disclosure is a necessary, but not sufficient, component of a regulatory scheme.

The current practice of CCRCs with respect to the disclosure element of regulation suggests that comprehensive disclosure requirements will not impose additional expensive burdens on most CCRCs. All 10 statutes analyzed in Chapter 12 include some form of disclosure within their extensive regulatory schemes. The disclosure provisions in these statutes were divided into three general types:

Those that allow general public inspection, on request, of financial statements and annual reports filed with the administering agency. Such a right is available to prospective residents, current residents, and the general public.

Those that require CCRC providers to furnish copies of specified disclosure material of varying content to all prospective residents or their advisers before execution of the contract.

Those that require CCRC providers to furnish annual disclosure statements to current residents.

As part of this research, a sample of representative CCRCs was assessed as to the extent of disclosure to residents at this time.[11] These communities were surveyed with a seven-question questionnaire that yielded the following results:

98 percent of the CCRCs surveyed formally disclosed some information to their residents.

CCRCs currently use diverse methods to disclose this information:

a. 90 percent disclose information at residents' meetings.

b. 88 percent disclose information in writing.

c. 81 percent disclose information through resident representatives.

d. 60 percent disclose information through regular newsletters.

e. 45 percent disclose information in a specialized disclosure statement.

f. 24 percent disclose information through other means, usually more informal than the above-noted methods.

The nature of the material disclosed to residents by CCRCs is also quite diverse:

a. 88 percent of the communities surveyed disclose financial statements to residents. Of these, 70 percent disclose those statements annually, 16 percent quarterly, and 11 percent monthly.

b. 100 percent of the communities surveyed disclose planned changes in fees to the residents. Of these, 60 percent disclose this information at least a month before the planned change, 29 percent at least two months before, and 7 percent on an annual basis.

c. 90 percent of the communities surveyed disclosed planned changes in services to their residents. Of these, 66 percent disclose these changes at least a month beforehand, 32 percent at least two months beforehand, and 3 percent on some other basis.

---

[11] Our sample community profile included 50 CCRCs with the following diverse characteristics:

Fifteen were constructed before 1970.
Fifteen were smaller than 300 residents.
Five were from the Northeast.
Twelve were from the North Central.
Seven were from the South.
Six were from the West.
Seventeen offered unlimited health care guarantees.
Thirteen offered limited health care guarantees.
Seventeen were in regulated states.
Thirty-seven were in nonregulated states.

d. 71 percent of the communities in our sample disclose planned changes in community size to their residents. A clear majority of these communities make this disclosure as far in advance as is practicable; only 17 percent of these communities have any specified time within which they disclose planned changes.

e. 83 percent of the communities surveyed disclose planned changes in construction to their residents. Again, as with planned changes in community size, the overwhelming majority disclose the plans as far in advance as is practicable.

52 percent of the CCRCs in our sample provide a narrative describing the financial condition of the community to residents. Of these, 77 percent provide the narrative annually, 5 percent quarterly, and 9 percent monthly.

Only 17 percent of the CCRCs surveyed disclosed to residents the salaries of their administrators, and only 12 percent disclosed any compensation paid to board members as a result of their service on the board.[12]

A clear majority of the CCRCs surveyed provide residents with background information on their owners (71 percent), administrators (88 percent), and members of the board (76 percent).

31 percent of the CCRCs in our sample disclosed to their residents information on the ownership interest of any owner, administrator, or member of the board in any company that did business with the particular community (e.g., management consulting companies).[13]

In sum, if the survey of CCRCs and existing statutes is any test at all, financial disclosure to residents is something that virtually every person associated with the continuing care industry can agree on. The authors are no exception. We have made the judgment that the financial disclosure element of regulation is an essential part of legislation.

The form and contents of disclosure are critical. States should require the use of a disclosure form that provides a complete summary of the CCRC's current and long-range financial picture. The form should be completed and submitted to the administering agency annually. All prospective residents should be given a copy of a simplified disclosure form including a clear narrative description of the financial condition of

---

[12] Fifty-five percent of the CCRCs surveyed, however, noted that the board members were not paid.

[13] This somewhat low figure is partially explained by the fact that 36 percent of the CCRCs surveyed marked this question "not applicable" or appeared to misunderstand the nature of the information requested by the question.

the CCRC to supplement all raw data supplied as a matter of course before execution of a continuing care contract. Current residents should be provided with copies of the simplified form annually and on request. Finally, residents and their advisers should be permitted access to the community's full financial and income statements, as well as to reports of any feasibility studies conducted. This right of inspection should be stated clearly and conspicuously on the simplified disclosure form.

The subject matter that the authors recommend be disclosed to the regulating agency draws heavily on the AAHA Model Continuing Care Provider Registration and Disclosure Act and includes the following:

The name, business address, and corporate form of the provider.

The names of the individual owners, including the names of all officers, directors, trustees, or managing partners of the provider.

With respect to any individual named above, as well as with respect to any proposed manager of the community, a description of the business experience of the person, the identity of any other business in which the person has a substantial ownership interest with which the community would do business, and a statement of any crime or civil fraud committed by such person.[14]

If the CCRC is to be or is operated by a management services company, full disclosure as to all persons affiliated with that management services company as above.

Statement of the experience of the provider in operating CCRCs.

Statement as to any affiliation with a religious, charitable, or other nonprofit organization, as well as an explanation of the extent of that organization's financial responsibility for the CCRC's operations.

Statement of the location and description of the properties of the provider relating to the CCRC.

Certified financial statements of the provider.

If operation of the CCRC has not yet begun, statement of the anticipated source and application of funds used or to be used in the purchase and construction of the CCRC.

A pro forma income statement for the CCRC for the next fiscal year.

A copy of the simplified disclosure form discussed elsewhere in this section.

---

[14] This last element will be confidential and not subject to public inspection.

The simplified disclosure form distributed annually to all residents and to prospective residents must contain at least the following information:

Simplified financial statements of the CCRC for the past year.

Simple narrative statement explaining the financial position of the CCRC.

The names of the individual owners, including the names of all officers, directors, trustees, or managing partners of the provider.

With respect to any individual named above, as well as with respect to any proposed manager of the community, a description of the business experience of the person, and the identity of any other business in which the person has a substantial ownership interest with which the community would do business.

If the CCRC is to be or is operated by a management services company, full disclosure as to all persons affiliated with that management services company as above.

Form and Contents of the Contract

A regulatory provision governing the contents of the continuing care agreement would, like regulations mandating full disclosure, attempt to equalize bargaining power between providers and prospective residents. By regulating the form of contracts (e.g., size of print and plain English requirements) and the contents of agreements (e.g., fees, refunds, and termination rights), the state can, in a relatively unintrusive way, ensure that the agreement reached and signed between the CCRC and the resident contains some basic protection for the resident and approximates a contract that would be reached between negotiators of equal bargaining strength. Further, regulation of certain substantive terms has the incidental benefit of reducing uncertainty and, therefore, simplifying much of the litigation surrounding continuing care.

Arguments that the form and contents of continuing care agreements should not be regulated in any way are rarely encountered. There are certainly potential administrative difficulties, and the possibility exists that state regulations in this area would have to be quite complete for fear that certain communities would include in their contract only the provisions required by the statute. Most significantly, and with some justification, there has been an increasing resistance to state legislation that, in effect, provides a standard form contract that each CCRC is forced to adopt.

Chapter 12 detailed quite extensively the method by which each of the statutes analyzed dealt with this element of regulation. Seven of the 10 statutes under consideration regulated the form and/or the contents of continuing care contracts to some extent. The form of each statute varies considerably.

The authors selected 25 CCRCs to serve as a sample of current practice vis-à-vis continuing care contract forms.[15] The following represents a breakdown of the percentage of continuing care retirement communities from the sample whose contracts contain provisions on the following list of items:

		Percent
I.	*Fees and accommodations*	
	A. Size and payment schedule for entrance fees and monthly fees	100%
	B. Provision governing increases in monthly fees	84
	C. Health and financial conditions required to gain entrance to the community and to stay in the community	76
	D. Type of accommodations	72
	E. Provision covering the contingency of two residents in any one unit	60
	F. Provision governing how long the resident can keep his or her individual unit upon transfer to a health center	80
	G. Services provided and surcharges	100
	H. Provision noting that no property interest is granted by the contract; only an agreement for services	52
II.	*Refunds*	
	A. General provision on refunds	80
	B. More specific refund terms	
	1. For death or withdrawal before occupancy	32
	2. Probationary refund	48
	3. Refund upon withdrawal of resident at any time	88
	4. Address contingency of death after occupancy	80
	5. Timing of refund	48
III.	*Termination rights*	
	A. Preoccupancy cooling-off period	36
	B. Probationary period termination provision	48
	C. Resident cancellation rights	92
	D. Community's rights of dismissal	84
	E. Provision governing the contingency of inability to pay	68
	F. Provision mandating that the residents preserve assets	44

As a result of the study, an analysis of the current statutory provisions, and current practice in both regulated and unregulated jurisdictions, the authors have reached the following conclusions with respect to the form and contents of the continuing care contract element of regulation. First, we conclude that provisions governing the form and

---

[15] The characteristics of this 25-community sample are as follows:
Eleven were constructed before 1970.
Eleven had fewer than 300 residents.
Five were from the Northeast.
Eight were from the North Central.
Six were from the South.
Six were from the West.
Thirteen offered an unlimited health care guarantee.
Twelve offered a limited health care guarantee.
Eight were in regulated states.
Seventeen were in nonregulated states.

contents of CCRC contracts fit within the first set of regulations described in the introduction to this chapter—that is, that they are an absolutely essential element of regulation in all states.

Second, the state legislation should impose a "plain English" requirement on all contracts for continuing care providers. Such provisions can be modeled after similar provisions found in several pieces of consumer protection legislation enacted at both the federal and state levels over the past 5 to 10 years.

Third, the state legislation should require that all new CCRC contract forms be approved by the responsible administering agency. Thirty days following submission of the contract to the administering agency, the form of the contract should be deemed approved even if the CCRC has received no word from the agency. The legislation should also require existing CCRC contracts to be submitted to the responsible administering agency. The agency approval requirement, however, should apply only to future continuing care contracts; that is, existing contractual agreements should be "grandfathered."

Fourth, any contract that attempts to limit the permissible increases in monthly fees should be prohibited. Any continuing care contract submitted to the administering agency containing such a provision should be automatically rejected.

Finally, although the state legislation should not generally impose particular word-for-word provisions on continuing care contracts, it should require all continuing care contracts to contain provisions dealing with the following issues:

The value of all assets transferred to the CCRC, the initial amount of the monthly fees, and the manner of changing monthly fees should all be stated in the contract.

Any health or financial condition of a resident that can allow the community to terminate the contract of a resident should be set forth in detail.

The particular living unit contracted for by the applying resident should be disclosed in the contract.

A provision governing dual occupancy of residency units should be included in all contracts. This provision must specify what occurs when one of the two residents dies, withdraws, is dismissed, or needs to be transferred to the health facility.

Provisions governing the reoccupancy of residents' living units as a result of prolonged sickness should be included in the contract.

The contract should list all services to be provided and any surcharges that may be levied.

The contract should specify that it creates no property interest of any kind, that it is simply a service agreement.

The refund provisions should be clearly stated in the text of the contract, either in boldface type or in type larger than the rest of the body of the contract. Full refunds, less a nominal processing fee, should be mandated in the case of death or withdrawal before the resident takes occupancy of the unit. The refund policies of the community on either withdrawal by the resident or dismissal by the CCRC should be stated explicitly. As a recommended, but not required, provision, the state legislation might contain a section providing for a probationary refund. Finally, the contingency of death after occupancy should be addressed explicitly in each continuing care contract.

Each contract should provide for a preoccupancy cooling-off period of at least seven days following execution of the contract, during which the resident may elect to cancel the contract with a full refund, less some small administrative fee for processing the application.

As an optional, but not required, section, state legislation might include a provision establishing a 90-day probationary period during which either party to the contract may cancel the contract, with or without cause. In such an event, there should be a full refund to the resident of all fees paid to the CCRC less reasonable costs.

All rights of cancellation by the resident should be conspicuously stated in the contract.

Similarly, the CCRCs' rights of dismissal should be clearly stated in the contract. Any state statute should include a good-cause limitation on the dismissal power of the community. Residents should also be protected against eviction and retaliation for complaints against the community.

A provision explaining clearly what can happen to the resident who is unable to continue to afford the monthly payments should be in each continuing care contract.

A provision in which each resident promises to preserve his or her assets to the best of his or her ability should also be mandated by state legislation

Rights of Self-Organization

In order to combat some of the potential harms of institutionalization, as well as the theoretical disincentive to care that may be present in some CCRCs,[16] it has been argued that it is advisable to grant rights of

---

[16] *See* Comment, *Continuing-Care Communities for the Elderly: Potential Pitfalls and Proposed Regulation,* 128 U. Pa. L. Rev. 883, 884 n.7, 911–12, 912 n.142 (1980).

self-organization to residents. By giving residents a voice and a role in a community's governance, one is, in effect, charging them with partial responsibility for assuring that the community function smoothly and efficiently. Like disclosure, therefore, this element is designed to give residents the power and the information to safeguard their own interests. Further, residents can often bring great wisdom and insight to the governance of a CCRC.

One objection to this type of regulatory provision is that, if the residents are given a role in the governance of the community that enables them to gain effective control of the community's operations, the facility's tax-exempt status might be in jeopardy. The study, however, has disclosed no examples of this potential problem.

A second potential problem with granting residents rights of self-organization applies only to the issue whether it should be mandatory that residents sit on the CCRC's board of directors. An objection is that residents sitting on a board of directors might be unable to execute their responsibilities properly due to a sense of emotional, rather than administrative and financial, responsibility. For example, residents on a board might hesitate to raise rates or tend to negotiate lower increases because of their concern for the reaction of their fellow residents (because they will continue to live in the community) as well as their own financial self-interest.

The authors find this argument persuasive, and, therefore, no provision mandating a CCRC to have a resident on its board is recommended for any state legislation. Of course, individual communities may wish to place residents on their boards, and legislation should not prohibit this.

The current approach of the various states that regulate the continuing care industry was detailed in Chapter 12. Only three of the statutes, plus one state's regulations, recognize any right to resident self-organization. Notwithstanding this statutory framework, a recently published study[17] found that 70 percent of all nonprofit homes for the aging (including CCRCs) permit some form of resident participation in decision making. Most typically, this participation takes the form of a resident council or association.

The study found that CCRCs with a relatively large number of residents (approximately 150 or more), CCRCs that contain independent living units, and CCRCs that offer several different levels of care are most likely to have resident involvement in aspects of daily operations and long-range planning. Consistent with this finding, the authors concluded that CCRCs also have a relatively high degree of involvement by residents in the decision-making process of the board of directors.

---

[17] A. Trueblood-Raper, *Resident Participation in Governance of Homes for the Aging* (1981).

Thus, although only 10 percent of the entire sample permitted residents to sit as fully participating members of their boards of directors, 18 percent of the CCRCs identified by the study have residents on their boards.

The authors have concluded that a statutory provision guaranteeing residents a role in the governance of their individual communities is appropriate. Because CCRCs tend to attract people who are highly educated and have had professional and community experience, an unusual pool of talent, resources, and decision-making skills exists in the typical CCRC resident population. The Trueblood-Raper study concluded that one finds a broad base of resident participation in a typical CCRC: residents serve on numerous committees, produce newsletters, coordinate and sponsor activities and events, and raise funds to serve the community and other charitable purposes. CCRC residents also currently influence decision making in other formal and informal ways.

A regulatory provision on residents' rights to organize would, therefore, be appropriate in any state statute regulating the continuing care industry. But such a provision should not require that any residents serve on the facility's board of directors. A general statement delineating some of the residents' organizational rights should be provided, however, in addition to a provision requiring periodic meetings, but only if requested by the residents, between management and residents to discuss income, expenditures, financial problems, and proposed changes in policies or services. Such provisions will help facilitate the voluntary development of resident councils, committees, and associations.

Advertising Regulation

The primary public policy behind all types of advertising regulation is an attempt to reduce misinformation and minimize the significance of weak bargaining power on the part of residents by ensuring that CCRC advertising and solicitation materials are accurate and not subject to misinterpretation. Advertising regulation is a basic antifraud protection common in many industries.

Seven of the analyzed statutes contain some form of regulation pertaining to advertising and promotional literature. The analysis of current practice in the continuing care industry disclosed no obvious examples of extreme abuse in either advertising or solicitation literature.[18] Yet, the fear is often expressed that an unscrupulous opera-

---

[18] In the past, there have been several examples of less than model behavior in the distribution of advertising materials by certain providers. For example, Pacific Homes' advertising literature suggested strongly the existence of a financial link between the provider and the United Methodist Church, a connection that the church went all the way to the Supreme Court of the United States to deny.

tor could, through clever advertising suggesting a relationship between the community and some well-known entity, either intentionally or negligently mislead prospective residents.

Although it is a close question, the authors have concluded that some form of advertising regulation is an appropriate component in state legislation of the continuing care industry. We reach this conclusion with full recognition of the reluctance of some to encourage this form of meddlesome government intervention. We also recognize that all CCRCs would be subject to any state statute of general applicability prohibiting the use of fraudulent or misleading advertising. The authors believe, however, that, owing to the subtleties and complexities of continuing care, and the particular skills and interests required to review advertising in a meaningful manner, advertising regulation of the CCRC industry is merited. This conclusion was made easier by the lack of any problems experienced by states that presently regulate CCRC advertising.

Advertising should be a defined term in the statute. That term can be defined so as to include promotional and solicitation literature, media advertisements, and similar material, but so as to exclude such items as community newsletters and routine correspondence to current and prospective residents. Misleading advertising, especially advertising that implies the existence of financial connections between CCRCs and unrelated but well-known and respected organizations, should be expressly prohibited. All advertising, promotional, and solicitation literature should be submitted to the administering agency and checked against the extensive ownership disclosure data already on file. Any mention of outside, but unaffiliated, organizations in the literature should be required to be followed, in print at least the same size, by an explanation of the financial connection between those organizations and the community. Continuing care operators should not be permitted to distribute or print any of the literature submitted to the administering agency for 14 days to permit the agency to review and, if appropriate, reject the proposed literature. Once again, as with the contract form approval process, failure of the agency to respond within 14 days should be statutorily deemed to be approval of the advertising, and distribution can begin.[19]

Lien Provisions and Preferred Claims

Definitionally, a *lien* gives the residents something beyond their contracts to sue on. Most critically, a filed lien gives the residents *priority* over subsequent claimants even if the community goes under 10 years after the filing. A *preferred claim* is, in essence, a special lien used only

---

[19] The Florida experience with this sort of "deeming" provision appears to have created no problems.

in liquidation proceedings. Thus, despite the classification of lien provisions and preferred claims in the "Legal Regulation of Resident Relationships with the Community" section of this chapter, such provisions are basically designed as financial protections.

It is the authors' conclusion that no provisions for liens or preferred claims should be adopted by any state enacting legislation in the continuing care area. First, and potentially of the greatest significance, liens and preferred claims are, in all probability, invalid as statutory liens under the provisions of the new Bankruptcy Code. Assuming that this analysis is correct, legislation at the state level creating such liens would be wholly frustrated by the supremacy of federal bankruptcy laws.

Second, current legislative and administrative practice involving such provisions has demonstrated the ineffectiveness of both liens and preferred claims as protections for resident financial interests. For example, such liens and preferred claims would invariably have to be subordinated to existing encumbrances such as first mortgages. (If this were not the case, CCRCs would find it nearly impossible to finance initial construction costs.) Such encumbrances are usually the largest obligations a CCRC takes on; thus, the protection given residents is only a minimal one.

Further, most lien and preferred-claim provisions are subject to discretionary action on the part of the agency administering the state legislative scheme. The only example that could be located involving actual use of lien or preferred-claim provisions occurred in California during the Pacific Homes controversy. In that case, the California State Department of Social Welfare acted too late in filing the lien, and then compounded this error by later subordinating the lien to further borrowings, thereby reducing even further whatever minimal protection the lien or preferred claim might have had for residents.[20]

Finally, it is the authors' judgment that granting either a lien or a preferred claim to residents might make borrowing by CCRCs more expensive or even impossible.

STATE ADMINISTRATION OF THE STATUTE

Responsible Agency

Not much can be said at the policy level about this particular element of regulation. The key is to ensure that the responsible agency has both the expertise and the interest necessary to administer whatever regulatory program the state develops. In any event, once the decision has

---

[20] R. Matthews, *Report of the Trustee of Pacific Homes*, 52–53 (Oct. 15, 1979).

been made to enact a statute, it is essential that the statute include a provision vesting regulatory discretion in some administrative agency.

To review current practice, administrative discretion is vested in the departments of insurance of four states, in the department of social services of one state, in the office of aging of one state, and in the securities bureaus of two states, and one state has created a board of examiners of life care. This study takes no definitive position on which agency a state should vest with administrative discretion over CCRCs. A state department of insurance, however, would not appear to be an appropriate candidate. State departments of insurance tend to be extremely overloaded in a rather detailed form of regulation (involving fee-setting) that, despite the many analogies between the continuing care industry and the insurance industry, is not particularly well suited to proper regulation of the continuing care industry.

Optimally, what one suspects would be appropriate is some form of blend of social service, health, actuarial, and aging skills. It is the authors' conclusion, therefore, that each state should make its own determination as to which agency it wishes to vest with regulatory discretion over the continuing care industry. Further, the authors have concluded that, in order to aid the selected agency in acquiring and maintaining an appropriate level of expertise and interest, each state should create a CCRC advisory board made up of attorneys, residents, and administrators of CCRCs, actuaries, and other appropriate personnel.

Investigative, Enforcement, and Rehabilitative Powers

No matter what form a regulatory scheme takes, and regardless of whether it is administered by government or private sources, enforcement of its provisions is essential. Investigation and audit capabilities are crucial adjuncts to the enforcement power. The policy debates on this element, therefore, center mostly on the scope of the investigatory, enforcement, and rehabilitative powers and, more specifically, on the nature of the necessary enforcement and rehabilitative powers.

The authors have reached a mixed conclusion on this regulatory element. Although we believe that investigative and enforcement powers are essential elements of any state regulatory scheme, and, therefore, have classified those two aspects in our first category, we believe equally strongly that rehabilitative powers along the lines of those used in the states that have enacted comprehensive regulatory schemes are inappropriate. Thus, we believe state statutes should include detailed investigative and enforcement powers but no rehabilitative powers.

As to investigative and enforcement powers, full investigative authority should be vested in the administering agency. This authority should extend both to on-site inspections and to examinations and financial audits. Second, strong civil and criminal penalties should be included to ensure the compliance of CCRC administrators with the statutory requirements. Third, full subpoena power should be given to the administering agency. Fourth, the basic remedial authority of the administering agency should require that agency to notify the noncomplying provider of its violation and to give the provider an opportunity to correct the violation. The basic tools available to the administering agency should include the authority to impose a cease and desist order or seek injunctive relief in the courts, and the appointment of examiners to supervise compliance with court or agency orders.[21] Such methods permit the operator to continue to run the facility, a feature of some importance because of his specialized knowledge of that particular community.

It is the authors' view that the type of comprehensive statute proposed in this chapter, coupled with this investigative and enforcement scheme, is all that is necessary to ensure proper operation of CCRCs. In the past, however, some states have determined that it is necessary to go further than the proposed provisions noted above and have included a provision permitting the administering agency and the court to appoint an outside person to assume operation of a financially troubled CCRC. It is not beyond the realm of possibility that some states might choose to enact such rehabilitative mechanisms in the future as well.

For the benefit of those states, the authors offer the following comments on what we regard as a limited rehabilitative procedure. The use of rehabilitative procedures that displace the operator from the community should be sharply limited to cases of actual fraud or gross mismanagement, which presumably will be rare. Such restrictions on rehabilitation appear justified by the lack of evidence that a government-appointed administrator would be better able to handle the serious problems that arise once a community is in financial trouble; indeed, most of the commonsense evidence to date supports a contrary conclusion.

Such limited corrective mechanisms are analogous to the reorganization provisions of the new Bankruptcy Code. A comparison between the authors' proposal and bankruptcy reorganization requires a brief glimpse of the old bankruptcy procedure, however. The Bankruptcy Act of 1898, which still has limited application, has three business reorganization chapters: 10, 11, and 12. In chapter 10, the appointment of a trustee is mandatory when the bankrupt's liability exceeds

---

[21] The provisions and policies of the new Bankruptcy Code are mirrored in this study's proposal that, on request by the administering agency, a court appoint an examiner to investigate and supervise the affairs of a troubled CCRC provider. *See* 11 U.S.C. §1104(B); H.R. Rep. No. 95–595, 95th Cong., 2d Sess., *reprinted in* (1978) *U.S. Code Cong. & Ad. News,* 5963, 6193–94.

$250,000.[22] In chapters 11 and 12, however, appointment of a trustee is optional,[23] and the bankrupt usually remains in control of the business.[24] This disparity results from two apparently irreconcilable policies behind business reorganizations: protection of creditors and the public (the chapter 10 policy) and facilitation of an effective reorganization to benefit both creditors and the bankrupt (the chapters 11 and 12 policy).

The Bankruptcy Reform Act of 1978 struck a different balance between these two policies. First, all business reorganizations are handled under a new chapter 11. Second, the debtor remains in possession of his business, unless a request for appointment of a trustee is made.[25] "The standard provided in the bill directs the court to order appointment of a trustee only if the protection afforded by a trustee is needed and the costs and expenses of a trustee would not be disproportionately higher than the protection afforded."[26]

The authors propose that courts be required to apply a similar standard in CCRC rehabilitation proceedings. The chances for successful rehabilitation are greatly enhanced if the CCRC provider remains in possession. Like the debtor going through reorganization, the provider is more familiar with his business than an outside trustee would be. If it remains, there will be no period of adjustment while the outside trustee familiarizes itself with the unique features of the particular facility. Finally, the cost of an outside trustee is avoided.[27] Consistent with the new Bankruptcy Code,[28] the authors recommend appointment of a trustee only in the event of fraud or gross mismanagement. But short of this result of regulatory failure, there is no reason to resort to the drastic remedy of appointing an outside trustee.

THE PROPRIETARY/NONPROFIT DISTINCTION

As noted in Chapter 12, a provision barring proprietary operators from offering continuing care contracts appears to be based on the notion that profit seeking has an adverse effect on the quality of care and services. One state (Michigan) appears to have attempted to bar such

---

[22] 11 U.S.C. §556 (1976).

[23] *Id.* §§742, 832.

[24] *See* D. Epstein & M. Scheinfeld, *Teaching Materials on Business Reorganization under the Bankruptcy Code,* 52 (1980).

[25] 11 U.S.C. §1104 (Supp. II 1978).

[26] H.R. Rep. No. 95–595, 95th Cong., 2d Sess. 234, *reprinted in* (1978) *U.S. Code Cong. & Ad. News,* 5963, 6193.

[27] *See id.* 233, *reprinted in* (1978) *U.S. Code Cong. & Ad. News,* 5963, 6192.

[28] *See* 11 U.S.C. §1104(A)(1) (Supp. II 1978).

operators from the life care industry; another (Pennsylvania) has considered a move in that direction, at least if one can believe the state legislature's press clippings.

Unfortunately, regardless of one's views on the desirability of such a policy, a provision excluding proprietary operators would not effectively advance this aim. Any proprietary operator who wished to circumvent the statute could establish a nonprofit corporate shell to run the CCRC and distribute the profits to himself by having the nonprofit shell contract with his own proprietary management and services company. The authors believe, therefore, that no provision prohibiting proprietary operators from offering continuing care contracts should be included in any state statute. To the extent that any state is concerned about the fraud, conflict of interest, and self-dealing abuses that it has been argued inhere in such arrangements, the appropriate vehicle with which to regulate such abuses is the state nonprofit corporation law. ■

Chapter Fourteen

Summary and Conclusions

■ This chapter contains an overview of the research presented in this book and summarizes the authors' recommendations in three subject areas. In addition, the chapter lists several areas for further research. The three areas covered in this book are: (1) an empirical survey of CCRCs that describes the various characteristics of existing communities; (2) a financial analysis of CCRCs that includes current financial management practices along with an extensive analysis of how actuarial science can be applied to develop appropriate fees and monitor the long-term financial health of CCRCs; and (3) a legal analysis that first describes the current status of CCRC regulation among the various states and then sets forth the areas where the authors believe that regulation is and is not appropriate.

The following summary cannot possibly serve as an adequate substitute for a thorough reading of each chapter. In many instances, especially in the financial and legal areas, there are no clear-cut answers to the many issues raised and discussed, requiring that the management of CCRCs exercise judgment as to the approaches that should be taken for their community. In those areas where judgment is required, the authors' best judgment is represented in the conclusions and recommendations provided below. The chapters themselves, however, set forth the various points of view so that conscientious readers will be in an excellent position to form their own conclusions.

EMPIRICAL SURVEY

Size of Industry

The study was able to identify 274 communities throughout the United States that met the following definition of a CCRC:

The facility consists of independent living units and generally has one or more of the following facilities: (1) congregate living, (2) personal care, (3) intermediate nursing care, and (4) skilled nursing care.

The community guarantees shelter and various health care services to residents under a contract that lasts for more than one year.

The additional fees for resident health care, if any, are less than the full cost of such services, implying a risk pooling of health care costs among residents.

The study also identified another 120 communities that offered services similar to CCRCs but did not precisely meet the characteristics listed above. For example, a number of communities that would have been classified as CCRCs in prior years have changed their contract so that residents now pay the full cost of any required health care services. These communities are not considered CCRCs as defined by this study.

The survey conducted as a part of this study collected an extensive amount of information on 207 of the 274 identified CCRCs. This represents a response rate of 76 percent, implying that the characteristics summarized here and discussed in detail in Chapters 2 and 3 are quite accurate for the industry as a whole. While it is true that the 24 percent not responding may have a systematic characteristic (for example, they may be predominantly financially distressed communities that did not wish to be examined), the authors believe that little or no such systematic bias exists in the sample.[1]

The 207 communities identified in the study currently serve 55,000 individuals, all of whom are over age 65 and whose ages range predominantly from 75 to 85, the average age being about 81. This is a relatively small fraction of the total number of individuals over 65 in the United States (0.2 percent) and of the number of individuals expected to fall within this age range during the next several decades. Therefore, the authors believe there is a tremendous potential for increasing the number of CCRCs to serve aged Americans. Moreover, as discussed later in this summary, the cost of entering and living in a CCRC appears to be well within the reach of a large number of such individuals.

---

[1] One fact leading to this conclusion is that the communities participating only after extensive follow-up efforts showed no characteristics distinctively different from those that participated after the initial contact.

About 20 percent of all CCRCs were formed prior to 1960; 40 percent were built between 1960 and 1970; and the remaining 40 percent were constructed since 1970. The median age of all communities is 14 years; however, numerous communities constructed prior to 1960 have offered continuing care contracts for decades.

Physical Aspects of Communities

The survey results indicated quite a range in the physical characteristics of CCRC facilities. Half of the communities have only a skilled nursing facility in conjunction with their independent living units, while the other half also have a personal care facility. The authors believe that the latter type of configuration, providing a continuum of health care services, is probably the most desirable approach in terms of the quality, appropriateness, and economic efficiency of delivering health care services to CCRC residents.

The number of independent living units per community is uniformly distributed from 50 to 300 units; however, a distinct trend toward a larger number of units exists in newer communities. The authors believe it desirable, from an economic viewpoint, to build CCRCs with at least 250 independent living units. This size provides economies of scale in management and allows the construction of a skilled nursing facility that meets the needs of the population on the one hand while complying with state regulations on the other.

CCRCs are evenly split between garden apartment, or low-rise, structures and high-rise structures. The main determinant of the type of structure is the suburban versus urban location of the facility. None of the analyses suggested that one type is perferable over the other.

The geographic distribution of CCRCs throughout the United States follows the distribution of aged individuals, with one important exception. The exception is the state of New York, where CCRCs as defined in this study are not permitted under law. Based on the research findings contained in this book that CCRCs are not only financially viable but also within the financial reach of a large number of aged individuals, the authors believe strongly that the laws in New York should be changed to accommodate CCRCs. Fifty percent of the CCRCs are located in the following states, listed in order of the number of communities per state: California, Florida, Pennsylvania, Ohio, and Illinois.

Fee Levels. The average entry fee for CCRCs as of December 1981 was $35,000, with $2,000 being added for the second of two individuals sharing an apartment. The average entry fee per square foot of independent living unit is $60. The range in entry fees is fairly wide, with 80 percent of all communities having entry fees falling in the range of $13,000 to $65,000.

The average monthly fee among CCRCs as of December 1981 was $550, with 80 percent of such fees falling in the range of $300 to $900 per month. The increase in monthly fees for a second person living in an apartment unit was found to be $250, an increment much greater, percentagewise, than the corresponding increment in entry fees.

Although a convincing actuarial argument can be made that entry fees and monthly fees should vary by such factors as the resident's entry age, sex, and health status, CCRCs tend to vary fees by the apartment type that the resident selects and by whether a second person is involved. This implies that the management of such communities are socializing not only health care expenses but also the expenses associated with other factors that affect the cost of providing future shelter and health care throughout the lifetimes of residents.

The fee ranges charged by CCRCs appear to be within the financial grasp of a large number of individuals over age 70. This is an important finding, since it suggests that CCRCs are not exclusively for the wealthy aged individuals in the United States.

Interestingly, 75 percent of CCRCs provide financial aid to residents whose financial resources become depleted. Although most CCRCs reserve the right to terminate the contracts of individuals who lack the financial resources to pay their monthly service fee, the survey did not find one instance where this had occurred. This reinforces the point that CCRCs are affordable by a large number of aged individuals in the United States. Even in cases where an individual's longevity coupled with inflation-related increases in monthly fees causes financial difficulties, such institutions are able to continue, through financial assistance, the care that the individual expected upon entering the community.

CCRCs are evenly split on the issue of offering partial entry fee refunds at the death of the resident. With respect to the half that provide such refunds, the methods used in determining the dollar amount vary significantly, there being no common approach among the communities.

Services Provided. CCRCs are evenly divided between those that offer an extensive health care guarantee and those that offer a limited guarantee. The differences between the two are as follows:

> *Extensive guarantee:* Residents pay the same monthly service fee while in the health care center as they paid while living in their apartment unit (or, if the monthly fee differs, the health care monthly fee is less than 80 percent of the per diem rate for such services).

> *Limited guarantee:* Residents pay the per diem rate while in the health care center; however, the higher fees do not begin until after a specified period of health care center residency, such as 180 days.

Thus, contrary to the belief that once an individual enters a CCRC, health care services are a free good, the basic insurance principle of "co-pay" is widely used among CCRCs. Surprisingly, however, the data indicated *less* health care utilization among residents in CCRCs with extensive health care guarantees. Perhaps this can be explained by the fact that the management of such CCRCs has a greater financial incentive to monitor and manage health care utilization. This is an area deserving of additional research, since the results are at odds with the general belief that the lower the cost of health care services, the more such services will be used.

With respect to the number of meals offered under continuing care contracts, again communities were found to be evenly split between those offering three meals per day as a part of the basic fee structure and those offering one meal with residents paying additionally if more than one meal per day is prepared for them by the community. However, there is a trend among newer communities to include only one meal, thus giving residents more freedom in structuring services to best meet their needs.

Affiliation and Management. Virtually all CCRCs are nonprofit organizations with religious affiliations. One third of the communities purchase management services from an outside organization, generally a for-profit organization, while the remaining two thirds are self-managed.

FINANCIAL ANALYSIS

The financial analysis of CCRCs comprises eight chapters in this book, Chapters 4 through 11. Chapter 4 provides an overview of the subject matter; Chapter 5 discusses the types of actuarial assumptions required to perform appropriate financial analyses of CCRCs; Chapter 6 describes how the future resident population of a CCRC can be projected with confidence, a process that represents the first step in financially analyzing the future of a CCRC; Chapter 7 discusses the actuarial theory for establishing appropriate fees for new entrants to a community; Chapter 8 provides a methodology to assist management in selecting the appropriate annual fee increases that are required to maintain the long-term financial soundness of the community; Chapter 9 illustrates the cash flow of a CCRC over a 20-year period and shows why conventional accounting procedures are not adequate for financially monitoring such communities; Chapter 10 gives an overview of the fundamentals with respect to financial statements in general and as they are typically applied to CCRCs; and Chapter 11 discusses the modifications that need to be made to traditional accounting statements so that the management of CCRCs has the proper information for maintaining their long-term financial success. An overview of the findings and recommendations presented in these eight chapters is given below.

Actuarial Assumptions. Several types of actuarial assumptions are required in performing financial analyses of CCRCs, two of the more important ones being mortality rates and morbidity rates. One of the recommendations of the study is that the CCRC industry must begin to develop a national data base for use in developing community-specific rates. Although it is true that mortality and morbidity experience varies among communities, a national data base would provide the basis for monitoring each community's experience and would also provide valuable information to individuals who are planning a new facility.[2]

As a part of this study, the mortality and morbidity experience of seven communities was studied. This data base, which consists of 25,000 life years (where one life year represents an individual living in a community for one year), indicates that the life expectancy of CCRC residents is significantly longer than the life expectancy of individuals of the same age in the general population. In fact, the life expectancy of CCRC residents is comparable to the life expectancy of individuals who purchase annuities from insurance companies. Overall, the life expectancy of both groups is about 20 percent greater than that of the general population. The greater life expectancy of CCRC residents could, in fact, be due to the same reason as that of annuitants— namely, such individuals tend to be in good health at the start of the contract. However, some individuals believe that additional factors may be associated with the greater life expectancy of CCRC residents, such as ready access to good health care, closeness to one's spouse if a resident is transferred to the health care center, the communal spirit among residents, and the opportunity to remain quite active in various recreational activities. Whether such factors make a difference in the life expectancy of CCRC residents must be studied in future research.

The data base also suggests that potential savings may be associated with the lower hospital utilization of CCRC residents as compared to that of the general population. Although the data base was too thin to draw definitive conclusions, this finding could have important implications relating to the cost of delivering health care to older Americans, and the authors suggest that this is a rich subject for further research.

The final point with respect to actuarial assumptions concerns the manner in which such assumptions are being used by those performing financial analyses of CCRCs versus the manner in which such assumptions should be used. One serious mistake in applying actuarial as-

---

[2] The insurance industry has pooled the experience of large companies in developing mortality rates for many years. The authors are suggesting that this same degree of cooperation would be beneficial to the life care industry as well.

sumptions is to use life expectancies for amortizing lump-sum entry fees into the community's income stream. This subject will be mentioned again at a later point in this summary.

A second serious mistake is that financial planners do not distinguish between mortality rates applicable while the individual is living in an apartment and the corresponding (and higher) mortality rates applicable while the individual is living in the health care center. While it is true that the overall mortality rates of CCRC residents follow those of an annuitant mortality table, the table itself is of little value in performing financial analyses. The annuitant mortality table must be decomposed into two tables, with lower rates applicable to apartment lives and higher rates applicable to health care center lives. This split in rates is important because the cost of caring for individuals differs significantly depending on their living status. Applying one table to all residents means that death rates for apartment dwellers will be too high (implying that projected apartment turnover rates and hence projected entry fee income will be overstated) and death rates for health care center residents will be too low (implying that the projected cost of health care will be too high). This misapplication can cause serious errors in the financial analyses of CCRCs.

Population Projections

In order to perform a financial analysis of a CCRC, whether a new or existing community, it is necessary to project the resident population on a year-by-year basis for a period of years into the future, calculating each year the expected number of apartment releases, the number of individuals expected to be transferred to the health care center, and so forth. Among the significant deficiencies observed in the industry are that existing communities, by and large, do not engage in this type of projection and that the projection period associated with financial feasibility studies for developing communities is generally limited to five or seven years. The authors recommend that all communities engage in such forecasts periodically and that such forecasts extend for a period of 20 years or more, especially for new communities, whose expected health care utilization is expected to be lower than the ultimate expected utilization during their maturation (the first 10 to 15 years of operation).

This research discusses and illustrates the problem of random deviations associated with projecting a population of only a few hundred individuals. Even if the underlying mortality and morbidity assumptions are precisely correct, a deterministic projection of the population will not reveal the likely variations in rates of death and morbidity, and the impact of these variations on the financial health of the community. Compounding this problem is the fact that the underlying rates themselves may be somewhat off the true rates. These two difficulties poses a significant barrier to adequate financial planning with respect to CCRCs. Therefore, two of the major conclusions of this research are: (1) that multiple projections must be made using various sets of pessimistic and optimistic rates in order to assess the implications of making an error in the underlying assumptions (i.e., a sensitivity analysis must be performed) and (2) that the projection must incorporate stochastic (or Monte Carlo) methodology. Under stochastic methodology, the population projection includes random deviations. Thus, estimates can be made of the best and worst financial events that are likely to occur, enabling management to plan accordingly.

The simulations presented in connection with the population projection analysis showed that it takes 15 years or more for a new CCRC to reach maturity, where maturity is defined by such statistics as a relative stable year-to-year average age of residents, a relatively constant number of residents living in the health care center on a permanent basis, a relatively stable apartment turnover rate (ignoring random deviations), and so forth. Thus, long-term projections are critical to the proper financial planning and management of CCRCs.

The simulations revealed some interesting statistics in addition to the data on the length of time it takes for a new CCRC to reach a mature state. For example, the density ratio (i.e., the ratio of apartment residents to the number of apartment units) is likely to decrease to some ultimate level from the ratio at the time the community is first opened. The initial density ratio, of course, is dependent on the number of couples in the start-up resident population. Similarly, the ultimate density ratio is dependent on the number of couples assumed to enter in future years and on the community's policy with regard to the transfer of an individual to a smaller apartment unit upon the death or permanent transfer of his or her spouse. Depending on the pricing structure of the community, the density ratio can have an important financial impact.

The simulations also showed, for the set of assumptions used, that the expected period of time spent in the health care center for all entrants will average two to three years. Moreover, since only half of the entrants will ever reside permanently in the health care center, this statistic implies that the average length of stay for those who do transfer is four to six years. Given this tenure, and given the high cost of caring for an individual in the health care center, it is essential that management take such data into account in developing fees. The research also found that a significant role in determining the community's health care costs is played by both management policies and the community's health care delivery system (i.e., whether there is only a skilled nursing facility as opposed to a continuum of care possibly represented by a home nursing program, a personal care facility, an intermediate care facility, and a skilled nursing facility). Those communities that strive to avoid transfers to the skilled nursing facility until this is absolutely necessary have lower health care costs but also have lower apartment release rates (and hence lower entry fee revenues), and vice versa. Since these factors are important, it is essential that the population methodology, along with the underlying actuarial assumptions, reflect both management policies and the community's health care program.

Finally, over the years a number of rules of thumb have been developed regarding such important items as apartment turnover rates, health care utilization, and density ratios. This research has found that, at best, these rules are not very good in performing financial analyses of CCRCs. There are too many differences among communities, such as differences in management policies, in health requirements for new entrants, and in health care programs, for such rules to be relied on when financially analyzing a community. Therefore, the authors strongly recommend against relying on such rules of thumb in establishing fees and/or projecting the population of a CCRC.

New Entrant Pricing

The actuarial theory for establishing fees for new entrants to a CCRC is set forth in Chapter 7. As a precursor to developing fees, however, the authors introduce what is undoubtedly a new concept to the CCRC industry, the concept of an actuarial liability for new entrants. This actuarial liability is equal to the present value of all future expenses expected to be incurred on behalf of the individual throughout his or her lifetime in the community. For example, the actuarial liability for an age-75 female entrant, given the hypothetical community and the hypothetical set of assumptions used in the research, was calculated to be $150,000. Put another way, if this amount were paid by each such individual at entry (a pricing policy *not* being recommended by the authors), then along with interest earnings on the unused balance it would be sufficient to pay all of the expected expenses for the individual (provided that all of the assumptions were realized).

The actuarial liability for an individual is dependent on four sets of factors: (1) *demographic factors,* such as the entrant's age, sex, and health status; (2) *contractual factors,* such as the community's death refund provision and the extensiveness of its health care guarantee; (3) *accounting factors,* such as the manner in which the cost of fixed assets (e.g., building and furniture) is allocated over time and the manner in which operating expenses are allocated (e.g., on a per capita versus a square footage basis); and (4) *economic factors,* such as future inflation and interest rates. Although many of these factors are technical, the point is that each individual entering the community has an associated actuarial liability depending on a large number of factors, and it is this liability which is the basis for determining fees.

Once the actuarial liability has been determined for an individual or a group of individuals, the next step is to decide what portion of the liability is to be paid by entry fees and what portion is to be paid by monthly fees. Theoretically, the mix between the two can range from 100 percent entry fees to 100 percent monthly fees; however, neither extreme is recommended by the authors. For reasons detailed in Chapter 7, the authors believe that entry fees should not exceed 30 to 40 percent of the actuarial liability.

Another approach to determining the entry fee/monthly fee mix is to assume that entry fees cover capital costs, while monthly fees cover all other costs. This generally results in an entry fee that does not exceed 40 percent of the actuarial liability, and such an approach supposedly has appeal to prospective residents. There is nothing sacrosanct about this approach (sometimes called the real estate/actuarial approach to setting fees), since it is simply one of an infinite number of ways to split the actuarial liability between entry fees and monthly fees.

Assuming that the actuarial liability and the mix between entry fees and monthly fees have been determined, it is still necessary for management to decide whether fees will reflect all of the factors that affect the actuarial liability itself. In other words, since the actuarial liability is higher for females and younger entrants, for example, should fees also be higher for such individuals? Similarly, since the actuarial liability differs by the type of apartment and by the number of individuals entering the apartment (i.e., single versus couple), should fees differ by these factors as well? Management must decide which of these dimensions the fee structure should reflect. Most CCRCs have fees that differ by apartment type and by the number of individuals occupying an apartment. This type of pricing structure, therefore, socializes the cost of numerous dimensions, a management policy that is perfectly acceptable, provided that the overall fee structure is equal to or greater than the overall actuarial liability of the new entrants. The authors have no recommendation regarding the distribution of costs among residents as long as the actuarial test is met.

Finally, with respect to the development of fees for new entrants, the authors set forth two objectives that appear to be reasonable and desirable for CCRCs:

Group equity: Fees for a group of entrants should be self-supporting, implying that the fees associated with future groups should not be required to pay for the services used by prior groups.

Inflation-constrained increases in monthly fees: The annual increases in monthly fees should not exceed the community's internal inflation exposure, implying that the increased cost of greater health care utilization during the community's maturation period must be advance-funded.

The authors recognize that some CCRC managements may not share these objectives, in which case the pricing structure of their communities could differ significantly from the structure that logically follows from the objectives.

Actuarial Valuations

An actuarial valuation involves the application of actuarial science to determining whether a community's aggregate assets (current assets plus prospective fees) are equal to its aggregate liabilities (current liabilities plus prospective costs for all residents). If such an equality exists, then the current fee structure is adequate, whereas if the asset-liability relationship is not equal, then fees should be changed to bring about the balance. One of the most important recommendations of this research is that CCRCs, and especially new CCRCs, should have an actuarial valuation performed periodically, such as annually or every two or three years. In addition to determining whether a community's assets are in balance with its liabilities, an actuarial valuation provides information on how fees should be adjusted from year to year to achieve and maintain such a balance. In other words, even if a community is in actuarial balance currently, random deviations during the following year will inevitably cause the balance to be altered. An actuarial valuation informs management of the financial implications of such deviations and provides guidance on the fee changes that should be made to restore the balance.

An actuarial valuation does not, however, provide management with information on the proper level of liquid assets, or working capital. However, this research clearly demonstrates that a community with an actuarially based fee structure will inevitably generate far more liquid assets than the minimums that various accounting techniques (or cash management techniques) would suggest. The fact that a community with actuarially based fees will generate significant amounts of cash, all of which is required to meet the long-term health care liability and other future commitments of the community, reinforces the need for actuarial valuations. This is the case because the managements of non-profit organizations are often reluctant to allow such funds to build up and/or because residents object to fee increases when sizable amounts of funds are on hand. An actuarial valuation not only determines the total amount of assets that a community must have but allocates such assets to various liabilities, such as the health care liability, thereby showing management and residents that such funds are *not* redundant and that fees should continue to increase with the community's inflation experience.

If an actuarial valuation of a community shows an unfunded actuarial liability (i.e., aggregate assets are less than aggregate liabilities), management has several options for funding it, such as a one-time percentage increase in fees over and above the current year's inflation increase, a temporary percentage increase over and above inflation for a period of years, or a flat dollar surcharge on fees for a period of time. The only requirement is that the additional increase in fees pay off the unfunded liability either in the current year or over a period of years. The authors recommend that such unfunded liabilities be funded over as short a period as possible, subject to marketing constraints and the ability of residents to pay the increased fees.

With respect to year-to-year random deviations, two methods for dealing with the corresponding change in the unfunded liability are discussed. One method is to adjust fees each year to fully account for the deviations. The other method is to build up a buffer or contingency fund, against which unfavorable deviations are charged and favorable deviations are credited. Under this approach, the size of the fund can be evaluated periodically and adjusted to the proper level if it has grown too small or too large. Either approach is acceptable from the authors' viewpoint.

Case Study Results

All of the actuarial techniques developed in the study were applied to six CCRC case studies. The communities that participated in this portion of the study were not selected on a random basis; therefore, it is *not* possible to generalize from the results. Nevertheless, it was interesting to discover that the fees charged by five of the six communities placed them in reasonable actuarial balance. The fees for these communities fell in the following ranges:

Weighted average entry fee range: $25,000–$55,000.

Weighted average monthly fee range: $400–$800.

Given the fact that these fee ranges produce reasonable actuarial balances, it appears that CCRCs are well within the financial grasp of a large number of Americans over age 65 and that the CCRC concept is financially viable.

One of the communities studied was found to be in severe financial distress; however, it was later learned that imprudent practices by previous management contributed to this situation. Therefore, it was not possible to tell whether the current pricing structure of the community would have supported the community's continuation if these practices had not occurred.

Financial Management Statements

As noted previously, the cash flow of an actuarially priced community will generally be quite strong. The problems associated with a CCRC accumulating significant amounts of cash were also mentioned. Moreover, accounting statements prepared according to generally acceptable accounting practices (GAAP) were found to contribute to this problem because such statements do not reflect the future long-term liability of the community. Generally speaking, the authors found three areas where GAAP statements could be modified to better represent the financial picture of a CCRC:

> *Entry fee earnings:* The current practice is to earn entry fees over the life expectancy of an individual or a group of individuals. This approach was found to bring too much money into the community's income statement too fast. Therefore, the authors recommend that entry fees should be earned over an individual's lifetime on an increasing-dollar basis, an approach that better matches revenues with expenses.

> *Expensing fixed assets:* Expensing fixed assets according to a cost-based depreciation schedule charges too little for such assets in an inflationary environment. Therefore, the authors recommend that such statements should be based on a replacement-basis depreciation method.

> *Health care fund accounting:* Most accounting statements commingle the apartment side of the CCRC with the health care center side. This adds confusion and often masks the true financial picture of the community. Therefore, the authors recommend that fund accounting be employed to generate separate statements, one for apartment cost center revenues and expenses and another for health care cost center revenues and expenses.

LEGAL ANALYSIS

The legal analysis of CCRCs is presented in Chapters 12 and 13 of this book. An overview of that material is given in the following subsections.

Current Regulation

The study contains a descriptive analysis of existing formal legal regulation of CCRCs. This material serves as a foundation for the study's analysis. For analytical purposes, the study divided its discussion of the current regulatory status of the continuing care industry into three parts:

Detailed state regulatory schemes: The study first discussed the responses of nine states and at least one organization—detailed regulation of CCRCs. The issues covered in this analysis include the definition of communities to be regulated, government certification/private accreditation, regulation of financial status, protection of residents' rights, and the legal structure of the community.

Limited state regulatory schemes: The study also discussed the responses of at least three states—selected regulation of one or two of the problems of the continuing care industry most susceptible to legal regulation.

Nonregulation: The third division of the study discussed the responses of the remaining 36 states, the District of Columbia, and the federal government—virtually total nonregulation. Included in this discussion are comments on proposed, but as yet unenacted, legislation and judicial attitudes toward CCRCs.

Evaluation of Legislative Options

The core of the study's legal analysis of CCRCs is presented in Chapter 13. That chapter contains the study's conclusions, underlying analysis, and recommendations for future legislative action concerning the continuing care industry.

The full contours and rationale underlying all the judgments reached by the study in its legal analysis cannot be explained in general terms; rather, the conclusions can be justified only through analysis of the value judgments drawn with respect to each element of regulation. As a result, both chapters of the legal analysis are organized according to the various elements of regulation identified by the study. Some of the highlights of the study's conclusions and recommendations are as follows:

Type of legislation: Foremost among the judgments drawn by the study is its judgment that legislation at the state, rather than federal, level will be appropriate in many states. The most substantial justification underlying this judgment is the study's view that, because CCRCs are still relatively new, it would be advantageous to encourage the variety of legislative programs that would develop at the decentralized state level.

Certification: The study concluded that certification requirements should be adopted by all states implementing continuing care legislation. This conclusion is tempered by the study's recommendation that each state approve private self-accreditation programs that meet certain specified standards and, once these programs have been approved, perform the accreditation function for the state.

Escrow: For existing communities, the study recommends that legislation require all entrance fees, including refundable deposits in excess of 5 percent of the then existing entrance fee for the unit requested, to be held in a cash escrow account to be released to the community on the day that the unit becomes available for occupancy by the resident. For new communities, the study recommends that state legislation require all entrance fees and refundable deposits to be held in a cash escrow account until the CCRC becomes 50 percent subscribed, commitment has been secured for both construction and long-term financing, and aggregate entrance fees received by or pledged to the provider plus anticipated proceeds from financing equal not less than 100 percent of the aggregate cost of construction or of purchasing, equipping, and furnishing the community plus not less than 100 percent of the funds necessary to fund start-up losses of the community.

Reserve funds: Although the study makes no specific recommendation at the present time on reserves, the authors feel strongly that mandating actuarially sound reserves is the best long-term legislative solution. More research is necessary on this issue, however. At the very least, periodical actuarial reviews should be required.

Financial disclosure: The study recommends that all states regulating the continuing care industry mandate financial disclosure to residents. The study's recommendation is both for a complete disclosure form to be filed with the state and for a simplified disclosure form, including a clear narrative description of the financial condition of the community, to be supplied to all prospective and current residents.

Contract regulation: The study concluded that both the form and the content of the continuing care contract should be regulated by the state. The state, however, should not regulate the precise wording of continuing care contracts; rather, the optimal statute would simply mandate the subject areas that each continuing care contract should cover.

Advertising regulation: Although the study concedes that this is a close question, the authors have concluded that some form of advertising regulation is an essential component in any legislation of the continuing care industry. Misleading advertising, therefore, should be expressly forbidden. In addition, the study would require that all advertising, promotional, and solicitation literature be submitted to the administering agency for approval. Failure of the agency to respond within 14 days should be statutorily deemed to be approval of the literature.

There is a need to develop and further test various methodologies for determining whether fees are set to maintain long-term financial viability; however, the fee-setting mechanisms should avoid the disadvantages of trying to apply a simple mechanistic formula to all cases.

Among the other recommendations made by the study were expanding and strengthening preconstruction requirements to protect bondholders' interests and establishing a formal disclosure criterion to minimize possible abuse through conflict of interest among management and board members.

AREAS FOR FUTURE RESEARCH

During the two years of study leading to this book, it became clear that there were a number of issues related to continuing care that required additional research and evaluation.

Although these issues were outside the scope of the study, the authors and members of the Advisory Committee feel strongly that consideration should be given to such issues, which include the following:

How large is the demand for continuing care, and how widely can the continuing care concept be applied successfully?

Do CCRCs help to prolong life, and if so, what specific factors produce this longer life expectancy? Based solely on a review of life expectancies in this study, CCRC entrants tend to live longer than the general population.

Contrary to the general belief that more health care services are used when the cost is lower, the study data indicated *less* health care utilization among residents of CCRCs. Why?

Comparative studies are needed to determine not only what differences exist in the cost of health care but also what is being bought with the health care dollar: physician usage, usage of skilled nurses and of nurse practitioners, drugs, laboratory tests, and additional recognized services such as podiatry and dental care. Data are also needed on health care expenditures by CCRC residents compared to expenditures by comparable groups living outside CCRCs.

Does the immediate availability of health services in a CCRC produce better health among residents?

What are the economies of scale in a CCRC?

There is a definite need for development of a national, or regional, data base from which guidelines can be drawn in selecting the assumptions to be used for financial analyses of CCRCs. Development of CCRC mortality rates is especially needed because it is impossible to reflect the financial consequences of a continuing care contract with accuracy using only life expectancies and mortality rates.

How will CCRCs be affected by federal and state tax laws?

What bioethical and legal questions will arise as a result of the increasing age of CCRC residents?

Is discrimination on the basis of age, race, or religious affiliation being practiced by any CCRCs?

Who will determine the allocation of decreasing resources?

What are the legal impacts of Medicare and Medicaid decisions? ∎

Appendix A

CCRC Universe (as of December 31, 1981)

Kirkwood by the River	Birmingham, Ala.
Mount Royal Towers, Inc.	Birmingham, Ala.
*Friendship Village	Tempe, Ariz.
Orangewood Retirement Community	Phoenix, Ariz.
Aldersly, Inc.	San Rafael, Calif.
The Alhambra	Alhambra, Calif.
Brethren Hillcrest Homes, Inc.	La Verne, Calif.
Canterbury Woods	Pacific Grove, Calif.
Carlsbad-by-the-Sea	Carlsbad, Calif.
Carmel Valley Manor, Inc.	Carmel, Calif.
Casa Dorinda	Montecito, Calif.
Channing House	Palo Alto, Calif.
Covenant Village	Turlock, Calif.
Forest Hill Manor	Pacific Grove, Calif.
Grand Lake Gardens	Oakland, Calif.
The Heritage	San Francisco, Calif.
Lake Park Retirement Home	Oakland, Calif.
Los Gatos Meadows	Los Gatos, Calif.
Mount Miguel Covenant Village	Spring Valley, Calif.
Mt. San Antonio Gardens	Pomona, Calif.
Piedmont Gardens	Oakland, Calif.
Pilgrim Haven	Los Altos, Calif.
*Plymouth Village of Redlands	Redlands, Calif.
*Rosewood Retirement Community	Bakersfield, Calif.
Quaker Gardens	Stanton, Calif.
Regents Point	Irvine, Calif.
Royal Oaks Manor	Duarte, Calif.
St. Paul's Towers	Oakland, Calif.
The Samarkand of Santa Barbara, Inc.	Santa Barbara, Calif.
San Joaquin Gardens	Fresno, Calif.
The Scripps Home	Altadena, Calif.
The Sequoias—Portola Valley	Portola Valley, Calif.
The Sequoias—San Francisco	San Francisco, Calif.
*Solheim Lutheran Home	Los Angeles, Calif.
Sunny View Lutheran Home	Cupertino, Calif.
The Tamalpais	Greenbrae, Calif.
The Valle Verde Retirement Center	Santa Barbara, Calif.
*White Sands of La Jolla	La Jolla, Calif.
Windsor Manor	Glendale, Calif.
Frasier Meadows Manor	Boulder, Colo.
*Medalion Retirement Center	Colorado Springs, Colo.
*Medalion West	Colorado Springs, Colo.

* = not included in data base for empirical analysis.

*Sunny Acres Villa.................................. Denver, Colo.
*Villa Pueblo Towers .... Pueblo, Colo.

*Covenant Village and Pilgrim Manor .... Cromwell, Conn.
Thirty Thirty Park.................................. Bridgeport, Conn.
Whitney Center, Inc. .... Hamden, Conn.

Cokesbury Village.................................. Hockessin, Del.

Lisner-Louise Home................................ Washington, D.C.
*Presbyterian Home of D.C......................... Washington, D.C.
*Thomas House...................................... Washington, D.C.

Abbey Delray....................................... Delray Beach, Fla.
Asbury Towers .... Brandenton, Fla.
Azalea Trace .... Pensacola, Fla.
Bay Village of Sarasota, Inc. .... Sarasota, Fla.
Bradenton Manor .... Bradenton, Fla.
Calusa Retirement Center .... Fort Myers, Fla.
Canterbury Tower, Inc.............................. Tampa, Fla.
*Congregational House .... Clearwater, Fla.
Covenant Palms of Miami........................... Miami, Fla.
Covenant Village of Florida .... Plantation, Fla.
East Ridge Retirement Village, Inc. .... Miami, Fla.
Evergreen Woods .... Springhill, Fla.
Jacksonville Regency House......................... Jacksonville, Fla.
*John Knox Village of Central Florida................. Orange City, Fla.
John Knox Village of Florida, Inc. .... Pompano Beach, Fla.
*John Knox Village of Margate .... Margate, Fla.
*John Knox Village of Tampa Bay .... Tampa, Fla.
Leisure Manor...................................... St. Petersburg, Fla.
Moorings Park .... Naples, Fla.
Oak Bluffs Retirement Center .... Clearwater, Fla.
Oak Cove Retirement and Health Center.............. Clearwater, Fla.
Orlando Lutheran Towers........................... Orlando, Fla.
Palm Shores Retirement Center..................... St. Petersburg, Fla.
Plymouth Harbor, Inc.............................. Sarasota, Fla.
St. Andrews Estates................................ Boca Raton, Fla.
*St. Mark Village .... Palm Harbor, Fla.
Shell Point Village................................. Fort Myers, Fla.
The Shores .... Bradenton, Fla.
*Trinity Lakes .... Sun City Center, Fla.
The Waterford .... Juno Beach, Fla.
Westminster Oaks.................................. Tallahassee, Fla.
Westminster Towers................................ Orlando, Fla.
Winter Park Towers and Village .... Winter Park, Fla.

*Arcadia Retirement Residence .... Honolulu, Hawaii

Apartment Community of Our Lady of the Snows .... Belleville, Ill.
Bensenville Home Society........................... Bensenville, Ill.
*Bethany Home and Hospital........................ Chicago, Ill.
Covenant Village—Northbrook .... Northbrook, Ill.
*Danish Old People's Home......................... Chicago, Ill.
Evenglow Lodge .... Pontiac, Ill.
Friendship Manor .... Rock Island, Ill.
*Friendship Village of Schaumburg.................... Schaumburg, Ill.
The Georgian .... Evanston, Ill.
The Holmstad...................................... Batavia, Ill.
Plymouth Place, Inc. .... La Grange Park, Ill.
The Presbyterian Home .... Evanston, Ill.

*The Scottish Home .... North Riverside, Ill.
Wesley Willows .... Rockford, Ill.
*Westminster Place .... Evanston, Ill.
Westminster Village—Bloomington .... Bloomington, Ill.

Altenheim Community .... Indianapolis, Ind.
Asbury Towers .... Greencastle, Ind.
The Four Seasons Retirement Center .... Columbus, Ind.
*Franklin United Methodist Home .... Franklin, Ind.
*Friends' Fellowship Community .... Richmond, Ind.
Hoosier Village Retirement Center .... Indianapolis, Ind.
Topsfield Terrace Retirement Community .... South Bend, Ind.
The Towne House .... Fort Wayne, Ind.
United Methodist Memorial Home .... Warren, Ind.

Calvin Manor .... Des Moines, Iowa
*Cedar Falls Lutheran Church .... Cedar Falls, Iowa
Friendship Village—Waterloo .... Waterloo, Iowa
Heather Manor .... Des Moines, Iowa
Heritage House .... Atlantic, Iowa
Meth-Wick Manor .... Cedar Rapids, Iowa
Northcrest Community .... Ames, Iowa
*Oaknoll Retirement Residence .... Iowa City, Iowa
Ridgecrest Retirement Village .... Davenport, Iowa
United Presbyterian Home .... Washington, Iowa
Valley View Village .... Des Moines, Iowa
Wesley Acres .... Des Moines, Iowa

*Aldersgate Village ....,.......... Topeka, Kans.
Arkansas City Presbyterian Manor .... Arkansas City, Kans.
Brewster Place .... Topeka, Kans.
Lakeview Village .... Lenexa, Kans.
Lawrence Presbyterian Manor .... Lawrence, Kans.
Presbyterian Manor of Kansas City .... Kansas City, Kans.
Salina Presbyterian Manor, Inc .... Salina, Kans.
Sterling Presbyterian Manor .... Sterling, Kans.
Wesley Towers, Inc. .... Hutchinson, Kans.
Wichita Presbyterian Manor .... Wichita, Kans.

*St. James Place .... Baton Rouge, La.

*Asbury Methodist Home .... Gaithersburg, Md.
*Augsburg Lutheran Home .... Baltimore, Md.
*Broadmead .... Cockeysville, Md.
Fairhaven .... Sykesville, Md.

Friendship Village Kalamazoo .... Kalamazoo, Mich.
Glacier Hills .... Ann Arbor, Mich.
Independence Village .... Frankenmuth, Mich.
Inter-City Christian Manor .... Allen Park, Mich.
Vista Grande Villa .... Jackson, Mich.

Covenant Manor Retirement Community .... Minneapolis, Minn.
Friendship Village of Bloomington .... Bloomington, Minn.
Madonna Towers .... Rochester, Minn.
Thorne-Crest Retirement Center .... Albert Lea, Minn.

The Charless Home .... St. Louis, Mo.
*Friendship Village of South County .... St. Louis, Mo.
Friendship Village of West County .... Chesterfield, Mo.
Fulton Presbyterian Manor .... Fulton, Mo.
John Knox Village .... Lee's Summit, Mo.

*John Knox Village East .... Higginsville, Mo.
*John Knox Village of the Ozarks .... Waynesville, Mo.
*Presbyterian Manor at Farmington .... Farmington, Mo.
Rolla Presbyterian Manor .... Rolla, Mo.
St. Louis Altenheim .... St. Louis, Mo.
Vista del Rio .... Kansas City, Mo.

*Eastmont Towers .... Lincoln, Neb.
Gateway Manor, Inc. .... Lincoln, Neb.
Northfield Villa, Inc. .... Gering, Neb.
*Skyline Manor .... Omaha, Neb.

Home for Aged Women .... Portsmouth, N.H.

Cadbury .... Cherry Hill, N.J.
Meadow Lakes .... Princeton, N.J.
Medford Leas .... Medford, N.J.
Navesink House .... Red Bank, N.J.
Workmen's Circle Home for the Aged .... Elizabeth, N.J.

*El Castillo Retirement Residence .... Santa Fe, N.Mex.
Landsun Homes, Inc. .... Carlsbad, N.Mex.

J. W. Abernethy Center .... Newtown, N.C.
Carol Woods Retirement Community .... Chapel Hill, N.C.
*Carolina Village .... Hendersonville, N.C.
*Episcopal Home for the Aging .... Southern Pines, N.C.
The Methodist Home .... Charlotte, N.C.
*Moravian Home, Inc. .... Winston-Salem, N.C.
The Presbyterian Home, Inc. .... High Point, N.C.
*The Presbyterian Home at Charlotte .... Charlotte, N.C.

Bethesda Scarlet Oaks Retirement Community .... Cincinnati, Ohio
Breckenridge Village .... Willoughby, Ohio
Copeland Oaks .... Sebring, Ohio
Dorothy Love Retirement Community .... Sidney, Ohio
*First Community Village .... Columbus, Ohio
*Friends Care Center of Yellow Springs .... Yellow Springs, Ohio
Friendship Village of Columbus .... Columbus, Ohio
*Friendship Village of Dayton .... Dayton, Ohio
Friendship Village of Dublin .... Dublin, Ohio
*Hill View Retirement Center .... Portsmouth, Ohio
Judson Park .... Cleveland Heights, Ohio
Maple Knoll Village .... Springdale, Ohio
The Marjorie P. Lee Home .... Cincinnati, Ohio
Methodist Home on College Hill .... Cincinnati, Ohio
Otterbein Home .... Lebanon, Ohio
Mt. Pleasant Retirement Village .... Monroe, Ohio
Park Vista Presbyterian Home .... Youngstown, Ohio
Portage Valley Retirement Village .... Pemberville, Ohio
Rockynol .... Akron, Ohio
*Trinity Home .... Dayton, Ohio
Wesley Glen, Inc. .... Columbus, Ohio
Westminster Thurber Community .... Columbus, Ohio

Oklahoma Christian Home/Apartments .... Edmond, Okla.

Cascade Manor .... Eugene, Ore.
Friendsview Manor .... Newberg, Ore.
Holladay Park Plaza .... Portland, Ore.
Rogue Valley Manor, Inc. .... Medford, Ore.
*Rose Villa, Inc. .... Portland, Ore.
*Willamette View Manor .... Portland, Ore.

Calvary Fellowship Homes, Inc. . . . . Lancaster, Pa.
Cathedral Village . . . . Philadelphia, Pa.
Cross Keys Village . . . . New Oxford, Pa.
Crosslands. . . . . Kennett Square, Pa.
Dunwoody Village. . . . . Newtown Square, Pa.
*Gloria Dei Village . . . . Holland, Pa.
Fiddler's Woods . . . . Philadelphia, Pa.
Fort Washington Estates . . . . Fort Washington, Pa.
Foulkeways at Gwynedd . . . . Gwynedd, Pa.
Friendship Village of South Hill. . . . . Upper St. Clair, Pa.
Green Ridge Village . . . . Dillsburg, Pa.
Gwynedd Estates. . . . . Springhouse, Pa.
*Heritage Towers . . . . Doylestown, Pa.
Kendal at Longwood . . . . Kennett Square, Pa.
Lima Estates . . . . Lima, Pa.
*Martin's Run . . . . Marple Township, Pa.
Messiah Village . . . . Mechanicsburg, Pa.
Paul's Run. . . . . Philadelphia, Pa.
Pennswood Village, Inc. . . . . Newtown, Pa.
Philadelphia Protestant Home. . . . . Philadelphia, Pa.
Pine Run . . . . Doylestown, Pa.
Rosemont Presbyterian Village. . . . . Rosemont, Pa.
Rydal Park . . . . Rydal, Pa.
Sarah A. Reed Home—Retirement Center . . . . Erie, Pa.
*Sherwood Oaks . . . . Wexford, Pa.
*Simpson House . . . . Philadelphia, Pa.
Southampton Estates . . . . Southampton, Pa.
Spring House Estates . . . . Springhouse, Pa.
*Springfield Retirement Residence . . . . Wyndmoor, Pa.
The Village at St. Barnabas . . . . Gibsonia, Pa.
*Wood River Village. . . . . Bensalem, Pa.

McKendree Manor, Inc. . . . . Hermitage, Tenn.
*Shannondale. . . . . Knoxville, Tenn.
The Trezevant Episcopal Home. . . . . Memphis, Tenn.

*Bayou Manor . . . . Houston, Tex.
*The Hallmark . . . . Houston, Tex.
*John Knox Village of Metroplex . . . . Denton, Tex.
John Knox Village of the Rio Grand Valley . . . . Weslaco, Tex.
John Knox Village of West Texas . . . . Lubbock, Tex.
Presbyterian Village North, Inc. . . . . Dallas, Tex.
*Westminster Manor. . . . . Austin, Tex.

Goodwin House. . . . . Alexandria, Va.
Hermitage Home of Richmond. . . . . Richmond, Va.
*Hermitage in Northern Virginia . . . . Alexandria, Va.
*Hermitage on the Eastern Shore . . . . Onancock, Va.
Lakewood Manor . . . . Richmond, Va.
*Masonic Home of Virginia . . . . Richmond, Va.
United Methodist Home in Roanoke. . . . . Roanoke, Va.
Virginia Baptist Homes—Culpeper . . . . Culpeper, Va.
Westminster Canterbury Corporation . . . . Richmond, Va.
Westminster-Canterbury in Virginia Beach . . . . Virginia Beach, Va.
Westminster-Canterbury of Lynchburg, Inc. . . . . Lynchburg, Va.

Bayview Manor . . . . Seattle, Wash.
Covenant Shores, Inc. . . . . Mercer Island, Wash.
The Frank Tobey Jones Home. . . . . Tacoma, Wash.
The Hearthstone . . . . Seattle, Wash.
Horizon House, Inc. . . . . Seattle, Wash.

*Judson Park Retirement Residence .... Seattle, Wash.
Riverview Terrace................................. Spokane, Wash.

Alexian Village of Milwaukee........................ Milwaukee, Wis.
Evergreen Manor, Inc.............................. Oshkosh, Wis.
Fairhaven Corporation .... Whitewater, Wis.
*Friendship Village of Milwaukee .... Milwaukee, Wis.
Methodist Manor, Inc.............................. West Allis, Wis.
Milwaukee Catholic Home, Inc. .... Milwaukee, Wis.
Milwaukee Protestant Home for the Aged.............. Milwaukee, Wis.
St. John's Home of Milwaukee .... Milwaukee, Wis.
Tudor Oaks Retirement Community .... Hales Corners, Wis.

Appendix B
Actuarial Assumptions

Mortality Rates for Illustrative Financial Analysis
(rates per 100 residents)

Age	Mortality rates for apartment residents		Mortality rates for health care residents	
	Female	Male	Female	Male
65	0.5 deaths	0.9 deaths	1.9 deaths	5.2 deaths
66	0.5	1.0	2.0	5.6
67	0.5	1.1	2.1	6.1
68	0.6	1.1	2.3	6.6
69	0.6	1.2	2.5	7.2
70	0.7	1.3	2.8	7.8
71	0.8	1.4	3.1	8.5
72	0.9	1.5	3.5	9.3
73	1.0	1.7	3.9	10.1
74	1.1	1.8	4.5	11.1
75	1.3	2.0	5.0	12.1
76	1.4	2.2	5.7	13.3
77	1.6	2.4	6.4	14.6
78	1.8	2.7	7.2	16.1
79	2.0	2.9	8.2	17.6
80	2.3	3.2	9.3	19.4
81	2.6	3.5	10.5	21.3
82	3.0	3.9	11.9	23.3
83	3.4	4.2	13.4	25.5
84	3.8	4.6	15.2	27.9
85	4.3	5.1	17.2	30.5
86	4.8	5.6	19.4	33.5
87	5.5	6.2	21.9	36.9
88	6.1	6.8	24.6	40.8
89	6.9	7.5	27.5	45.3

TABLE B–1B
Mortality Rates for Illustrative Financial Analyses
(rates per 100 residents)

Age	Mortality rates for apartment residents		Mortality rates for health care residents	
	Female	Male	Female	Male
90	7.6 deaths	8.4 deaths	30.5 deaths	50.4 deaths
91	8.4	9.4	33.5	56.1
92	9.1	10.4	36.4	62.5
93	9.8	11.6	39.1	69.6
94	10.4	12.9	41.6	77.1
95	11.0	14.2	44.0	85.2
96	11.6	15.6	46.2	93.5
97	12.1	17.0	48.4	100.0
98	12.7	18.5	50.8	—
99	13.3	20.1	53.3	—
100	14.0	21.6	56.1	—
101	14.8	23.2	59.3	—
102	15.7	24.8	62.9	—
103	16.8	26.4	67.0	—
104	17.9	28.1	71.7	—
105	19.3	29.7	77.0	—
106	20.8	31.4	83.0	—
107	22.5	33.0	89.9	—
108	24.4	34.7	97.5	—
109	26.3	36.3	100.0	—
110	100.0	100.0	—	—

TABLE B-1C ————————————

Morbidity Rates for Illustrative Financial Analyses

(rates per 100 residents)

Age	Permanent transfer morbidity rates		Temporary transfer morbidity rates	
	Female	**Male**	**Female**	**Male**
65	0.9 transfers	1.2 transfers	400 days	0 days
66	1.0	1.3	500	0
67	1.1	1.4	600	0
68	1.2	1.6	700	0
69	1.3	1.7	800	100
70	1.4	1.8	900	200
71	1.6	2.0	1,000	300
72	1.8	2.2	1,100	400
73	2.0	2.4	1,200	500
74	2.2	2.6	1,300	600
75	2.5	2.8	1,400	700
76	2.8	3.1	1,500	800
77	3.2	3.4	1,600	900
78	3.6	3.7	1,700	1,000
79	4.1	4.1	1,800	1,100
80	4.6	4.5	1,900	1,200
81	5.3	5.0	2,000	1,300
82	5.9	5.4	2,100	1,400
83	6.7	5.9	2,200	1,500
84	7.6	6.5	2,300	1,600
85	8.6	7.1	2,400	1,700
86	9.7	7.8	2,500	1,800
87	10.9	8.6	2,600	1,900
88	12.3	9.5	2,700	2,000
89	13.8	10.6	2,800	2,100

TABLE B–1D —————————————————————————
Morbidity Rates for Illustrative Financial Analyses
(rates per 100 residents)

	Permanent transfer morbidity rates		Temporary transfer morbidity rates	
Age	Female	Male	Female	Male
90	15.2 transfers	11.8 transfers	2,900 days	2,200 days
91	16.7	13.1	3,000	2,300
92	18.2	14.6	3,100	2,400
93	19.6	16.2	3,200	2,500
94	20.8	18.0	3,300	2,600
95	22.0	19.9	3,400	2,700
96	23.1	21.9	3,500	2,800
97	24.2	23.8	3,600	2,900
98	25.4	25.9	3,700	3,000
99	26.6	28.9	3,800	3,100
100	28.1	30.2	3,900	3,200
101	29.6	32.4	4,000	3,300
102	31.5	34.7	4,100	3,400
103	33.5	37.0	4,200	3,500
104	35.9	39.3	4,300	3,600
105	38.5	41.6	4,400	3,700
106	41.5	44.0	4,500	3,800
107	44.9	46.5	4,600	3,900
108	48.8	48.5	4,700	4,000
109	53.1	50.8	4,800	4,100
110	0.0	0.0	4,900	4,200

TABLE B–2 —————————————————————————
New Entrant Assumptions for Illustrative Financial Analyses*

Assumption	Female	Male
Entry age distribution:		
64 and younger	0%	0%
65–74	30	30
75–84	60	60
85 and older	10	10
Average	77 years	77 years
Gender distribution:		
Single entrants	90%	10%
Paired entrants (percent same sex)	10%	
Double-occupancy percentage:		
Studio	0%	
One bedroom	50	
Two bedrooms	100	

* These assumptions are applied to all entrants after the initial move-in of first generation.

TABLE B–3

Economic Assumptions for Illustrative Financial Analyses*

Time period	Inflation rates	Interest rates
Short-term rates:		
1983	10%	12%
1984	10	12
1985	10	12
1986	10	12
1987	10	12
Long-term rates:		
1988 and thereafter	10%	12%

* Format of this table is used to illustrate that short-term assumptions could differ from long-term assumptions.

Appendix C

Expense and Valuation Assumptions

EXPENSE ASSUMPTIONS

The four steps required to develop expense assumptions are: (1) defining expense items and their aggregate values for the initial year; (2) projecting aggregate expenses for at least as many years as the difference between the age of the youngest resident and the assumed end of the human life span; (3) defining expense allocation factors that specify the portion of each aggregate expense allocated to the apartment center versus the health care center, the portion of each cost center expense allocated on a per capita (per person) basis versus a per unit (square footage) basis, and the number of residents over whom each expense is to be shared; and (4) specifying annual expenses by living status for an individual resident.

Table C–1 contains the base year assumptions for eight operating expense categories and six capital expense categories. These values were derived from projected expenses for three similar communities whose first full year of operation begins in 1983. This facility is assumed to contain 295 apartment units and 60 health care beds. The notes to Table C–1 describe the assumptions used to calculate actuarial expenses for fixed assets. These assumptions result in total actuarial expenses for the base year of approximately $5 million.

Tables C–2 and C–3 contain the expense allocation assumptions used to determine the proportion of each expense category allocated to individual residents. Table C–3 presents the allocation assumptions that define the amount of each expense category allocated between the apartment center and the health care center. For example, 85 percent of the $451,000 administrative expenses in the base year, or $383,350, is allocated to the apartment center, and 15 percent, or $67,650, is allocated to the health care center. Table C–3 presents the allocation assumptions that specify the portion of each expense estimated to vary as the number of residents changes (per capita allocation) and the portion that does not vary as the number of residents changes (per unit allocation).[1] Apartment center expenses that are allocated on a per unit basis are assumed to be shared among 280 units (95 percent occupancy) consisting of three types: studio, one-bedroom, and two-bedroom. The relative sizes of the units follow a ratio of 1 to 1.5 to 2, and the percentage mix of unit types is 20 percent studio, 60 percent one-bedroom, and 20 percent two-bedroom. By way of example, the per unit allocations imply that residents of studio apartments will be allocated 13 percent of the apartment per unit expenses, residents of one-bedroom apartments will be allocated 60 percent, and residents of two-bedroom apartments will be allocated 27 percent.

---

[1] The apartment center per capita expenses are assumed to be shared among 350 residents (1.25 residents per occupied apartment). The health care center expenses are also allocated on a per capita basis over 57 residents (95 percent occupancy). Any portion of the health care center expenses that would be allocated on a per unit basis would be the same as per capita because all health care beds are assumed to occupy the same square footage.

TABLE C–1
Base Year Expense Assumptions for Actuarial Liability Calculation

Operating expenses:

Administrative	$ 451,000
Food service	568,000
Housekeeping	196,000
Maintenance	249,000
Utilities	374,000
Nursing care	584,950
Resident services	125,000
Taxes and insurance	80,000
Total operating expenses	2,627,950

Capital expenses:

Building	1,624,602
Land	60,000
Original equipment and furnishings	189,626
Equipment and furnishings replacement	18,963
Refurbishments	17,930
Original start-up costs	406,151
Total capital expenses	2,317,272
Total expenses	$4,945,222

Notes:

1. Interest rate used to expense all fixed assets is 12 percent.
2. Building cost is assumed to be $15 million: with an assumed useful lifetime equal to 40 years.
3. Cost of land was $500,000; actuarial methodology treats land expense as a perpetuity. (Since land is assumed to have an infinite useful lifetime, the actuarial expensing methodology implies that the proper expense for land should last forever.)
4. Cost of fully equipping and furnishing the facility is $1,200,000; these short-term assets are assumed to have an average useful lifetime equal to 10 years.
5. Equipment and furnishings replacement expenditures are assumed to be $120,000 ($1,200,000 ÷ 10) initially and are increased by 10 percent annually. These expenditures are expensed over 10 years, and future expenses will be added to the initial value, generating a 10-year layer of expense for each calendar year.
6. The initial refurbishment expenditure is equal to 1 percent of the building cost, $150,000, and is assumed to increase 10 percent annually. The annual expenditures are expensed over 20 years, and future expenses will be added to the preceding year's expense, generating a 20-year layer of expense for each calendar year.
7. Original start-up costs include architects' fees, legal fees, marketing costs, development fees, sewer construction, and financing costs, which are assumed to be 25 percent of the construction cost, or $3,750,000; these costs are expensed over the assumed useful lifetime of the facility (40 years).

TABLE C–2 ─────────────────────────────
Expense Allocation Factors for Apartment and Health Care Cost Centers

	Allocation percentage		Expense amount allocated to	
	Apartment center	Health care center	Apartment center	Health care center
Operating expenses:				
Administrative	85%	15%	$ 383,350	$ 67,650
Food service....................	85	15	482,800	85,200
Housekeeping...................	80	20	156,800	39,200
Maintenance....................	85	15	211,650	37,350
Utilities	85	15	317,900	56,100
Nursing care....................	0	100	0	584,950
Resident services................	80	20	100,000	25,000
Taxes and insurance..............	85	15	68,000	12,000
Total operating expenses......			1,720,500	907,450
Capital expenses:				
Building........................	85	15	1,380,912	243,690
Land...........................	85	15	51,000	9,000
Original equipment and furnishings....................	65	35	123,257	66,369
Equipment and furnishings replacement	65	35	12,326	6,637
Refurbishments	65	35	11,654	6,276
Original start-up costs	85	15	345,228	60,923
Total capital expenses			1,924,377	392,895
Total expenses...................			$3,644,877	$1,300,345

TABLE C-3
Expense Allocation Factors for Per Capita and Per Unit Allocations to Apartment and Health Care Center Residents

	Apartment center per capita percentage	Apartment center per unit percentage	Apartment center expense amount — Allocated on a per capita basis	Apartment center expense amount — Allocated on a per unit basis	Health care expense amount allocated on a per capita basis
Operating expenses:					
Administrative	60%	40%	$ 230,010	$ 153,340	$ 67,650
Food service	100	0	482,800	0	85,200
Housekeeping	40	60	62,720	94,080	39,200
Maintenance	20	80	42,330	169,320	37,350
Utilities	20	80	63,580	254,320	56,100
Nursing care	100	0	0	0	584,950
Resident services	100	0	100,000	0	25,000
Taxes and insurance	20	80	13,600	54,400	12,000
Total operating expenses			995,040	725,460	907,450
Capital expenses:					
Building	20	80	276,183	1,104,729	243,690
Land	20	80	10,200	40,800	9,000
Original equipment and furnishings	20	80	24,651	98,606	66,369
Equipment and furnishings replacement	20	80	2,465	9,861	6,637
Refurbishments	20	80	2,331	9,323	6,276
Original start-up costs	20	80	69,046	276,182	60,923
Total capital expenses			384,876	1,539,501	392,895
Total expenses			$1,379,916	$2,264,961	$1,300,345

TABLE C-4
Valuation Assumptions

Occupancy distribution

	Occupied units	Residents
Studio	56	56
One bedroom	168	210
Two bedrooms	56	84
Total	280	350

Fees as of January 1, 1983

	Entry fees		Monthly fees	
	One person	**Two persons**	**One person**	**Two persons**
Studio	$40,781	—	$659	—
One bedroom	52,129	$72,512	720	$1,157
Two bedrooms	63,475	85,901	781	1,222

Average age of residents.. 77.0 years

Percentage female 75.7%

Revenue and expense inflation rate 10%

Interest discount rate... 12%

Mortgage interest rate... 12%

TABLE C-5
Statement of Estimated Uses and Sources of Funds

Uses of funds:

Construction..........................		$15,000,000
Land.................................		500,000
Equipment............................		1,200,000
Contingency		500,000
Working capital		700,000
Start-up:		
Architect...........................	$ 750,000	
Sewer..............................	350,000	
Development	300,000	
Marketing	1,000,000	
Legal	375,000	
Financing...........................	975,000	3,750,000
Debt service reserve...................		1,800,000
Funded interest		3,150,000
Total uses of funds		$26,600,000

Sources of funds

Debt..............................	$15,000,000
Entry fees*..........................	11,600,000
Total sources of funds	$26,600,000

* Total entry fees received are $16,079,917.

Appendix D

Technical Description of Actuarial Pricing Methodology

METHODOLOGY FOR DETERMINING ACTUARIAL LIABILITIES AND FEES

The purpose of this appendix is to present the technical details of the methodology used to determine actuarial liabilities and corresponding fees for funding those liabilities. This methodology was used to generate the numerical values presented in Chapters 7 and 8. The discussion begins with the basic pricing equation that equates monthly fee revenues and entry fee earnings with expenses. This equation is modified to incorporate the time value of money (present values), probability of survival, and health care cost differentials. The final result is a generalized pricing equation that can be used to develop actuarial liabilities for a specific set of demographic (age, sex, health status), contractual (limited or extensive health care guarantee and alternative refund provisions), accounting policy (per capita and per unit allocations and timing of capital expenses), and economic (inflation and interest) assumptions, as well as to determine various fee setting methods under alternative pricing philosophies that may or may not vary fees on some or all of the characteristics affecting costs.

Basic Pricing Equation

The fundamental pricing equation for any continuing care contract is that the revenues expected to be collected from a group of residents must equal their expected expenses. Not only must total revenues equal total expenses for the group, but annual revenues must also "match" annual expenses (in order to prevent intergroup subsidies). Algebraically, this equivalency can be represented by the following equation:

$$R_0 + R_1 + R_2 + \cdots = E_0 + E_1 + E_2 + \cdots$$

where

R_t = Expected revenues in year t
E_t = Expected expenses in year t

This formula, which will be referred to as the actuarial pricing equation, is the basis for developing a theoretically equitable and adequate pricing structure.

In order to introduce the "inflation-constrained increase in monthly fees" objective, the revenue (left-hand) side of the equation must be separated into two components. One is monthly fee revenues, and the other is the amortization of entry fees (or entry fee earnings).

$$(MF_0 + EFE_0) + (MF_1 + EFE_1) + (MF_2 + EFE)_2 + \cdots$$
$$= E_0 + E_1 + E_2 + \cdots$$

where

MF_t = Monthly fees during year t
EFE_t = Entry fee earnings during year t

Entry fee earnings represent the portion of the original entry fee plus interest on the unearned balance recognized as revenue each year. The inflation-constrained monthly fees increase objective implies that the maximum change in monthly fees in any one year is limited; hence, entry fee earnings must equal the difference between total expenses and monthly fee revenues for the cohort group of residents. This condition has an important impact both on the method by which entry fees are determined and on how they are earned on an income statement.

Figure D–1 presents the ideal relationship between expenses, monthly fees, and entry fee earnings. Expenses and monthly fees are assumed to increase by 10 percent annually for inflation, and all residents are assumed to live for 20 years.[1] For purposes of this illustration, all values are given in terms of monthly fees that total to $1 annually, that is, monthly fees of $0.08 ($1 ÷ 12). In the first year, annual monthly fees are assumed to be $1 and expenses are assumed to be $1.20. By the end of 20 years, monthly fees (on an annual basis) are projected to increase to $6.73 and expenses to $8.07, reflecting 20 years of 10 percent inflation.

The amortization of entry fees, which are defined to be the difference between expenses and monthly fees, are also given in this graph. Initially, entry fee earnings are $0.20 ($1.20 − $1.00). By the end of 20 years, entry fee earnings are $1.34 ($8.07 − $6.73). In this example, these earnings increase at the same rate as expenses and monthly fees;

---

[1] This unrealistic assumption is used at this point for pedagogic purposes. The assumption will be relaxed in further developments of the pricing structure.

FIGURE D-1 _____

Inflation-Adjusted Expense, Monthly Fee, and Entry Fee Earnings

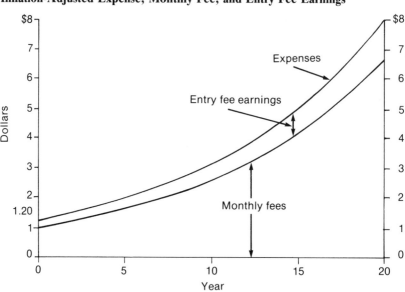

however, as shown later in this appendix, they will increase faster than inflation.[2]

Time Value of Money

Revenues and expenses for a group of continuing care contractholders are spread over a period of years. In order to equate the value of these future dollars, it is necessary to determine their value today. This requires that the "time value" of money be incorporated into the actuarial pricing equation. The time value of money reflects the fact that $1 today is worth more than $1 payable in the future since interest can be earned by investing today's dollar.

The actuarial pricing equation modified to reflect the time value of money is given below:

$$(MF_0v_0 + EFE_1v_1) + (MF_1v_1 + EFE_1v_1) + \cdots$$
$$= E_0v_0 + E_1v_1 + E_2v_2 + \cdots$$

where

v_t = Present value of $1 promised in t years

---

[2] The correct method for earning entry fees is a major point of controversy for the financial statements used by CCRCs. The manner in which entry fees should be earned bears a direct relationship to the philosophy used to establish fees. Since there is no universally accepted philosophy for determining fees, there is no one entry fee earnings schedule that is correct for all communities.

By way of example, assume that money invested today earns 12 percent interest compounded annually. Column 2 of Table D–1 contains the present value of $1 payable in future years. The present value of $1 today is $1. The present value of $1 promised at year 1 is $0.89. In other words, if one invested $0.89 in a fund that yields 12 percent per year, the original investment would accumulate to $1 at the end of one year. Similarly, $1 promised at year 4 has a present value of $0.64; the present value of $1 at year 19 is $0.12; and so forth.

Table D–1 applies these present values to discount the projected annual expenses and revenues, both of which are assumed to increase by 10 percent inflation, as shown previously in Figure D–1. Column 3 shows the projected annual expense, and column 4 gives the present value of those expenses (i.e., column 2 times column 3). The present value of future expense is $1.12 at year 4, while at year 9 the present value is $1.02. The sum of the present value of future expenses over the 20 years is $20.33. The present value of future monthly fees and entry fee earnings is given in columns 6 and 8, respectively.

Entry fee earnings, equal to the difference between projected expenses and projected monthly fees, sum to $11.47. The present value of entry fee earnings is derived by subtracting the present value of monthly fees, $16.94, from the present value of future expenses, $20.33, and is equal to $3.39, one third of the sum of entry fee earnings.[3]

Probability of Survival

The preceding example was based on the assumption that all residents survived for 20 years. A more realistic scenario is that only a portion of the cohort will survive to each future year. In order to properly match expenses and revenues, these dollar payment streams must additionally be discounted for death. The survivors from a closed group of residents can be estimated by using an actuarial model, known as a life table, which specifies the probability of survival (or death) in each year.

In actuarial terminology, the probability of surviving to future years is specified by a l_x column, in which the "l" refers to the number of lives and the "x" refers to a specific age. By way of example, consider 100 females at age 75. Table D–2 shows the expected number of survivors from this group over the next 20 years.[4] Column 2 shows that

---

[3] This implies that an actuarially correct method of earning entry fees would have total earnings that would exceed the initial entry fee due to interest earnings on the unearned balance.

[4] These probabilities were developed from the mortality assumptions presented in Appendix B.

TABLE D-1
Calculation of Interest-Discounted Expenses and Revenues

Year t	Present value of $1 promised in year t	Projected expenses	Interest-discounted expenses	Projected monthly fees	Interest-discounted monthly fees	Projected entry fee earnings	Interest-discounted entry fee earnings
0	1.00000	$ 1.20	$ 1.20	$ 1.00	$ 1.00	$ 0.20	$0.20
1	0.89286	1.32	1.18	1.10	0.98	0.22	0.20
2	0.79719	1.45	1.16	1.21	0.96	0.24	0.19
3	0.71178	1.60	1.14	1.33	0.95	0.27	0.19
4	0.63552	1.76	1.12	1.46	0.93	0.30	0.19
5	0.56743	1.93	1.10	1.61	0.91	0.32	0.18
6	0.50663	2.13	1.08	1.77	0.90	0.36	0.18
7	0.45235	2.34	1.06	1.95	0.88	0.39	0.18
8	0.40388	2.57	1.04	2.14	0.87	0.43	0.17
9	0.36061	2.83	1.02	2.36	0.85	0.47	0.17
10	0.32197	3.11	1.00	2.59	0.84	0.52	0.17
11	0.28748	3.42	0.98	2.85	0.82	0.57	0.16
12	0.25668	3.77	0.97	3.14	0.81	0.63	0.16
13	0.22917	4.14	0.95	3.45	0.79	0.69	0.16
14	0.20462	4.56	0.93	3.80	0.78	0.76	0.16
15	0.18270	5.01	0.92	4.18	0.76	0.84	0.15
16	0.16312	5.51	0.90	4.59	0.75	0.92	0.15
17	0.14564	6.07	0.88	5.05	0.74	1.01	0.15
18	0.13004	6.67	0.87	5.56	0.72	1.11	0.14
19	0.11611	7.34	0.85	6.12	0.71	1.22	0.14
Sum*	8.36578	$68.73	$20.33	$57.26	$16.94	$11.47	$3.39

* Some columns may not sum exactly due to rounding errors.

TABLE D-2
Discounting Expenses and Revenues for the Probability of Survival

Year t	Age x	Number of survivors to age x	Probability of survival to age x	Survival-discounted expenses	Survival-discounted monthly fees	Survival-discounted entry fees
0	75	100.000	1.00000	$ 1.20	$ 1.00	$0.20
1	76	98.697	.98697	1.30	1.09	0.22
2	77	97.147	.97147	1.41	1.18	0.24
3	78	95.307	.95307	1.52	1.27	0.25
4	79	93.130	.93130	1.64	1.36	0.27
5	80	90.563	.90563	1.75	1.46	0.29
6	81	87.551	.87551	1.86	1.55	0.31
7	82	84.053	.84053	1.97	1.64	0.33
8	83	80.028	.80028	2.06	1.72	0.34
9	84	75.453	.75453	2.13	1.78	0.36
10	85	70.318	.70318	2.19	1.82	0.36
11	86	64.638	.64638	2.21	1.84	0.37
12	87	58.463	.58463	2.20	1.83	0.37
13	88	51.886	.51886	2.15	1.79	0.36
14	89	45.058	.45058	2.05	1.71	0.34
15	90	38.188	.38188	1.91	1.60	0.32
16	91	31.526	.31526	1.74	1.45	0.29
17	92	25.321	.25321	1.54	1.28	0.26
18	93	19.782	.19782	1.32	1.10	0.22
19	94	15.041	.15041	1.10	0.92	0.18
Sum*		1,357.948	13.57948	$38.82	$32.35	$6.47

* The sums are based on projections to age 110.

98.697^5 of the original 100 females are expected to survive to age 76. This indicates that the probability of survival for one year is 98.7 percent for a female age 75. The probability of surviving two years is 97.1 percent. Other probabilities are determined by dividing the number of survivors at a given time by the initial number of residents.[6]

Taking the probability of survival into consideration, the basic pricing formula now becomes:

$$(MF_0 v_0 p_0 + EFE_0 v_0 p_0) + (MF_1 v_1 p_1 + EFE_1 v_1 p_1) + \cdots$$
$$= E_0 v_0 p_0 + E_1 p_1 p_1 + E_2 v_2 p_2$$

[5] Fractional deaths are used to make precise actuarial calculations, even though in real-life situations only whole numbers of persons survive.

[6] The projected number of survivors extends past the 20 years presented in this table. In deriving fees, actuarial projections of survivors are extended to the assumed end of the human life span (in our example, this is age 110). The total number of years lived by the original group of residents is derived by summing the number of survivors over all future years and deducting one-half year per resident for the assumption that deaths occur midway through the year. This sum is 1,308 [1,358 ($-\frac{1}{2} \times 100$)]. The life expectancy is equal to the sum of years lived divided by the number of original residents, 13.1 (1,308 ÷ 100) years. Due to the characteristics of the mortality curve, the life expectancy, or mean of the death distribution, will approximately equal the median of that distribution. Hence, the life expectancy can be thought of as the maximum number of years that the survivors for a closed group will equal 50 percent of the original number.

where

p_t = Probability of surviving t years

Columns 5 through 7 of Table D–2 contain the survival-discounted value of expenses, monthly fees, and entry fees over the next 20 years, respectively. The sum of survival-discounted expenses to the end of the human life span (assumed to be 100) is $38.82. This amount represents, in today's dollars, the expenses for services provided to survivors from the current group of residents. The sum of the expected monthly fees and entry fees is $32.35 and $6.47, respectively. This table shows that even though the number of surviving residents decreases annually, their expenses increase for 11 years before declining.

Health Care Cost Differential

The preceding examples do not reflect the consequences of changes in the residents' living status during their stay in the community. Such changes have a significant impact on projecting future *expenses*. Typically, nursing care costs are 2 to 3 times greater than apartment costs. Therefore, in order to reflect properly the future costs of offering a continuing care contract, it is necessary to define the probability of survival by living status, and to adjust projected expenses to reflect changes in living status.

This projection can be made by using a multiple decrement model to estimate the future living status of survivors. This also means that the mortality assumptions used for pricing decisions must be differentiated by living status (i.e., apartment versus health care). In addition, morbidity (health care utilization) assumptions are required to estimate the probability of permanent transfer from the apartment center to the health care center and of temporary utilization of the health care center.

Figure D–2 shows the impact of higher health care costs. Health care center expenses are initially assumed to be twice apartment center expenses, and are assumed to increase 10 percent annually for inflation. The expected expense curve is weighted according to costs of living in the apartment center versus the health care center according to the relative probability of survival in each living status. For this example, however, neither the expense curve nor the revenue curve is discounted for survivorship. The monthly fee curve is the same as in Figure D–1 since monthly fees are not assumed to change with living status. However, both the expense curve and the entry fee earnings curve change substantially. The expense curve is found to increase faster than the underlying inflation assumption because of increasing expected health care utilization with its proportionately higher costs. The expense curve increases to $12.51 from $1.20 in 20 years—an

FIGURE D-2
Living Status Weighted Expense, Monthly Fee, and Entry Fee Earnings

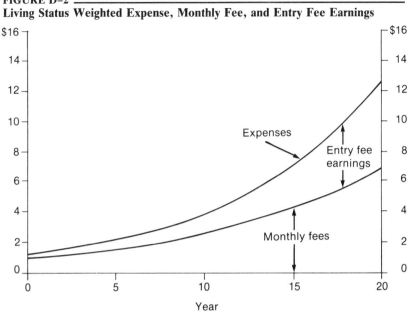

average annual rate of 12 percent, or two percentage points more than the underlying inflation rate. (The example in Figure D-1 shows that total expenses increase to $8.07 in 20 years.)

Entry fee earnings also increase faster than inflation since they must equal the difference between expenses and monthly fees. Entry fee earnings start at $0.20 and increase to $5.78 in 20 years (compared to $1.35 in the Figure D-1 example), an average annual rate of 18 percent.

Table D-3 shows the results of a multiple decrement projection incorporating survival probabilities with living status cost differentials. Column 3 contains the number of surviving apartment residents; initially, this number is assumed to be 100. During the first year, 2.496 are expected to transfer permanently to the health care center (column 4), leaving 96.264 survivors in their apartments at the end of the year. The number of deaths in apartments, 1.240 residents, is equal to the original number of apartment residents minus the number of survivors at the end of the year plus the permanent transfers (this value is not given in the table). Of the 2.496 transfers to the health care center, 2.434 (column 5) are expected to live to the end of the year. In the first year, 1.337 residents are expected to die while residing in their apartments and 2.712 residents are expected to transfer permanently to the health care center. Hence, there are 92.215 apartment survivors at year 2 and 4.932 in the health care center. This sequence is continued for each successive year. At year 10 there are 70.318 surviving residents, 29.7

TABLE D-3 ———
Probability of Survival by Living Status and Survival Discounted Revenues and Expenses by Living Status

Year t	Age x	Number of apartment residents	Number of permanent transfers	Number of health care residents	Survival-discounted apartment expenses	Survival-discounted health care expenses	Total survival-discounted expenses
0	75	100.000	2.496	0.000	$ 1.20	$ 0.00	$ 1.20
1	76	96.264	2.712	2.434	1.27	0.06	1.33
2	77	92.215	2.932	4.932	1.34	0.14	1.48
3	78	87.848	3.154	7.459	1.40	0.24	1.64
4	79	83.160	3.373	9.970	1.46	0.35	1.81
5	80	78.154	3.584	12.409	1.51	0.48	1.99
6	81	72.843	3.776	14.708	1.55	0.63	2.17
7	82	67.259	3.938	16.793	1.57	0.79	2.36
8	83	61.449	4.060	18.579	1.58	0.96	2.54
9	84	55.473	4.134	19.980	1.57	1.13	2.70
10	85	49.403	4.151	20.915	1.54	1.30	2.84
11	86	43.323	4.102	21.315	1.48	1.46	2.94
12	87	37.332	3.977	21.131	1.41	1.59	3.00
13	88	31.538	3.767	20.348	1.31	1.69	2.99
14	89	26.066	3.469	18.991	1.19	1.73	2.92
15	90	21.041	3.095	17.147	1.05	1.72	2.77
16	91	16.572	2.667	14.954	0.91	1.65	2.56
17	92	12.732	2.218	12.589	0.77	1.53	2.30
18	93	9.548	2.782	10.234	0.64	1.37	2.00
19	94	6.997	1.387	8.044	0.51	1.18	1.69
Sum*		1,064.675		293.274	$26.79	$24.05	$50.84

* The sums are based on projections to age 110.

percent of whom reside in the health care center. 50 percent of the survivors are in the health care center by the end of year 18.[7]

Table D–3 also shows the development of survival-discounted expenses based on different apartment and health care center expenses. Column 6 contains the survival-discounted apartment expenses (these are initially assumed to be $1.20, increased by 10 percent per year). Column 7 contains survival-discounted health care expenses (health care expenses are twice projected apartment expenses). The total survival-discounted expenses, given in column 8, are the sum of columns 6 and 7.

Figure D–3 shows the relationship between survival-discounted expenses and revenues. It can be observed from this graph that expected expenses are at their highest value after 12 years, while monthly fee

---

[7] It should be noted that apartment center mortality rates are significantly less than those for health care center residents. This may not be apparent from Table D–3 since the total number of health care residents increases for a period while apartment residents decrease. This is due to the fact that the number of permanent transfers to the health care center exceeds the number of deaths during the first 13 years.

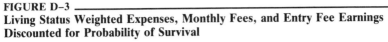

FIGURE D-3
Living Status Weighted Expenses, Monthly Fees, and Entry Fee Earnings
Discounted for Probability of Survival

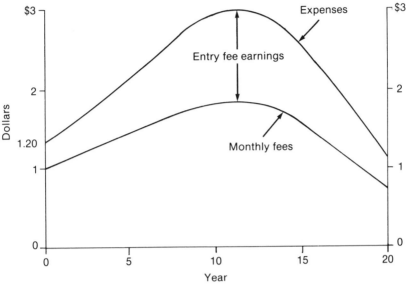

revenues and entry fee earnings reach their highest levels in 11 and 14 years, respectively.[8]

Table D-4 shows the expected expenses and revenues discounted for both interest and the probability of survival, with expenses weighted according to the differential costs of apartment center versus health care center. This table shows that the present value of future expenses, based on expense projections and survival to the assumed end of the life span, is equal to $16.86, which is 33 percent ($16.86 ÷ $50.84) of projected expenses not discounted for interest. The present value of future monthly fees is $11.76, and the entry fee (the present value of entry fee earnings) must now be $5.11 to make up the difference. Hence, by incorporating interest discounts, probability of survival, and cost differentials, the true actuarial liability of a continuing care contract can be estimated. In other words, today's value of expected expenses is $16.86, while the cash flow associated with those expenses will be 3 times more than the present value.

---

[8] This graph also illustrates several key considerations in developing a theoretically sound methodology for earning entry fees. Under the proposed pricing philosophy, initially very small portions of the entry fees should be earned in order to match revenues with expenses correctly. Maximum entry fee earnings should occur some 10 to 12 years after entry into the community. Also, the earnings schedule should not be limited to a fixed time period, such as life expectancy, which is 13 years in this case, since expenses exceed monthly fees after that point.

TABLE D-4
Present Value of Future Expenses and Revenues Discounted for Interest and Survival

Year t	Age x	Present value of expenses discounted for interest and survival	Present value of monthly fees discounted for interest and survival	Present value of entry fee earnings discounted for interest and survival
0	75	$ 1.20	$ 1.00	$0.20
1	76	1.19	0.97	0.22
2	77	1.18	0.94	0.24
3	78	1.17	0.90	0.27
4	79	1.15	0.87	0.28
5	80	1.13	0.83	0.28
6	81	1.10	0.79	0.32
7	82	1.07	0.74	0.33
8	83	1.02	0.69	0.33
9	84	0.97	0.64	0.33
10	85	0.91	0.59	0.33
11	86	0.85	0.53	0.32
12	87	0.77	0.47	0.30
13	88	0.69	0.41	0.28
14	89	0.60	0.35	0.25
15	90	0.51	0.29	0.22
16	91	0.42	0.24	0.18
17	92	0.33	0.19	0.15
18	93	0.26	0.14	0.12
19	94	0.20	0.11	0.09
Sum*		$16.86	$11.76	$5.11

* These sums are based on projections to age 110.

Generalized Actuarial Pricing Equation

The generalized actuarial pricing equation, incorporating interest discount, probability of surviving by living status, and living status cost differentials, is as follows:

$$(MF_0 v_0 p_0 + EFE_0 v_0 p_0) + (MF_1 v_1 p_1 + EFE_1 v_1 p_1) + \cdots$$
$$= (E_0^a v_0 p_0^a + E_0^h v_0 p_0^h) + (E_1^a v_1 p_1^a + E_1^h v_1 p_1^h) + \cdots$$

where

p_t = Probability of being alive in year t
p_t^a = Probability of residing in the apartment center in year t
p_t^h = Probability of residing in the health care center in year t
E_t^a = Apartment center expenses in year t
E_t^h = Health care center expenses in year t

By regrouping values on the left-hand side of the generalized actuarial pricing equation, we get

$$(EFE_0 v_0 p_0 + EFE p_1 v_1 p_1) + (MF_0 v_0 p_0 + MF_1 v_1 p_1) + \cdots$$
$$= (E_0^a v_0 p_0^a + E_0^h v_0 p_0^h) + (E_1^a v_1 p_1^a + E_1^h v_1 p_1^h) + \cdots$$

The above equation is summarized as:

$$PVEF + PVMF = PVFE$$

or

$$PVFR = PVFE$$

where

PVEF = Present value of entry fee earnings
PVMF = Present value of monthly fees
PVFE = Present value of future expenses
PVFR = Present value of future revenues

Even though this formula appears to be somewhat complex, it is a straightforward extension of the initial actuarial pricing equation developed at the beginning of this appendix. With appropriate assumptions for determining expenses and revenues, this equation can be used to develop pricing structures that meet the pricing objectives set forth in Chapter 7. Other refinements to this general pricing equation include the development of probabilities for the temporary utilization of the health care center and the expenses associated with such utilization and the development of survival probabilities that vary by age, sex, number of occupants in a particular unit, and mortality improvements.

Appendix E

Illustrative CCRC Financial Statements

Statements of Changes in Financial Position
of Unrestricted Funds
For the Years Ended March 31, 1981 and 1980

	1981	1980
Sources of working capital:		
Resident entry fees received..............................	$1,202,400	$1,432,150
Increase (decrease) in advance deposits......................	(1,000)	22,000
Equipment donated...	20,241	13,746
Transfer from restricted funds	6,296	—
Working capital provided............................	1,227,937	1,467,896
Uses of working capital:		
Excess of (revenues) expenses	7,006	(417,752)
Items not providing (requiring) working capital:		
Depreciation and amortization	(1,040,837)	(1,033,122)
Resident entry fee amortization	1,538,458	2,141,182
Working capital used in operations	504,627	690,308
Additions to land, buildings and equipment....................	141,683	42,132
Repayments and current maturities of long-term debt:		
Scheduled	271,205	290,310
Advanced payment	—	600,000
Transfer of loan...	150,000	—
Entry fee refunds..	64,620	52,228
Working capital used	1,132,135	1,674,978
Increase (decrease) in working capital	$ 95,802	$ (207,082)
Working capital changes—increase (decrease):		
Cash, certificates of deposit, and short-term investments	$ 303,056	$ (383,462)
Accounts receivable......................................	(94,451)	165,906
Accrued interest receivable................................	(59,012)	68,151
Inventory and prepaid expenses.............................	13,783	16,900
Current portion of long-term debt	20,008	8,106
Accounts payable and accrued expenses	(26,518)	5,225
Advance billings for residents' care	(61,064)	(87,908)
Increase (decrease) in working capital	$ 95,802	$ (207,082)

Statements of Changes in Fund Balances
For the Years Ended March 31, 1981 and 1980

	Unrestricted operating	Restricted										
		Plant replacement and expansion fund and other restricted funds										
		Plant	Other	Reserve fund I	Reserve fund II	Financial assistance fund I	Financial assistance fund II	Funds I and II	Life income fund I	Life income fund II	Addition fund	Independent housing project fund
Balances, March 31, 1979	$ 664,505	$ 9,560	$ 400	$112,069	$36,827	$24,003	$11,000	—	$281,516			
Excess of revenues over expenses	417,752											
Restricted contributions			7,985	35,718	9,581	1,000		$10,000				
Donated equipment	11,142											
Investment income		1,090	47	13,794	5,121	1,309	563	1,026				
Unrealized depreciation of investments in common stocks									(18,672)			
Noncapital expenditures of restricted funds			(569)									
Transfers of restricted funds for capital additions		(1,004)	(1,600)									
Loss on sale of investment									(13,611)			
Balances, March 31, 1980	1,096,003	9,646	6,263	161,581	51,529	26,312	11,563	11,026	249,233			
Excess of expenses over revenues	(7,006)											
Restricted contributions			21,199	30,258	18,579				30,375	$25,000	$230,832	$25,339
Income:												
Investment income		1,194	56	19,821	6,626	1,230	202	1,298	22,415	655	37,435	1,450
Other												
Change in unrealized depreciation of investments in common stocks									15,637			
Noncapital transfer of restricted funds	6,296		(6,296)									
Transfers of restricted funds for capital additions	20,241		(20,241)									
Loss on sale of investments									(1,340)			
Distributions to beneficiaries									(23,609)			
Interest expense											(10,239)	(6,539)
Balances, March 31, 1981	$1,115,534	$10,840	$ 981	$211,660	$76,734	$27,542	$11,765	$12,324	$292,711	$25,655	$258,028	$20,250

Statements of Revenues and Expenses
of Unrestricted Funds
For the Years Ended March 31, 1981 and 1980

	1981	**1980***
Revenues:		
Resident care fees	$5,210,137	$4,517,295
Amortization of entry fees	1,538,458	2,141,182
Medical center fees:		
Resident	1,025,357	844,836
Medicare and other insurance reimbursement	453,261	343,927
Nonresident	146,826	226,439
Registration fees	13,000	19,700
Interest income	253,955	233,549
Other	27,244	20,266
Total revenues	$8,668,238	$8,347,194
Expenses:		
General and administrative	$1,044,267	$ 861,213
Housekeeping	528,213	468,020
Maintenance	697,687	633,384
Food service	1,731,152	1,598,093
Medical center	1,750,849	1,487,369
Utilities	784,527	668,584
Real estate taxes	360,599	318,674
Depreciation	972,219	964,482
Amortization of preopening expenses	68,618	68,641
Interest expense	732,199	843,932
Other	4,914	17,050
Total expenses	8,675,244	7,929,442
Excess of revenues (expenses)	$ (7,006)	$ 417,752

* Reclassified to conform to 1981 presentation.

Appendix F

Sources of Additional Information Regarding State Statutes

Arizona	Department of Insurance 1601 West Jefferson Phoenix, Arizona 85007
California	Department of Social Services 744 P Street Sacramento, California 95814
Colorado	Department of Insurance 201 East Colfax Avenue Denver, Colorado 80203
Florida	Department of Insurance Office of the Treasurer State of Florida Tallahassee, Florida 32304
Indiana	Department of Securities Room 102, Statehouse Indianapolis, Indiana 46204
Maryland	Office on Aging 301 West Preston Street Room 1004 Baltimore, Maryland 21201
Michigan	Corporation Securities Bureau Department of Commerce PO Box 30220 Lansing, Michigan 48909
Minnesota	none
Missouri	Division of Insurance Department of Consumer Affairs 515 East High Street Jefferson City, Missouri 65101

AAHA   American Association of Homes for the Aging
Suite 770
1050 17th Street NW
Washington, D.C. 20036

LCSC   Life Care Services Corporation
800 Second Avenue
Des Moines, Iowa 50309

Index

This book has been set Linotron 202 in 10 and 9 point Times Roman, leaded 2 points. Part and chapter numbers are 24 point Times Roman Regular. Part and chapter titles are 30 point Times Roman Regular. The size of the type page is 26 picas by 47 picas.